T0212764

Lecture Notes of the Institute for Computer Sciences, Social Informatics and Telecommunications Engineering 420

More information about this series at https://link.springer.com/bookseries/8197

Masood Ur Rehman · Ahmed Zoha (Eds.)

Body Area Networks

Smart IoT and Big Data for Intelligent Health Management

16th EAI International Conference, BODYNETS 2021
Virtual Event, October 25–26, 2021
Proceedings

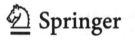 Springer

Editors
Masood Ur Rehman 🆔
University of Glasgow
Glasgow, UK

Ahmed Zoha 🆔
University of Glasgow
Glasgow, UK

ISSN 1867-8211 ISSN 1867-822X (electronic)
Lecture Notes of the Institute for Computer Sciences, Social Informatics
and Telecommunications Engineering
ISBN 978-3-030-95592-2 ISBN 978-3-030-95593-9 (eBook)
https://doi.org/10.1007/978-3-030-95593-9

This Springer imprint is published by the registered company Springer Nature Switzerland AG
The registered company address is: Gewerbestrasse 11, 6330 Cham, Switzerland

Preface

We are delighted to introduce the proceedings of the sixteenth edition of the European Alliance for Innovation (EAI) International Conference on Body Area Networks (BodyNets 2021). This conference provided a lively platform for discussing ideas, comparing practices, encouraging adoption, and sharing experience among researchers and practitioners from academia and industry working in the fields of wireless communication, computer science, electrical engineering, biomedical engineering, and medicine. The theme of BodyNets 2021 was "Smart IoT and big data for intelligent health management".

The technical program of BodyNets 2021 consisted of 21 full papers, including two invited papers, in oral presentation sessions at the main conference tracks: Track 1 - Human Activity Recognition; Track 2 - Sensing for Healthcare; Track 3 - Innovating the Future Healthcare Systems; and Track 4 - Data Analytics for Healthcare Systems. Besides the high-quality technical paper presentations, the technical program also featured six keynote speeches and one invited talk. The keynote speeches were delivered by Cecilia Mascolo from University of Cambridge (UK), Mehmet Rasit Yuce from Monash University (Australia), Chun Tung Chou from the University of New South Wales (Australia), Alessandra Costanzo from the University of Bologna (Italy), Wen Jung Li from City University of Hong Kong (China), and Konstantina Nikita from the National Technical University of Athens (Greece). The invited talk was presented by Dena Ahmed S. Al-Thani from Hamad Bin Khalifa University (Qatar).

Coordination with the General Chairs, Muhammad Ali Imran and Qammer H Abbasi, was essential for the success of the conference. We sincerely appreciate their constant support and guidance. It was also a great pleasure to work with such an excellent organizing committee for their hard work in organizing and supporting the conference. In particular, we are grateful to the Technical Program Committee who have handled the peer-review process for the technical papers excellently and helped to put together a high-quality technical program. We are also grateful to Conference Manager Lucia Sladeckova for her support and all the authors who presented their fine contributions at the BodyNets 2021.

We strongly believe that the BodyNets conference provides a vibrant platform for sharing ideas among researchers, developers, and practitioners from both industry and academia working on state-of-the-art research and development in body area networks. We also expect that the future BodyNets conferences will be as successful and stimulating as this year's, as indicated by the contributions presented in this volume.

November 2021

Masood Ur Rehman
Ahmed Zoha
Akram Alomainy
Asimina Kiourti

Conference Organization

Organizing Committee

General Chairs

Muhammad Ali Imran   University of Glasgow, UK
Qammer H. Abbasi   University of Glasgow, UK

Technical Program Committee Chairs

Masood Ur Rehman   University of Glasgow, UK
Ahmed Zoha   University of Glasgow, UK
Akram Alomainy   Queen Mary University of London, UK
Asimina Kiourti   Ohio State University, USA

Sponsorship and Exhibit Chair

Imran Ansari   University of Glasgow, UK

Local Chair

Lina Mohjazi   University of Glasgow, UK

Workshops Chair

Nikolaos Thomos   University of Essex, UK

Publicity and Social Media Chairs

Syed Aziz Shah   Coventry University, UK
Mohsin Raza   Edgehill University, UK

Publications Chair

Hasan Tahir Abbas   University of Glasgow, UK

Web Chair

Sajjad Hussain   University of Glasgow, UK

Posters and PhD Track Chair

Muhammad Babar Ali Abbasi   Queen's University Belfast, UK

Panels Chair

Sema Dumanli   Bogazici University, Turkey

Demos Chair

Kamran Ali   Middlesex University, UK

Tutorials Chair

Muhammad Mahtab Alam   Tallinn University of Technology, Estonia

Technical Program Committee

Adnan Zahid Khan	Heriot Watt University, UK
Ahmed Taha	University of Glasgow, UK
Syeda Fizzah Jillani	Aberystwyth University, UK
Xiaoce Feng	Wayne State University, USA
Syed Ali Hassan	National University of Sciences and Technology, Pakistan
Eric Benoit	Université Savoie Mont Blanc, France
Ismail Mabrouk	Al Ain University, UAE
Aifeng Ren	Xidian University, China
Abdelrahim Mohamed	University of Surrey, UK
Xiaopeng Yang	Beijing Institute of Technology, China
Sultan Shoaib	Wrexham Glyndwr University, UK
Ameena Saad Al-Sumaiti	Khalifa University, UAE
Naveed Ul Hassan	Lahore University of Management Sciences, Pakistan
Hakim Ghazzai	Stevens Institute of Technology, USA
Arman Farhang	Trinity College Dublin, Ireland
Michael Samwel Mollel	Nelson Mandela African Institution of Science and Technology, Tanzania
Yusuf Dogan	Gumushane University, Turkey
Ahmad Jawad	Edinburgh Napier University, UK

Contents

Sensing for Healthcare

Data Analytics for Healthcare Systems

Innovating the Future Healthcare Systems

Human Activity Recognition

Data Fusion for Human Activity Recognition Based on RF Sensing and IMU Sensor

Zheqi Yu[1]([🖂]), Adnan Zahid[2], William Taylor[1], Hasan Abbas[1], Hadi Heidari[1], Muhammad A. Imran[1], and Qammer H. Abbasi[1]

[1] James Watt School of Engineering, University of Glasgow, Glasgow G12 8QQ, UK
`z.yu.2@research.gla.ac.uk`, `2536400T@student.gla.ac.uk`,
`{hasan.abbas,hadi.heidari,muhammad.imran,`
`Qammer.Abbasi}@glasgow.ac.uk`
[2] School of Engineering and Physical Sciences, Heriot Watt University, Edinburgh EH14 4AS, UK
`a.zahid@hw.ac.uk`

Abstract. This paper proposes a new data fusion method, which uses the designed construction matrix to fuse sensor and USRP data to realise Human Activity Recognition. At this point, Inertial Measurement Unit sensors and Universal Software-defined Radio Peripherals are used to collect human activities signals separately. In order to avoid the incompatibility problem with different collection devices, such as different sampling frequency caused inconsistency time axis. The Principal Component Analysis processing the fused data to dimension reduction without time that is performed to extract the time unrelated 5×5 feature matrix to represent corresponding activities. There are explores data fusion method between multiple devices and ensures accuracy without dropping. The technique can be extended to other types of hardware signal for data fusion.

Keywords: Data fusion · Human activity recognition · Artificial intelligence · Signal processing

1 Introduction

Currently, there are four main types of technologies to achieve Human Activity Recognition (HAR), which are sensors [16], radar[28], RF signals [30] and camera [2]. Due to cost constraints, most applications mainly use the first two methods that are sensors and radar hardware to capture and identify human movements of activity. Their principles are different: radar mainly obtains the distance, speed and angle of the object by sending electromagnetic waves and receiving echoes. Sensors based on wearable devices to collect physical quantities of human movement. Such as angular velocity [4], linear velocity relative to the ground [13], acceleration [3], vibration [29] and direction based on contact [12].

© ICST Institute for Computer Sciences, Social Informatics and Telecommunications Engineering 2022
Published by Springer Nature Switzerland AG 2022. All Rights Reserved
M. Ur Rehman and A. Zoha (Eds.): BODYNETS 2021, LNICST 420, pp. 3–14, 2022.
https://doi.org/10.1007/978-3-030-95593-9_1

These two technologies have their own advantages and disadvantages. In general, wearable sensors have low cost [11], easy to use [22] and less limited by usage scenarios [27]. It is now necessary hardware for mobile portable devices to realise motion recognition. However, its range and accuracy are not as good as radar, which performance limited by other hardware such as batteries and microprocessors. The radar can realise the object detection with higher precision through the principle of Doppler shift [19]. Moreover, it is not constrained by power, and the hardware performance can be better released. However, it is generally used in a fixed scenario that can not move around quickly, which means the capture of the object signal is easily affected by factors such as occlusion and angle limited.

Therefore, a new solution is proposed, which integrates the sensor and radar cooperate to form a human motion perception system, it is complementing each other to achieve a more stable and reliable human motion recognition function [18]. After adopting the fusion method, the sensor and radar will acquire different perception information and complement each other quite well. However, there may also be contradictions by some special conditions. For example, under a single signal data, sometimes conflicting activity recognition results are obtained, it is caused by feedback the incompatible acquired information. Conflicting information may affect the recognition judgment of the results [23]. Therefore, in order for the perception system to receive consistent and clear activity results, it is necessary to fuse the data of sensor and radar by suitable calculation.

The basic principle of data fusion between sensors and radar signal, it is similar to the integrated processing of information from multiple organs such as eyes, nose and ears by the human brain. It mainly integrates data and information obtained by multiway hardware, which calculates redundant and complementary information of multiple type data in space or time, and then obtains a consistent description of activity feature. Following the early human activity recognition research to extend on the data fusion of multiple sensors [37]. At this point, we propose a data fusion method for sensors and radar signal, and processing it with neuromorphic computing to finally achieve a perception system for human activity recognition.

In recent years, the application of multi-hardware data fusion technology has become more and more widely, such as industrial control [5], robotics [21], object detection [20], traffic control [26], inertial navigation [31], remote sensing [32], medical diagnosis [38], image processing [33], pattern recognition [15] and other fields. Compared with a single-sensor system, the use of multi-hardware data fusion technology helps solve problems of detection, tracking and recognition. It can improve the reliability and robustness, enhance the credibility and accuracy of data, extend the time of the entire system, Space coverage, and increase the real-time performance and utilization of data.

In the traditional machine learning method [34], Muhammad *et al.* [24] proposed a data fusion for ensemble computing with a Random Forest algorithm to predict multiple sensors. The multiple sensor data is integrated with the fog computing environment to perform processing in a decentralised manner, and then feeding into the global classifier after performing data fusion, it can achieve more than 90% of average accuracy. Li *et al.* [17] use the Sequential Forward Selection method to fuse IMU and Radar information to form time series data. It can be used as features to train the Support Vector Machine (SVM) [36] and Artificial Neural Network (ANN) algorithm for classification computing, which improves about 6% higher than a single type of data. In view of the uneven data quality of different hardware [35], Huang *et al.* [14] propose three sparsity-invariant operations to utilise multi-scale features effectively. The sparsity-invariant of the hierarchical multi-scale encoder-decoder Neural Network is used to process sparse input and sparse feature maps for multi-hardware data. The features of multiple sensors can be fused further to improve the performance of deep learning work. However, multi-hardware of data fusion needs to run synchronously, ensuring the time axis is unified in the coordinate system. It puts forward higher requirements for multi-modal data acquiring, and not conducive to the system's future expandability.

This paper explores a new multi-hardware data fusion method that makes use of IMU sensors and Universal Software Radio Peripheral (USRP) for human motion recognition. Our approach is based on using building a constructing feature matrix to fusing different hardware information as unify data. Different hardware signals are difficult to match due to the signal shapes between the object. The difference in location and time axis is the main disadvantage of these data fusion. In order to overcome this limitation, we constructed matrices from vectors based on principal component analysis to combine IMU and USRP signals, then helps multi-hardware data fusion, and finally achieve better classification and recognition effect than traditional data fusion results.

The organization structure of this paper is as follows: In Sect. 2, we introduce the signal processing process of IMU and USRP hardware for human motion capture, and the feature details of data fusion. In Sect. 3, we propose the feature matrix details of data fusion with PCA algorithm, and quantitatively evaluate the recognition accuracy. In Sect. 4, we discuss the proposed data fusion processing methods, potentials, limitations and compare the results with related work. Finally, Sect. 5 summarizes this work, and it also describes our future direction of data fusion in different hardware.

2   Materials and Methods

We collect human activity signals through the Inertial Measurement Unit (IMU) sensor [9] and the Universal Software-defined Radio Peripheral (USRP) [10]. The IMU sensor is worn on the wrist of volunteers. On the side, the USRP keeps a distance of 2 meters from humans to collect electromagnetic signals in a fixed way. We tested a total of 20 volunteers for two activities with three repeat times, which are sitting down and standing up. The raw signal data of the sensor and the USRP is shown in Fig. 1.

2.1   IMU State Modeling

Inertial Measurement Unit (IMU) is a device for measuring the attitude angle of an object. The main components include a gyroscope, accelerometer and magnetometer. The gyroscope detects the angular velocity signals relative to the three degrees of freedom (X, Y and Z) in the coordinate navigation system, and the accelerometer monitors the acceleration signals of the independent three axes of the object carrier coordinate system in X, Y and Z directions. The magnetometer can obtain the surrounding magnetic field information. It can calculate the angle between the module with the north direction through the geomagnetic vector and help correct the angular velocity parameters of the gyroscope. The final real-time output of three-dimensional angular velocity signal, acceleration signal, and magnetic field information is used to calculate the object's current posture.

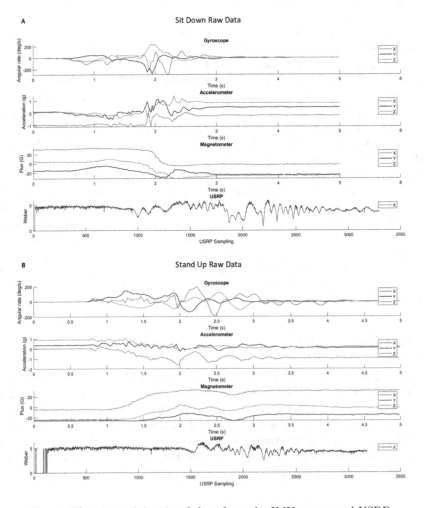

Fig. 1. The raw activity signal data from the IMU sensor and USRP.

The gyroscope directly measures the angular velocity rather than the angle, which is converted into angular velocity by acquiring the Coriolis force. Coriolis force as physical information comes from the inertia of the motion of the object. This is a description of the deviation on the linear motion, and it is a particle moving in a rotating system due to relative inertia. In the sensor, the object keeps moving in a direction. The angular velocity of rotation will produce Coriolis force in the vertical direction, which results in a change of capacitance difference. The change in capacitance is proportional to the rotation angular velocity, and then the rotation angle can be obtained from the corresponding capacitance. The principle of an accelerometer is more straightforward than a gyroscope. It measures acceleration directly through specific force, which is the overall acceleration without gravity or the non-gravitational force acting on the unit mass. The sensor of the mass block will move under the action of acceleration affected. The capacitors on both sides measure the mass block's position and calculate the magnitude of the acceleration. The magnetometer uses the Hall effect to measure the strength of the magnetic field. Under the magnetic field's action, the electrons will run in the vertical direction to generate an electric field on the side. Therefore, the magnetic strength can indirectly measure the strength and the positive and negative sign of the electric field. At this point, the IMU hardware's primary work is to obtain more accurate activity information from the three sensors' data.

2.2 USRP State Modeling

The USRP is a device that allows for radio frequency communication between a transmitter and a receiver antenna and allows for a wide range of parameters to be defined with the use of software. These devices are commonly used within research labs and universities. The device connects to a PC where software is used to control the USRP hardware for transmission and receiving RF signals.

In this paper the USRP is set up to communicate using Orthogonal frequency-division multiplexing (OFDM). Channel Estimation is an important feature of OFDM as it monitors the state of the channel for the purpose of improving performance. Channel estimation does this by using a specified set of symbols known as pilot symbols. These symbols are used in the transmission of the data and once the receiver antenna receives the data the received pilot symbols are compared to the expected pilot symbols and this provides details of the State of the channel.

This paper observes the channel state information while the activities of Sitting, Standing and no activity take place between the transmitter and receiver antennas. This is carried out through several samples. These samples can then be used in Machine Learning applications to see if the patterns can be recognised. The samples in this paper include 64 subcarriers. An average of each subcarrier is taken, and this represents the signal propagation while an action takes place between the transmitter and receiver. Each activity takes place while the USRP is communicating between the transmitter and receiver for 5 s. Then the data can be stored in CSV format. Then all the activities are complied into a single dataset for processing in machine learning.

3   The Proposed Structure Matrix to Data Fusion

Data fusion utilises comprehensive and complete information about the object and environment obtained by multiple hardware devices, which is mainly reflected in the data fusion algorithm. Therefore, the signal processing's core point on a multi-hardware system is to construct a suitable data fusion algorithm. For multi-type sensor hardware, which acquired information is diverse and complex. Moreover, the basic requirements for information data fusion methods are robustness and parallel processing capabilities. There are also requests for the speed and accuracy of the method, and the previous preprocessing calculations and subsequent recognition algorithms Interface compatibility that to coordinate with different technologies and methods; reduce information sample requirements, etc. In general, data fusion methods are based on nonlinear mathematical computing. It can achieve fault tolerance, adaptability, associative memory, and parallel processing capabilities.

The raw data obtained by the separately single hardware about the two activities, but how to fuse the two hardware's signal information becomes the key. They cannot be directly performed the calculation because their sampling rate makes the time axis incompatible with the coordinates system. At this point, the raw data need to reduce the time dimension of the activity feature. The Principal Component Analysis (PCA) [1] algorithm used for data dimension reduction can be achieved a time-independent activity features. Furthermore, after analysing the two types of signal, we can find that the sensor data has more dimensions than USRP data. Therefore, we designed a big sub-matrix to represent the sensor signal of human activity after data dimension reduction and a small sub-matrix representing the USRP signal after data dimension reduction.

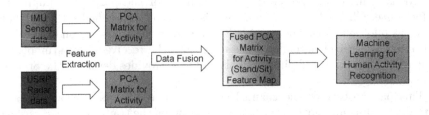

Fig. 2. The entire calculation workflow of feature extraction to human activity recognition.

Meanwhile, this design also facilitates subsequent machine learning, which requests normalise the fused data to obtain a standard feature map pattern [25] of each activity, and then loaded the feature map template into the Neural network algorithm for training. It gets the combination matrix of the feature map pattern. Its activity feature matrix of the sensor and USRP is combined by a direct row arrangement method of previous sub-matrices. Finally, the neural network obtains the classification function of the two activities based on the training. The neural network as a classifier to output recognition result. Figure 2 shows the entire calculation workflow from feature extraction to recognition.

3.1   Principal Component Analysis for Feature Extraction

The PCA algorithm for data dimensionality reduction calculates the covariance matrix of one dimension with sample information, and then solves the feature value and corresponding feature vector of the covariance matrix. It arranges these feature vectors according to their corresponding feature values from large to small as a new projection matrix. In this case, the projection matrix as the feature vector pattern after sample data transformation. It maps n-dimension features to k-dimension space, which is a brand new orthogonal feature as the principal component. It is a re-constructed k-dimension feature based on the original n-dimension features. Following the first K-dimension vectors are the essential features of the high-dimension data retained to remove noise and unimportant interference factors to improve data information quality.

4   Experimental Evaluation

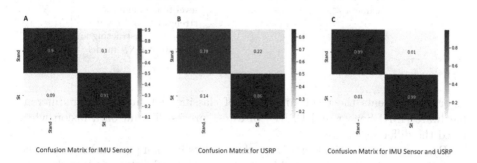

Fig. 3. The ANN algorithm classification confusion matrix of IMU sensor, USRP and IMU sensor fused USRP data.

After PCA feature extraction of the hardware signal, it is evaluated the training and testing performance following by the Artificial Neural Network (ANN). Figure 3 illustrates the recognition accuracy of sensors data applied to the machine learning algorithm. The evaluation for the performance of a single sensor and fused data modality in activity recognition. It is the two layers ANN algorithm classification results of the confusion matrix for Sit down and Stand Up activities. Following feature extraction through the PCA algorithm, the ANN

Table 1. Comparison table with other data fusion methods.

Project	Hardware	Algorithm	Data fusion	Accuracy
Our	IMU sensor (magnetometer + accelerometer + gyroscope) + USRP	Artificial Neural Network	Using PCA algorithm for feature fusion	99.2%
Chen et al. [7]	IMU sensor (accelerometer + gyroscope)	K Nearest Neighbor	two-stage genetic algorithm-based feature selection algorithm with a fixed activation number	99.1%
		Random Forest		99.1%
		Support Vector Machine		98.9%
Chung et al. [8]	IMU sensor (magnetometer + accelerometer + gyroscope)	LSTM network	Using various combinations of sensors, and two voting ensemble techniques adopting all sensor modalities	94.47%
Calvo et al. [6]	Kinect + IMU + EMG	Hidden Markov Model Classification	From each sensor, it is keep track of a succession of primitive movements over a time window, and combine them to uniquely describe the overall activity performed by the human	98.81%
Zou et al. [39]	WiFi-enabled IoT devices and camera	C3D model and CNN model ensemble DNN model	Performs multimodal fusion at the decision level to combine the strength of WiFi and vision by constructing an ensembled DNN model	97.5%

algorithm presents the results in terms of classification accuracy for different hardware (IMU Sensor and USRP) of direct processing and data fusion when fused the different features.

By comparing the single hardware data's classification performance with the data fusion method on the machine learning of neural network algorithm, we designed the fusion method to increase the activity classification accuracy from single signal data of 90.5% from IMU sensor and 81.8% from USRP signal to 99.2% after the IMU and USRP data fusion. This evaluation proves that our solution can pass the method of constructing the matrix helps the data fusion between different hardware, and the fused data can obtain higher accuracy. When the sensors are used individually, the IMU Sensor is more suitable for measures human activity. For multi-hardware of both IMU sensor and USRP, it improves single type signal quality with more angle and dimensionality on the feature extraction.

Table 1 shows a comparison against traditional machine learning algorithms' accuracy and proves that better results are achieved through the proposed data fusion method. Such as Chen *et al.* worked on the IMU Sensor with accelerometer and gyroscope, and they used traditional machine learning algorithms (K Nearest Neighbor (KNN), Random Forest (RF) and Support Vector Machine (SVM)) to classify human activities. Furthermore, Chung *et al.* improve the data fusion method to suitable for 9 axes IMU Sensor (magnetometer, accelerometer and gyroscope) and achieve results from the LSTM network. Based on the Kinect, IMU and EMG of the multi-hardware platform, Calvo *et al.* implements the Hidden Markov Model Classifier to recognise human activity signal, and Zou *et al.* design a Deep Neural Network (DNN) framework to ensembled the C3D and Convolutional Neural Network (CNN) model to processing fused data of WiFi-enabled IoT devices and camera. However, through comparing accuracy, our implementation is more accurate than their classification. We believed that the recognition findings are preferable, demonstrating that the PCA model to fuse multi-hardware signal features effectively recognises human behavior. Furthermore, our proposed workflow has greater robustness and can adapt to more different types of matrix data.

5   Conclusion

This paper proposes a data fusion design, which simply and quickly fuses the different hardware signal data by constructing a matrix processing the extracted features. From the experimental results, the fused data's accuracy is average about 13% higher than that of a single hardware signal under the same classification algorithm. It is finally achieved 99.2% classification accuracy on multi-hardware and multi-activities signals. This shows that this method can effectively fuse data between different hardware, and help the different data types to obtain more dimensional features without affecting the classification accuracy. The above results have demonstrated the potential of multi-sensor fusion in human activity recognition. For future work, a more intelligent algorithm will be deployed, with a drive to perform a more flexible multi-hardware framework in different environments.

Acknowledgements. Zheqi Yu is funded by Joint industrial scholarship (Ref:308987) between the University of Glasgow and Transreport London Ltd. Authors would also like to thank Francesco Fioranelli and Haobo Li for supporting Human Activities Dataset.

References

1. Abdi, H., Williams, L.J.: Principal component analysis. Wiley Interdisc. Rev. Comput. Stat. **2**(4), 433–459 (2010)
2. Aggarwal, J.K., Xia, L.: Human activity recognition from 3d data: a review. Pattern Recognit. Lett. **48**, 70–80 (2014)

3. Ahmed, H., Tahir, M.: Improving the accuracy of human body orientation estimation with wearable IMU sensors. IEEE Trans. instrum. Meas. **66**(3), 535–542 (2017)

4. Aoki, T., Lin, J.F.S., Kulić, D., Venture, G.: Segmentation of human upper body movement using multiple IMU sensors. In: 2016 38th Annual International Conference of the IEEE Engineering in Medicine and Biology Society (EMBC), pp. 3163–3166. IEEE (2016)

5. Barde, A., Jain, S.: A survey of multi-sensor data fusion in wireless sensor networks. In: Proceedings of 3rd International Conference on Internet of Things and Connected Technologies (ICIoTCT), pp. 26–27 (2018)

6. Calvo, A.F., Holguin, G.A., Medeiros, H.: Human activity recognition using multimodal data fusion. In: Vera-Rodriguez, R., Fierrez, J., Morales, A. (eds.) CIARP 2018. LNCS, vol. 11401, pp. 946–953. Springer, Cham (2019). https://doi.org/10.1007/978-3-030-13469-3_109

7. Chen, J., Sun, Y., Sun, S.: Improving human activity recognition performance by data fusion and feature engineering. Sensors **21**(3), 692 (2021)

8. Chung, S., Lim, J., Noh, K.J., Kim, G., Jeong, H.: Sensor data acquisition and multimodal sensor fusion for human activity recognition using deep learning. Sensors **19**(7), 1716 (2019)

9. De Leonardis, G., et al.: Human activity recognition by wearable sensors: Comparison of different classifiers for real-time applications. In: 2018 IEEE International Symposium on Medical Measurements and Applications (MeMeA), pp. 1–6. IEEE (2018)

10. Ettus, M., Braun, M.: The universal software radio peripheral (USRP) family of low-cost SDRs. Oppor. Spectr. Shar. White Space Access Pract. Real., 3–23 (2015)

11. Fletcher, R.R., Poh, M.Z., Eydgahi, H.: Wearable sensors: opportunities and challenges for low-cost health care. In: 2010 Annual International Conference of the IEEE Engineering in Medicine and Biology, pp. 1763–1766. IEEE (2010)

12. Garofalo, G., Argones Rúa, E., Preuveneers, D., Joosen, W., et al.: A systematic comparison of age and gender prediction on IMU sensor-based gait traces. Sensors **19**(13), 2945 (2019)

13. Hua, M.D., Manerikar, N., Hamel, T., Samson, C.: Attitude, linear velocity and depth estimation of a camera observing a planar target using continuous homography and inertial data. In: 2018 IEEE International Conference on Robotics and Automation (ICRA), pp. 1429–1435. IEEE (2018)

14. Huang, Z., Fan, J., Cheng, S., Yi, S., Wang, X., Li, H.: HMS-Net: hierarchical multi-scale sparsity-invariant network for sparse depth completion. IEEE Trans. Image Process. **29**, 3429–3441 (2019)

15. Khuon, T., Rand, R.: Adaptive automatic object recognition in single and multimodal sensor data. In: 2014 IEEE Applied Imagery Pattern Recognition Workshop (AIPR), pp. 1–8. IEEE (2014)

16. Lara, O.D., Labrador, M.A.: A survey on human activity recognition using wearable sensors. IEEE Commun. Surv. Tutor. **15**(3), 1192–1209 (2012)

17. Li, H., Shrestha, A., Heidari, H., Le Kernec, J., Fioranelli, F.: Magnetic and radar sensing for multimodal remote health monitoring. IEEE Sens. J. **19**(20), 8979–8989 (2018)

18. Li, H., Shrestha, A., Heidari, H., Le Kernec, J., Fioranelli, F.: Bi-LSTM network for multimodal continuous human activity recognition and fall detection. IEEE Sens. J. **20**(3), 1191–1201 (2019)

19. Li, X., He, Y., Jing, X.: A survey of deep learning-based human activity recognition in radar. Remote Sens. **11**(9), 1068 (2019)

20. Liang, M., Yang, B., Chen, Y., Hu, R., Urtasun, R.: Multi-task multi-sensor fusion for 3d object detection. In: Proceedings of the IEEE/CVF Conference on Computer Vision and Pattern Recognition, pp. 7345–7353 (2019)
21. Majumder, S., Pratihar, D.K.: Multi-sensors data fusion through fuzzy clustering and predictive tools. Expert Syst. Appl. **107**, 165–172 (2018)
22. Majumder, S., Mondal, T., Deen, M.J.: Wearable sensors for remote health monitoring. Sensors **17**(1), 130 (2017)
23. Mönks, U., Dörksen, H., Lohweg, V., Hübner, M.: Information fusion of conflicting input data. Sensors **16**(11), 1798 (2016)
24. Muzammal, M., Talat, R., Sodhro, A.H., Pirbhulal, S.: A multi-sensor data fusion enabled ensemble approach for medical data from body sensor networks. Inf. Fusion **53**, 155–164 (2020)
25. Noshad, Z., et al.: Fault detection in wireless sensor networks through the random forest classifier. Sensors **19**(7), 1568 (2019)
26. Olivier, B., Pierre, G., Nicolas, H., Loïc, O., Olivier, T., Philippe, T.: Multi sensor data fusion architectures for Air Traffic Control Applications. Citeseer (2009)
27. Patel, S., Park, H., Bonato, P., Chan, L., Rodgers, M.: A review of wearable sensors and systems with application in rehabilitation. J. Neuroeng. Rehabil. **9**(1), 1–17 (2012)
28. Shah, S.A., Fioranelli, F.: Human activity recognition: preliminary results for dataset portability using FMCW radar. In: 2019 International Radar Conference (RADAR), pp. 1–4. IEEE (2019)
29. Spörri, J., Kröll, J., Fasel, B., Aminian, K., Müller, E.: The use of body worn sensors for detecting the vibrations acting on the lower back in alpine ski racing. Front. Physiol. **8**, 522 (2017)
30. Taylor, W., Shah, S.A., Dashtipour, K., Zahid, A., Abbasi, Q.H., Imran, M.A.: An intelligent non-invasive real-time human activity recognition system for next-generation healthcare. Sensors **20**(9), 2653 (2020)
31. Wang, L., Li, S.: Enhanced multi-sensor data fusion methodology based on multiple model estimation for integrated navigation system. Int. J. Control Autom. Syst. **16**(1), 295–305 (2018). https://doi.org/10.1007/s12555-016-0200-x
32. Xu, Y., et al.: Advanced multi-sensor optical remote sensing for urban land use and land cover classification: outcome of the 2018 IEEE GRSS data fusion contest. IEEE J. Sel. Top. Appl. Earth Obs. Remote Sens. **12**(6), 1709–1724 (2019)
33. Yang, S., Yu, Z.: A highly integrated hardware/software co-design and co-verification platform. IEEE Des. Test **36**(1), 23–30 (2018)
34. Yu, Z., Abdulghani, A.M., Zahid, A., Heidari, H., Imran, M.A., Abbasi, Q.H.: An overview of neuromorphic computing for artificial intelligence enabled hardware-based hopfield neural network. IEEE Access **8**, 67085–67099 (2020)
35. Yu, Z., et al.: Energy and performance trade-off optimization in heterogeneous computing via reinforcement learning. Electronics **9**(11), 1812 (2020)
36. Yu, Z., Yang, S., Sillitoe, I., Buckley, K.: Towards a scalable hardware/software co-design platform for real-time pedestrian tracking based on a ZYNQ-7000 device. In: 2017 IEEE International Conference on Consumer Electronics-Asia (ICCE-Asia), pp. 127–132. IEEE (2017)
37. Yu, Z., et al.: Hardware-based hopfield neuromorphic computing for fall detection. Sensors **20**(24), 7226 (2020)

38. Zhu, Y., Liu, D., Grosu, R., Wang, X., Duan, H., Wang, G.: A multi-sensor data fusion approach for atrial hypertrophy disease diagnosis based on characterized support vector hyperspheres. Sensors **17**(9), 2049 (2017)
39. Zou, H., Yang, J., Prasanna Das, H., Liu, H., Zhou, Y., Spanos, C.J.: WiFi and vision multimodal learning for accurate and robust device-free human activity recognition. In: Proceedings of the IEEE/CVF Conference on Computer Vision and Pattern Recognition Workshops (2019)

Indoor Activity Position and Direction Detection Using Software Defined Radios

Ahmad Taha[1]([✉])(ID), Yao Ge[1](ID), William Taylor[1](ID), Ahmed Zoha[1](ID),
Khaled Assaleh[2], Kamran Arshad[2], Qammer H. Abbasi[1](ID),
and Muhammad Ali Imran[1,3](ID)

[1] James Watt School of Engineering, College of Science and Engineering,
University of Glasgow, Glasgow G12 8QQ, UK
ahmad.taha@glasgow.ac.uk
[2] Faculty of Engineering and IT, Ajman University, 346, Ajman, UAE
[3] Artificial Intelligence Research Center (AIRC), Ajman University, Ajman, UAE

Abstract. The next generation of health activity monitoring is greatly
dependent on wireless sensing. By analysing variations in channel state
information, several studies were capable of detecting activities in an
indoor setting. This paper presents promising results of an experiment
conducted to identify the activity performed by a subject and where it
took place within the activity region. The system utilises two Universal
Software Radio Peripheral (USRP) devices, operating as software-defined
radios, to collect a total of 360 data samples that represent five different
activities and an empty room. The five activities were performed in three
different zones, resulting in 15 classes and a 16th class representing the
room whilst it is empty. Using the Random Forest classifier, the system
was capable of differentiating between the majority of activities, across
the 16 classes, with an accuracy of almost 94%. Moreover, it was capable
of detecting whether the room is occupied, with an accuracy of 100%,
and identify the walking directions of a human subject in three different
positions within the room, with an accuracy of 90%.

Keywords: Artificial intelligence · Indoor positioning · Human
activity recognition · Occupancy monitoring

1 Introduction

Localisation and detection of human motion and activity have been of great
interest to many researchers in recent years [3]. This reasons to the technological advancements in the fields of wireless communication, computing, and
sensing techniques, through which studies have emerged that made significant
contributions to the field. A system that is capable of identifying the activity
and the position of the subject has numerous applications in several domains
including healthcare, energy management, and security [20].

© ICST Institute for Computer Sciences, Social Informatics and Telecommunications Engineering 2022
Published by Springer Nature Switzerland AG 2022. All Rights Reserved
M. Ur Rehman and A. Zoha (Eds.): BODYNETS 2021, LNICST 420, pp. 15–27, 2022.
https://doi.org/10.1007/978-3-030-95593-9_2

Several studies have emerged over the past years that utilised Radio Frequency (RF) to detect small scale activities such as vitals [22, 24], large scale body movements [6, 19, 21], and for localisation and tracking [5, 15, 18, 25]. The studies reported the use of various types of radio devices including the Universal Software Radio Peripheral (URSP) device [12, 23], Commercial off-the-shelf (COTS) Wi-Fi devices [8, 11, 27], Frequency-Modulated Continuous Wave radar (FMCW) [26], and Impulse Radio Ultra-Wideband (IR-UWB) [10].

The systems presented in the literature performed a distinct functionality, that is, either localisation or small/large scale activity detection. For instance, the activity detection systems presented by [13, 23] reported accuracies of 91% and 94% respectively, with both using the USRP N210 model. Other studies that performed localisation and tracking such as [5, 18] reported accuracies of 81% and an error of 5 cm in a $20 \times 70\,\mathrm{cm}^2$ area.

This paper improves on the studies presented in the literature by presenting a single system that is capable of utilising RF signals to detect, similar and different, activities performed in different locations, within the same room. As well as identify occupancy and the direction of movement across the activity area. The proposed system makes use of the USRP, operating as a Software-Defined Radio (SDR), to differentiate between five different activities and when the room is empty. Each of the activities was performed in three different positions, marked within the experimental area. The contributions in this paper can be summarised to, the integration of Machine Learning (ML), namely the Random Forest classifier, and Channel State Information (CSI), from SDRs, to recognise, with high accuracy, five different activities and their position within a room. The contributions can be summarised to the following:

- Localisation of activities in three different zones within a room
- Identifying direction of movement in three different positions within a room
- Identifying an empty room from one that is occupied

2   Materials and Methods

Having introduced the aim and focus of this paper, this section goes on to present details of the methodology adopted to conduct the experiments. Section 2.1 details the hardware and software components that were designed and utilised to enable collecting CSI data, depicting human activity, from the sensing devices. Whilst, Sect. 2.2 outlines the details of the conducted experiments, including, experimental setup, data collection, and training of the ML algorithm.

2.1   Technical Specifications

SDR models, particularly the USRP devices [7], X300 and X310, were used as the activity sensing nodes. The hardware and software specifications associated with the system are detailed in the following subsections.

Hardware. The set-up for data collection involved using two USRP devices communicating with each other while the activity was taking place within the area covered by them (see Fig. 1). The USRP X300 was used as the transmitter and the X310 was used as the receiver, with each using the VERT2450 omnidirectional antenna. Both devices were connected to a separate Personal Computer (PC), through a 1G Small Form-Factor Pluggable (SFP) connector. The PCs were equipped with the Intel(R) Core (TM) i7-7700 3.60 GHz processors and each has a 16 GB RAM and had an Ubuntu 16.04 virtual machine running on it. The virtual machine hosted the python scripts used to configure the USRP devices as well as collect and process the data.

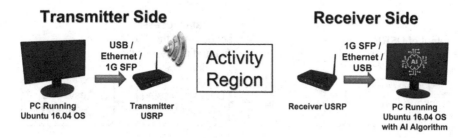

Fig. 1. System architecture.

Software. The software design stage involved two main activities, the first was the configuration of the USRP transmitter and receiver devices to communicate together. This was performed using the GNU radio python package to set parameters such as central frequency, which was 3.75 GHz, number of Orthogonal Frequency Division Multiplexing (OFDM) subcarriers, and power levels (see Table 1).

GNU Radio is a free and open-source software that is used in research for SDRs and signal processing [2]. GNU Radio comes with examples of OFDM signal processing where the CSI can be extracted. The GNU Radio software publishes the configuration in the format of a flow diagram which can be used to set up the blocks of the USRP and OFDM communication. The flow diagram can then be converted into a python script, which can be executed to begin OFDM communication.

Table 1. System parameters

Parameter	Value
Operating frequency	3.75 GHz
Number of OFDM subcarriers	52
Transmitter gain (dBm)	70
Receiver gain (dBm)	50

The second activity was to collect the CSI and create data sets from them in the form of "Comma-Separated Values" (CSV) files. The CSV files would hold the data sets that will be used for training and testing the ML algorithm. For this, another python script is used to process the raw data extracted by GNU radio from the receiver USRP, and filter out the CSI complex numbers. Python carries out mathematical functions to calculate the amplitude of the RF signal from the CSI complex numbers. The amplitude values are then saved to CSV format for ML and to visualise the signal propagation through line graphs. The "CSV file" creation process (see Fig. 2) was repeated for all the data collected in all the experiments.

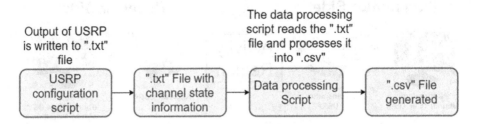

Fig. 2. Data flow diagram.

2.2 Experimental Design

The experiments presented in this paper were conducted at the University of Glasgow's James Watt South Building in a $3.8 \times 5.2\,\mathrm{m}^2$ room, where there is an active and approved ethical application. Three zones were marked in the room and all activities were repeated in them. The transmitter and receiver USRP devices were installed in the corners of the room, facing each other at an angle of 45°. The five activities performed were: Sitting, Standing, Walking along the 3.8 m side of the room from the transmitter to the receiver, Walking along the 3.8 m side of the room from the receiver to the transmitter, and Leaning forward.

Each of the five activities was repeated in three "Activity Zones", spaced by 1 m. Figure 3 shows the details of the experimental setup, including the activity areas, the location at which each activity was performed, and the positioning of the transmitter and receiver USRP devices.

Data Collection. The data collected for the proposed experiments were for a single subject performing the previously mentioned activities in three different zones within the room, as depicted in Fig. 3.

A total of 360 CSI samples were collected throughout the data collection stage, each consisted of approximately 1200 packets and this corresponds to about 3 s in time. The 360 CSI samples represent 16 different classifications, where each classification represents a data set, the "Empty Room" classification consists of 60 samples, that is, 20 samples collected to be used for every zone,

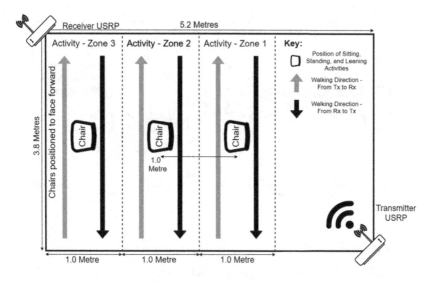

Fig. 3. Experimental setup.

and the remaining 15 classes each consists of 20 samples. A classification refers to a distinct class of data that represents an activity or the state of the room, for example, "Sitting" in "Zone One" is a classification, and "Sitting" in "Zone Two" is another. Given five activities are being captured in three different zones, this makes 15 out of the 16 classes. The 16th classification represented the CSI data captured for the room without the human subject present inside it. The choice to incorporate this class with the rest of the data was to see if the system can identify if the room is occupied and is one of the main contributions of this paper. Table 2 shows all the 16 classes and the number of samples collected for each. Furthermore, Fig. 4 shows the distinct variation in the wireless CSI patterns amongst all five activities and the "Empty Room".

Machine Learning. Having outlined the specifics of the data collection stage, using the USRP devices. This section provides an overview of the ML algorithm designed and used for classification in this paper. The choice of the algorithm was based on a study, previously conducted by the authorship team [21], where four ML algorithms were investigated, namely the Random Forest, K Nearest Neighbours (KNN) [14], Support Vector Machine (SVM) [16], and Neural Network [1,4,9]. In [21], the authors conducted two experiments to evaluate the accuracy of each algorithm, the first used 10-fold cross-validation and the second used train and test split. The 10-fold cross-validation takes the entire data set, and the data is split into 10 groups. One group is assigned as the test data and the other groups are assigned as the training data. The algorithm then uses the training data to create a model. The model is then applied to the test data to attempt to classify the data. This is then repeated until each group of data serves a turn as the test data. The predictions made each time are then compared to

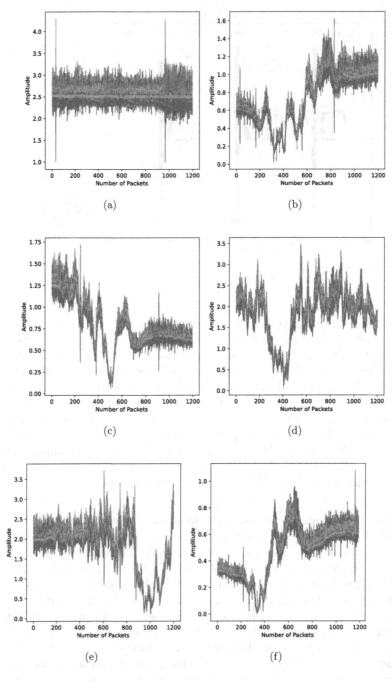

Fig. 4. Wireless CSI data samples representing various activity classes in activity Zone 1: a) Empty, b) Sitting, c) Standing, d) Walking from Tx to Rx, e) Walking from Rx to Tx and f) Leaning Forward.

Table 2. Data collection - The data classes and their description

Class	Class description	Number of samples
Empty Room	No human subject in the activity area	60
Sitting Zone 1	The action of "Sitting" at the designated location within Zone 1	20
Standing Zone 1	The action of "Standing" at the designated location within Zone 1	20
Walking Tx - Rx Zone 1	Walking from the USRP Tx side to the USRP Rx side within Zone 1	20
Walking Rx - Tx Zone 1	Walking from the USRP Rx side to the USRP Tx side within Zone 1	20
Leaning Forward Zone 1	Leaning forward with the upper body at the designated location within Zone 1	20
Sitting Zone 2	The action of "Sitting" at the designated location within Zone 2	20
Standing Zone 2	The action of "Standing" at the designated location within Zone 2	20
Walking Tx - Rx Zone 2	Walking from the USRP Tx side to the USRP Rx side within Zone 2	20
Walking Rx - Tx Zone 2	Walking from the USRP Rx side to the USRP Tx side within Zone 2	20
Leaning Forward Zone 2	Leaning forward with the upper body at the designated location within Zone 2	20
Sitting Zone 3	The action of "Sitting" at the designated location within Zone 3	20
Standing Zone 3	The action of "Standing" at the designated location within Zone 3	20
Walking Tx - Rx Zone 3	Walking from the USRP Tx side to the USRP Rx side within Zone 3	20
Walking Rx - Tx Zone 3	Walking from the USRP Rx side to the USRP Tx side within Zone 3	20
Leaning Forward Zone 3	Leaning forward with the upper body at the designated location within Zone 3	20

the correct labels from the data set and the performance can be measured. The train test split method only splits the data set between training and testing one predefined time. In the experiment in [21], the data set was split into 70% training data and the other 30% is set as the testing data. The algorithm performance was measured by comparing the Accuracy, Precision, Recall and F1-score. These performance metrics are calculated by looking at four classification values. The classification values are True Positive (TP), True Negative (TN), False Positive (FP) and False Negative (FN). The results of the evaluation, presented in [21], showed that the Random Forest algorithm had the highest accuracy of 92.47% with cross-validation and 96.70% using 70% training and 30% testing.

The Random Forest algorithm deploys a collection of decision trees where each tree predicts the output by looking for features found in the training phase. Each prediction is considered a vote and the majority of the votes decide on the overall Random Forest prediction [17].

System Testing. As mentioned earlier in Sect. 1, the paper aims to present a system that is capable of recognising with high accuracy the activity, its position within a room, and, where applicable, the direction of movement. The contributions of the paper are reiterated below:

1. Positioning of a human subject
2. Identifying the direction of movement in three different positions within a room
3. Identifying an empty room from one that is occupied
4. Establishing a relationship between the detection accuracy and the position of the activity

To do so, two different experiments were performed using the Random Forest classifier. The first involved applying ML to all classes representing each zone, individually. This means that ML was applied to data sets with the following labels: Empty, Sitting, Standing, Walking Tx-Rx, Walking Rx-Tx, and Leaning Forward, from each zone, to get three different outputs. The purpose of this experiment was to mainly meet the fourth contribution point mentioned above. The second experiment involved building a single data set with all 16 classes together. This experiment was to test the "Positioning", "Direction Detection", and "Occupancy" features of the system.

3   Results and Discussion

Two sets of results are presented in this section to showcase the contributions of this paper. The first set of results, which are from experiments performed for each "Activity Zone" separately and are presented in Sect. 3.1, focused on establishing a relationship between the activity position and the system's detection accuracy. However, they are also used to further validate the ability of the system to identify the direction of movement and occupancy.

The second set of results, which are from experiments performed for all "Activity Zones" combined and are presented in Sect. 3.2, are used to highlight the main contributions of the paper by measuring the system's ability to identify "Position of Activity", "Direction of Movement, and "Occupancy". The 10-fold cross-validation method was used to evaluate the system in all scenarios.

3.1   Detection Accuracy vs. Activity Position

This experiment was designed to evaluate the system's response to moving the activity area further away from the transmitter. Data for the following classes: 1) Empty, 2) Sitting, 3) Standing, 4) Walking Tx-Rx, 5) Walking Rx-Tx, 6) Leaning

Forward, were collected in all three "Activity Areas", and three separate data sets were built. The Random Forest 10-fold cross-validation was applied to each data set, and the results alongside the confusion matrices are shown in Table 3. As can be seen in Table 3, the accuracy for the data set from "Activity Zone One" was 100%, that is, the system was capable of fully differentiating between all 6 classes, without confusion. Whilst the accuracy was 97.5% and 95%, with the data sets from "Activity Zone Two" and "Activity Zone Three", respectively. The results presented by the confusion matrix clearly show a decrease in accuracy as the activity area moves further away from the transmitter, particularly with the "Leaning Forward", which was the most affected in "Zone Three". The reduction in the accuracy is believed to be linked to the CSI pattern which becomes less evident as the subject moves away from the transmitter. It can be seen in Fig. 5, that the wireless CSI pattern of a "Sitting" activity performed in "Zone One" (see Fig. 5a) is more evident than that of the same activity but performed in "Zone Three" (see Fig. 5b).

Although the focus of the experiment was to measure detection accuracy vs distance from the transmitter, the results also indicate the ability of the system to differentiate between when the room is "Empty" and "Occupied", that is, activity is being performed, and identifying the walking direction of the subject within each zone, as evident by the confusion matrices in Table 3.

Table 3. Three confusion matrices for each of the three zones with the Random Forest algorithm

Zone one - all activities (accuracy 100%)						
Class		Predicted class					
		Empty room	Leaning forward	Sitting	Standing	Walking Tx to Rx	Walking Rx to Tx
True class	Empty room	20	0	0	0	0	0
	Leaning forward	0	20	0	0	0	0
	Sitting	0	0	20	0	0	0
	Standing	0	0	0	20	0	0
	Walking Tx to Rx	0	0	0	0	20	0
	Walking Rx to Tx	0	0	0	0	0	20
Zone two - all activities (accuracy 97.5%)						
Class		Predicted class					
		Empty room	Leaning forward	Sitting	Standing	Walking Tx to Rx	Walking Rx to Tx
True class	Empty room	20	0	0	0	0	0
	Leaning forward	0	19	1	0	0	0
	Sitting	0	0	20	0	0	0
	Standing	0	0	0	19	1	0
	Walking Tx to Rx	0	1	0	0	19	0
	Walking Rx to Tx	0	0	0	0	0	20
Zone three - all activities (accuracy 95%)						
Class		Predicted class					
		Empty room	Leaning forward	Sitting	Standing	Walking Tx to Rx	Walking Rx to Tx
True class	Empty room	20	0	0	0	0	0
	Leaning forward	2	14	1	3	0	0
	Sitting	0	0	20	0	0	0
	Standing	0	0	0	20	0	0
	Walking Tx to Rx	0	0	0	0	20	0
	Walking Rx to Tx	0	0	0	0	0	20

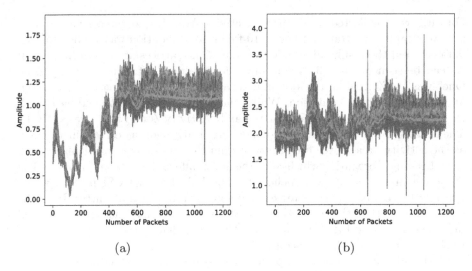

(a)   (b)

Fig. 5. Wireless CSI data samples for the Siting activity in: a) Zone 1, b) Zone 3.

3.2   Detecting Position, Direction of Movement, and Occupancy

To evaluate the system's ability to identify the position of the subject, whilst performing an activity, all 360 CSI data samples, that is, the data representing all 16 classes, were combined into one data set with 16 labels, presented earlier in Table 2. The results of applying the Random Forest 10-fold cross-validation and the confusion matrix, are shown in Table 4. The results show the capability of the system to differentiate between all 5 activities when performed in different positions of the room, with a high accuracy of 93.6%. The results can be further interpreted to tell the following:

- The system is capable of identifying walking directions in three different activity areas in the same room. This is evident by classes number 4 and 5, representing two walking directions in "Zone One", classes number 9 and 10, representing those in "Zone Two", and finally classes number 14 and 15 for "Zone Three". Approximately two data samples were miss-classified in each zone, giving an accuracy of almost 90%.
- The system was capable of successfully classifying 60 data samples representing an "Empty Room" correctly, with an accuracy of 100%, which gives this system an edge over other activity monitoring systems in the literature, as it can identify occupancy.

Table 4. Confusion matrix for all sixteen classes with the Random Forest algorithm

All sixteen classes - accuracy (93.6%)																		
Class			Predicted class															
			1	2	3	4	5	6	7	8	9	10	11	12	13	14	15	16
True class	1	Empty	**60**	0	0	0	0	0	0	0	0	0	0	0	0	0	0	0
	2	SitZ1	0	**20**	0	0	0	0	0	0	0	0	0	0	0	0	0	0
	3	StandZ1	0	0	**20**	0	0	0	0	0	0	0	0	0	0	0	0	0
	4	WalkTxRxZ1	0	0	0	**18**	0	0	1	0	0	0	0	0	0	0	1	0
	5	WalkRxTxZ1	0	0	0	0	**19**	0	0	0	1	0	0	0	0	0	0	0
	6	LeaningFZ1	0	0	0	0	0	**20**	0	0	0	0	0	0	0	0	0	0
	7	SitZ2	0	0	0	0	0	0	**18**	0	0	0	0	1	0	0	1	0
	8	StandZ2	0	0	0	0	1	0	0	**19**	0	0	0	0	0	0	0	0
	9	WalkTxRxZ2	1	0	0	0	1	0	0	0	**18**	0	0	0	0	0	0	0
	10	WalkRxTxZ2	0	0	0	0	0	0	0	0	0	**20**	0	0	0	0	0	0
	11	LeaningFZ2	0	0	0	0	0	0	1	0	0	0	**17**	0	1	1	0	0
	12	SitZ3	0	0	0	0	0	0	0	0	0	0	0	**20**	0	0	0	0
	13	StandZ3	0	0	0	0	0	0	0	0	0	0	2	0	**18**	0	0	0
	14	WalkTxRxZ3	0	0	0	0	0	0	0	0	0	0	0	0	0	**20**	0	0
	15	WalkRxTxZ3	0	0	0	0	1	0	0	0	0	1	0	0	0	0	**18**	0
	16	LeaningFZ3	0	0	0	0	0	0	2	0	0	0	3	0	3	0	0	**12**

4   Conclusion

This paper presented a novel system that utilises the USRP devices, working as SDRs, to detect multiple activities performed in different locations of the same room. The system aimed to offer a solution that is based on RF-sensing to identify, in an indoor setting, the position of a performed activity, the occupancy of a room, and, where applicable, the direction of particular activities. The conducted experiments resulted in interesting conclusion points, that still require further investigation through the collection of more data. Firstly, was the ability of the system to identify the position of the activity, with an accuracy of almost 94% (one of which was leaning which can be used to infer falling), the occupancy of the room with an accuracy of 100%, and the walking direction in three different positions within the room with an accuracy of 90%. Such capabilities can be used to develop systems for:

- Performing fall prediction and detection by inferring it based on the "Leaning" activity.
- Monitoring elderly people who live alone, without invading their privacy, to ensure they are active and conscious.
- The utilisation of the occupancy feature in energy saving systems, emergency evacuation, and security systems by monitoring the direction of movement of unauthorised subjects.

Secondly was the reduction in the system's activity detection accuracy when the activity is performed further away from the transmitter, as presented earlier in Table 3. However, further investigation is required due to the controlled nature of the experiment and the lack of a large data set that can be used to define a relationship between the accuracy of detection and the position of the activity.

Acknowledgements. This work was supported in parts by The Department for Digital, Culture, Media & Sport, 5G New Thinking project, the Engineering and Physical Sciences Research Council (EPSRC) grants, EP/R511705/1, EP/T021020/1, and EP/T021063/1, and the Ajman University Internal Research Grant.

References

1. Abbas Hassan, A., Sheta, A.F., Wahbi, T.M.: Intrusion detection system using weka data mining tool. Int. J. Sci. Res. (IJSR) (2015). https://doi.org/10.21275/1091703. www.ijsr.net
2. Adarsh, J., Vishak, P., Gandhiraj, R.: Adaptive noise cancellation using NLMS algorithm in GNU radio. In: 2017 4th International Conference on Advanced Computing and Communication Systems (ICACCS), pp. 1–4 (2017)
3. Al-qaness, M.A.A., Abd Elaziz, M., Kim, S., Ewees, A.A., Abbasi, A.A., Alhaj, Y.A., Hawbani, A.: Channel state information from pure communication to sense and track human motion: a survey. Sensors **19**(15) (2019). https://doi.org/10.3390/s19153329, https://www.mdpi.com/1424-8220/19/15/3329
4. Biswas, S.K.: Intrusion detection using machine learning: a comparison study. Int. J. Pure Appl. Math. **118**(19), 101–114 (2018)
5. Cao, X., Chen, Y., Liu, K.J.R.: High accuracy indoor localization: a WiFi-based approach, vol. 1, pp. 6220–6224. IEEE (2016)
6. Ding, S., Chen, Z., Zheng, T., Luo, J.: RF-net: a unified meta-learning framework for RF-enabled one-shot human activity recognition. In: SenSys 2020 - Proceedings of the 2020 18th ACM Conference on Embedded Networked Sensor Systems, pp. 517–530 (2020). https://doi.org/10.1145/3384419.3430735
7. Ettus, M., Braun, M.: The Universal Software Radio Peripheral (USRP) Family of Low-Cost SDRs, Chap. 1, pp. 3–23. Wiley, New York (2015). https://doi.org/10.1002/9781119057246.ch1. https://onlinelibrary.wiley.com/doi/abs/10.1002/9781119057246.ch1
8. Guo, X., Elikplim, N.R., Ansari, N., Li, L., Wang, L.: Robust WiFi localization by fusing derivative fingerprints of RSS and multiple classifiers. IEEE Trans. Ind. Inf. **16**(5), 3177–3186 (2020). https://doi.org/10.1109/TII.2019.2910664
9. Hamid, Y., Sugumaran, M., Balasaraswathi, V.: IDS using machine learning - current state of art and future directions. Curr. J. Appl. Sci. Technol. **15**(3), 1–22 (2016). https://doi.org/10.9734/bjast/2016/23668. https://www.journalcjast.com/index.php/CJAST/article/view/8556
10. Khan, F., Ghaffar, A., Khan, N., Cho, S.H.: An overview of signal processing techniques for remote health monitoring using impulse radio UWB transceiver. Sensors **20**(9), 2479 (2020). https://doi.org/10.3390/s20092479
11. Li, L., Guo, X., Ansari, N.: SmartLoc: smart wireless indoor localization empowered by machine learning. IEEE Trans. Ind. Electron. **67**(8), 6883–6893 (2020). https://doi.org/10.1109/TIE.2019.2931261
12. Patra, A., Simić, L., Petrova, M.: mmRTI: radio tomographic imaging using highly-directional millimeter-wave devices for accurate and robust indoor localization. In: IEEE International Symposium on Personal, Indoor and Mobile Radio Communications, PIMRC, 1–7 October 2017 (2018). https://doi.org/10.1109/PIMRC.2017.8292523

13. Pu, Q., Gupta, S., Gollakota, S., Patel, S.: Gesture recognition using wireless signals. GetMobile Mob. Comput. Commun. **18**(4), 15–18 (2015). https://doi.org/10.1145/2721914.2721919
14. Saçlı, B., et al.: Microwave dielectric property based classification of renal calculi: Application of a kNN algorithm. Comput. Biol. Med. **112**, 103366 (2019). https://doi.org/10.1016/j.compbiomed.2019.103366. https://www.sciencedirect.com/science/article/pii/S0010482519302434
15. Schmitz, J., Bartsch, F., Hernandez, M., Mathar, R.: Distributed software defined radio testbed for real-time emitter localization and trackingm pp. 1246–1252 (2017). https://doi.org/10.1109/ICCW.2017.7962829
16. Seehapoch, T., Wongthanavasu, S.: Speech emotion recognition using support vector Machines. In: 2013 5th International Conference on Knowledge and Smart Technology (KST), pp. 86–91 (2013). https://doi.org/10.1109/KST.2013.6512793
17. Shaikhina, T., Lowe, D., Daga, S., Briggs, D., Higgins, R., Khovanova, N.: Decision tree and random forest models for outcome prediction in antibody incompatible kidney transplantation. Biomed. Signal Process. Control **52**, 456–462 (2019). https://doi.org/10.1016/j.bspc.2017.01.012. https://www.sciencedirect.com/science/article/pii/S1746809417300204
18. Shi, S., Sigg, S., Chen, L., Ji, Y.: Accurate location tracking from CSI-based passive device-free probabilistic fingerprinting. IEEE Trans. Veh. Technol. **67**(6), 5217–5230 (2018). https://doi.org/10.1109/TVT.2018.2810307
19. Sigg, S., Scholz, M., Shi, S., Ji, Y., Beigl, M.: RF-sensing of activities from non-cooperative subjects in device-free recognition systems using ambient and local signals. IEEE Trans. Mob. Comput. **13**(4), 907–920 (2014). https://doi.org/10.1109/TMC.2013.28
20. Stella, M., Russo, M., Begušić, D.: RF localization in indoor environment. Radioengineering **21**(2), 557–567 (2012)
21. Taylor, W., Shah, S.A., Dashtipour, K., Zahid, A., Abbasi, Q.H., Imran, M.A.: An intelligent non-invasive real-time human activity recognition system for next-generation healthcare. Sensors **20**(9), 2653 (2020). www.mdpi.com/journal/sensors
22. Uysal, C., Filik, T.: RF-Based noncontact respiratory rate monitoring with parametric spectral estimation. IEEE Sens. J. **19**(21), 9841–9849 (2019). https://doi.org/10.1109/JSEN.2019.2927536
23. Wang, G., Zou, Y., Zhou, Z., Wu, K., Ni, L.M.: We can hear you with Wi-Fi! IEEE Trans. Mob. Comput. **15**(11), 2907–2920 (2016). https://doi.org/10.1109/TMC.2016.2517630
24. Wang, X., Yang, C., Mao, S.: On CSI-based vital sign monitoring using commodity WiFi. ACM Trans. Comput. Healthc. **1**(3), 1–27 (2020). https://doi.org/10.1145/3377165
25. Yang, M., Chuo, L.X., Suri, K., Liu, L., Zheng, H., Kim, H.S.: ILPS: Local Positioning System with Simultaneous Localization and Wireless Communication, vol. 2019, pp. 379–387. IEEE, April 2019. https://doi.org/10.1109/INFOCOM.2019.8737569
26. Zhao, M., et al.: RF-based 3D skeletons. In: SIGCOMM 2018 - Proceedings of the 2018 Conference of the ACM Special Interest Group on Data Communication, pp. 267–281 (2018). https://doi.org/10.1145/3230543.3230579
27. Zheng, Y., et al.: Zero-effort cross-domain gesture recognition with Wi-Fi, pp. 313–325 (2019)

Monitoring Discrete Activities of Daily Living of Young and Older Adults Using 5.8 GHz Frequency Modulated Continuous Wave Radar and ResNet Algorithm

Umer Saeed[1(✉)], Fehaid Alqahtani[2], Fatmah Baothman[3], Syed Yaseen Shah[4],
Syed Ikram Shah[5], Syed Salman Badshah[6], Muhammad Ali Imran[7],
Qammer H. Abbasi[7], and Syed Aziz Shah[1]

[1] Research Centre for Intelligent Healthcare, Coventry University,
Coventry CV1 5FB, UK
{saeedu3,syed.shah}@coventry.ac.uk

[2] Department of Computer Science, King Fahad Naval Academy,
Al Jubail 35512, Saudi Arabia
F-alqahtani@rsnf.gov.sa

[3] Faculty of Computing and Information Technology, King Abdul Aziz University,
Jeddah 21431, Saudi Arabia
fbaothman@kau.edu.sa

[4] School of Computing, Engineering and Built Environment,
Glasgow Caledonian University, Glasgow G4 0BA, UK
syedyaseen.shah@gcu.ac.uk

[5] College of Electrical and Mechanical Engineering, National University of Sciences
and Technology, Islamabad 44000, Pakistan
syed.shah15@ce.ceme.edu.pk

[6] School of Electronics Engineering, Xidian University, Xi'an 710071, China

[7] James Watt School of Engineering, University of Glasgow, Glasgow G12 8QQ, UK
{muhammad.imran,qammer.abbasi}@glasgow.ac.uk

Abstract. With numerous applications in distinct domains, especially healthcare, human activity detection is of utmost significance. The objective of this study is to monitor activities of daily living using the publicly available dataset recorded in nine different geometrical locations for ninety-nine volunteers including young and older adults (65+) using 5.8 GHz Frequency Modulated Continuous Wave (FMCW) radar. In this work, we experimented with discrete human activities, for instance, walking, sitting, standing, bending, and drinking, recorded for 10 s and 5 s. To detect the list of activities mentioned above, we obtained the Micro-Doppler signatures through Short-time Fourier transform using MAT-LAB tool and procured the spectrograms as images. The acquired data of the spectrograms are trained, validated, and tested exploiting a state-of-the-art deep learning approach known as Residual Neural Network

© ICST Institute for Computer Sciences, Social Informatics and Telecommunications Engineering 2022
Published by Springer Nature Switzerland AG 2022. All Rights Reserved
M. Ur Rehman and A. Zoha (Eds.): BODYNETS 2021, LNICST 420, pp. 28–38, 2022.
https://doi.org/10.1007/978-3-030-95593-9_3

(ResNet). Moreover, the confusion matrix, model loss, and classification accuracy are used as performance evaluation metrics for the trained ResNet model. The unique skip connection technique of ResNet minimises the overfitting and underfitting issue, consequently resulting accuracy rate up to 91%.

Keywords: Radar sensor · Non-invasive healthcare · Human activities identification · Deep learning · ResNet

1   Introduction

Activities of daily living (ADL) are essential and routine tasks that most healthy young and older adults can perform without assistance. The inability to perform these ADL might cause unsafe conditions and poor quality of life [1]. The healthcare team should be aware of the importance of assessing ADL in patients to help ensure that patients who require assistance and are identified [2]. Thus monitoring ADL is of utmost importance since any activity undetected can cause fatal injuries [3].

Recently, several sensing technologies have been implemented in this context to resolve these crucial issues and allow the identification of several human activities [4–12] or activities in order to detect critical events like falls [13–15]. Wearable sensors [16], thermal imaging [17], pressure sensors [18], and Radio Frequency (RF) sensors such as lightweight and low-cost radar schemes are among the technologies which can be effectively used for the identification of human activities [7,19,20]. To choose one or more technologies [20–24], we must analyze the benefits and drawbacks of each sensor when it comes to performance evaluation metrics like false alarms, model accuracy, proportion of failed identifications, cost, user compliance, and ease of deployment. Pressure and wearable sensors, for instance, have high detection accuracy, nevertheless, the gadget must be worn on the human's body, which can be uncomfortable at times, and the thermal imaging camera poses privacy issues. The radar sensor, on the other hand, provides an inexpensive, non-contact, and readily deployable solution for monitoring everyday activities [25].

This paper presents a deep learning-based solution utilizing Residual Neural Network (ResNet) for the identification of prevalent human activities like walking, sitting, standing, and other activities. To record human activities, we have used Frequency Modulated Continuous Wave (FMCW) radar exploiting Micro-Doppler (MD) signatures. Volunteers took part in the data collection process, which occurred in distinct locations. After data prepossessing, the deep learning model was trained to identify unknown human activities.

2   Methodology

2.1   Data Acquisition

We have used the dataset obtained for the recently finished project "Intelligent RF Sensing for Falls and Health Prediction - INSHEP" funded by Engineering and Physical Sciences Research Council (EPSRC).
(http://researchdata.gla.ac.uk/848/) [26].

This dataset was recorded using an FMCW radar functioning at C-band (5.8 GHz) over a bandwidth of 400 MHz and an output power of +18 dBm. The radar was connected to an antenna with +17 dBm gain. A total of 99 volunteers took part in the experimental campaign, with an age range of 21 years to 99 years at 9 different and separate locations and data was recorded for 10 s (walking) and rest of the activities for 5 s with 3 repetitions for each activity. The received signal was used to generate MD signatures using Short-time Fourier transform. The typical radar working principle is shown in Fig. 1(a), where a radio frequency signal is transmitted and received when encountering any object within its range. Figure 1(b) depicts the typical waveform of FMCW radar. Every movement of the body produces a distinct MD signature that can be employed to distinguish between various everyday activities [27–29]. Fundamentally, FMCW radar is a kind of radar sensor that, like a basic continuous-wave radar, emits continuous transmission power. FMCW radar, unlike continuous-wave radar, can adjust its working frequency throughout the measurements.

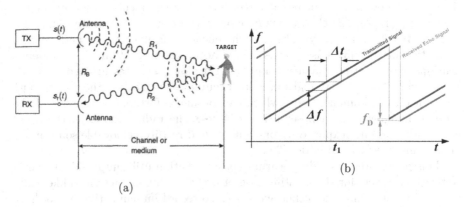

Fig. 1. (a) Typical radar working principle using reflected RF signal (b) FMCW radar waveform.

In this work, five distinct human activities were recorded using FMCW radar in separate locations, which were walking forward and back, sitting on a seat, standing from a seat, bending down to pick up an item, and drinking from a cup in standing position, as illustrated in Fig. 2 and listed in Table 1. Each human was asked to replicate the same task two or three times in order to collect data.

Figure 3 depicts the MD signatures of the data measurements. The spectrograms of a subject walking forward and back in front of radar are easily distinguishable from other activities. Activities like sitting on a seat and getting up from a seat are almost flipped images of each other. As shown in Fig. 3, when a subject bends down to pick up an item, the positive Doppler frequency changes significantly from 1.5–3 s. As the subject stood up again, a substantial alter in frequency was noted from 3.5–5 s.

Table 1. List of activities performed on humans.

Label	Activity
Activity 1	**Walking** (Forward and Back)
Activity 2	**Sitting** (On a Seat)
Activity 3	**Standing** (From a Seat)
Activity 4	**Bending** (Pick up Object)
Activity 5	**Drinking** (Standing Position)

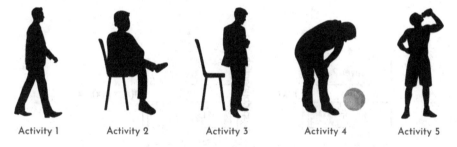

Activity 1   Activity 2   Activity 3   Activity 4   Activity 5

Fig. 2. Illustration of five distinct human activities. Activity 1 (Walking), Activity 2 (Sitting), Activity 3 (Standing), Activity 4 (Bending), Activity 5 (Drinking).

2.2 Classification Using Residual Neural Network

Machine learning-based techniques have been successfully employed in the past for different classification tasks [30–35]. In this paper, to classify distinct human activities through the obtained spectrograms, we have utilized a deep learning-based algorithm called Residual Neural Network or ResNet. The ability to train such a deep neural network (DNN) involves the use of skip connections. The input that feeds a layer is also applied to the output of a layer further up the stack. The aim of training a DNN is to get it to model a target function $h(x)$. If the network's output to the input is linked, for instance, adding a skip connection, the network would be strained to model $f(x) = h(x) - x$ instead of $h(x)$ [36,37]. This is referred to as "Residual Learning", as shown in Fig. 4.

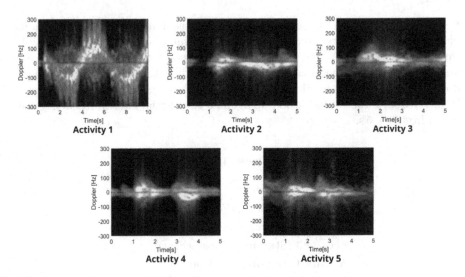

Fig. 3. Spectrograms of older adult with limited mobility - five different human activities.

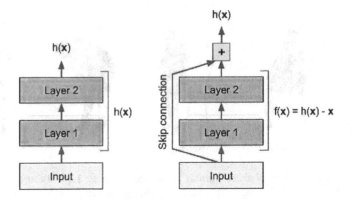

Fig. 4. ResNet learning framework.

The weights of a standard DNN are nearly zero when it is first initialised, so the network only outputs values near to zero. When a skip connection is added to the resulting network, it simply outputs a replica of its input, in other terms, it models the identity function at first. The training process can be significantly accelerated if the target function is close to the identity function which is frequently the case. Moreover, by adding a large number of skip connections, the network can begin to improve even though many layers are yet to learn. The signal can effectively traverse the whole network due to skip connections technique. The ResNet can be thought of as a pile of residual units, each of which is a diminutive neural network with a skip connection.

Furthermore, the establishment of a statistical relationship between the partial differential equation and the convolutional-residual-block assists to understand that why ResNet can be deeper to generate fine results in different tasks [38]. First, consider the following two-order partial differential equation:

$$\frac{\partial u(x,t)}{\partial t} = \frac{1}{2}\sigma^2 \frac{\partial^2 u(x,t)}{\partial x^2} + b\frac{\partial u(x,t)}{\partial x} + cu(x,t) \tag{1}$$

Equation 1 can be written in discrete form as:

$$u(x,\ t+1) - u(x,\ t) = \tfrac{1}{2}\sigma^2(u(x+1,t) - 2u(x,t) + u(x-1,t)) + \tfrac{b}{2}(u(x+1,t)$$
$$-u(x-1,t)) + cu(x,t) \tag{2}$$

Equation 2 can be rewritten in convolutional form as:

$$u(x,\ t+1) = u(x,\ t) + \left[\tfrac{1}{2}\left(\sigma^2 + b\right), c - \sigma^2, \tfrac{1}{2}\left(\sigma^2 - b\right)\right] * u(x,t) \tag{3}$$

As regard to the convolutional-kernel as $w(x,t)$, Eq. 3 has the same structure as residual-block:

$$u(x,\ t+1) = u(x,\ t) + w(x,\ t) * u(x,\ t) \tag{4}$$

According to the results of the aforementioned analysis, any two-order partial differential equation could be altered as residual-block through a convolutional-kernel size of three, and any higher-order partial differential equation could be transformed to a residual-block through a greater convolutional-kernel. The residual-block and the two-order partial differential equation have a correspondence since the ResNet kernel size is normally minimal. Furthermore, the Fourier Transform is commonly utilized in the solution of partial differential equation, and it can help explain why, as previously mentioned, deeper ResNet contributes to better results. We get the following statistics by applying the Fourier Transform to Eq. 1:

$$\hat{T}_x = \frac{1}{2}\sigma^2 \frac{\partial^2}{\partial x^2} + b\frac{\partial}{\partial x} + c \Longleftrightarrow \hat{T}_p = -\frac{1}{2}\sigma^2 p^2 + ibp + c \tag{5}$$

$$\hat{T}_p \tilde{u}(p,t) = \frac{d}{dt}\tilde{u}(p,t) \tag{6}$$

Solution of Eq. 6 is:

$$\tilde{u}(p,t) = e^{\hat{T}_p t}\tilde{u}(p,0) \tag{7}$$

If time t is minimal adequate, we get:

$$\tilde{u}(p,\ t) \approx \left(1 + \hat{T}_p t\right)\tilde{u}(p,0) \tag{8}$$

The following relationship can be obtained from the convolutional theorem by applying the inverse Fourier Transform to Eq. 8:

$$u(x,\ t) = u(x,0) + t\hat{T}_x\delta(x) * u(x,0) \tag{9}$$

Equations 4 and 9 are explicitly similar, and the convolutional-kernel $w(x,\ t)$ in continuous space corresponds to $t\hat{T}_x\delta(x)$. From a discrete point of view, Eq. 4 characterises the relation between the partial differential equation and the ResNet, while Eq. 9 captures the nature of the relation in the continuous domain. The numerals of the convolutional-kernels in residual-blocks are exceptionally minor. This is consistent with the fact that time t is short, since a short time span t means that the convolutional-kernel $t\hat{T}_x\delta(x)$ is mathematically small from Eq. 7–8. Furthermore, the lower size of the convolutional-kernels results in a low-order partial differential equation, which streamlines the iterative system's evolution. The analysis of the relation between the partial differential equation and residual-block provides insight into better comprehension of ResNet.

3   Results and Discussion

The ResNet algorithm considered in this study to identify distinct human activities was constructed in Python, primarily utilizing the TensorFlow and NumPy libraries. In this work, classification accuracy metric was taken into consideration to assess the performance of a trained model. The classification accuracy, in this case, human activity identification accuracy, can be described as the proportion of accurately identified human activities to the total number of human activities.

$$Identification\ Accuracy = \frac{Number\ of\ human\ activities\ identified}{Total\ number\ of\ human\ activities} \tag{10}$$

The dataset acquired consisted of five diverse human activities as listed in Table 1. Overall, 48×5 spectrograms were used for simulations, in which 22×5 were used for training, 4×5 for validation, and 22×5 for testing. Considering the size of a dataset, the number of epochs were set to 15 only and the DNN model ResNet was able to achieve accuracy up to 91%, as demonstrated in Fig. 5. Moreover, the model loss was recorded less than 0.5 as the number of epochs enhanced.

Additionally, Fig. 6 presents a confusion matrix of different human activities identified through the trained deep learning model. The ResNet was able to identify the walking activity with 100% accuracy. Moreover, there were only two misclassified instances for sitting and standing activities, hence exhibiting accuracy up to 90%. Whilst testing the trained model ResNet, the bending activity revealed maximum misclassified instances up to four against the drinking activity, therefore disclosing 81.8% accuracy. Lastly, the drinking activity unveiled 95% accuracy with only one misclassification against bending activity.

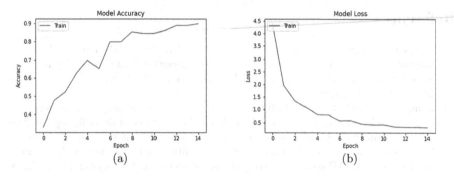

Fig. 5. (a) ResNet model accuracy and (b) model loss against the number of epochs.

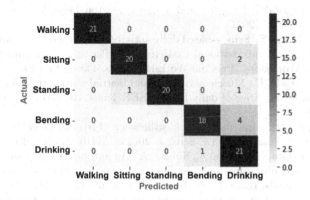

Fig. 6. Confusion matrix of five distinct human activities classified through ResNet.

4   Conclusions and Future Work

The idea behind this research is to exploit existing radar data to classify activities of daily living when data was obtained in nine different locations for ninety-nine volunteers. In this work, we provided preliminary findings for a simplified method that utilizes the FMCW radar to recognise distinct human activities such as walking, sitting, standing, bending, and drinking. As part of the experimental study, subjects were requested to undertake the five aforementioned human tasks at different geometrical positions. The radar system's MD signatures were then used as image data, and diverse features were extracted, validated, and trained using a well-known deep learning approach called ResNet. After training, the model was tested on various human activities spectrograms and simulation results revealed that ResNet attained up to 91% accuracy overall.

In the future, we aim to experiment with diverse diminutive human activities such as chest movement, lung movement, and minor gestures through hands or feet. Furthermore, we intend to utilize cutting-edge deep learning techniques such as Generative Adversarial Networks in order to regenerate lower acquired classes or instances from the datasets, hence increasing the performance of the trained algorithm.

References

1. Nguyen, H., Lebel, K., Bogard, S., Goubault, E., Boissy, P., Duval, C.: Using inertial sensors to automatically detect and segment activities of daily living in people with Parkinson's disease. IEEE Trans. Neural Syst. Rehabil. Engineering **26**(1), 197–204 (2018)
2. Soma, T., Lawanont, W., Yokemura, T., Inoue, M.: Monitoring system for detecting decrease of living motivation based on change in activities of daily living. In: 2020 IEEE International Conference on Consumer Electronics (ICCE), pp. 1–4 (2020)
3. Saeed, U., et al.: Discrete human activity recognition and fall detection by combining FMCW RADAR data of heterogeneous environments for independent assistive living. Electronics **10**(18), 2237 (2021)
4. Shah, S.A., et al.: Privacy-preserving wandering behavior sensing in dementia patients using modified logistic and dynamic newton Leipnik maps. IEEE Sens. J. **21**(3), 3669–3679 (2021)
5. Hossain, T., Inoue, S.: Sensor-based daily activity understanding in caregiving center. In: 2019 IEEE International Conference on Pervasive Computing and Communications Workshops (PerCom Workshops), pp. 439–440 (2019)
6. Totty, M.S., Wade, E.: Muscle activation and inertial motion data for noninvasive classification of activities of daily living. IEEE Trans. Biomed. Eng. **65**(5), 1069–1076 (2018)
7. Shah, S.A., et al.: Sensor fusion for identification of freezing of gait episodes using Wi-Fi and radar imaging. IEEE Sens. J. **20**(23), 14410–14422 (2020)
8. Tuncer, T., Ertam, F., Dogan, S., Subasi, A.: An automated daily sports activities and gender recognition method based on novel multikernel local diamond pattern using sensor signals. IEEE Trans. Instrum. Meas. **69**(12), 9441–9448 (2020)
9. Shah, S.A., et al.: Privacy-preserving non-wearable occupancy monitoring system exploiting Wi-Fi imaging for next-generation body centric communication. Micromachines **11**(4), 379 (2020)
10. Shah, S.A., Fioranelli., F.: RF sensing technologies for assisted daily living in healthcare: a comprehensive review. IEEE Aerosp. Electron. Syst. Mag. **34**(11), 26–44 (2019)
11. Shah, S.A., Fan, D., Ren, A., Zhao, N., Yang, X., Tanoli, S.A.K.: Seizure episodes detection via smart medical sensing system. J. Ambient Intell. Humaniz. Comput. **11**, 1–13 (2018). https://doi.org/10.1007/s12652-018-1142-3
12. Shah, S.A., et al.: Buried object sensing considering curved pipeline. IEEE Antennas Wirel. Propag. Lett. **16**, 2771–2775 (2017)
13. Taylor, W., Shah, S.A., Dashtipour, K., Zahid, A., Abbasi, Q.H., Imran, M.A.: An intelligent non-invasive real-time human activity recognition system for next-generation healthcare. Sensors **20**(9), 2653 (2020)
14. Mohankumar, P., Ajayan, J., Mohanraj, T., Yasodharan, R.: Recent developments in biosensors for healthcare and biomedical applications: a review. Measurement **167**, 108293 (2021)
15. Ali, F., et al.: An intelligent healthcare monitoring framework using wearable sensors and social networking data. Future Gener. Comput. Syst. **114**, 23–43 (2021)
16. Dua, N., Singh, S.N., Semwal, V.B.: Multi-input CNN-GRU based human activity recognition using wearable sensors. Computing **103**(7), 1461–1478 (2021). https://doi.org/10.1007/s00607-021-00928-8
17. Naik, K., Pandit, T., Naik, N., Shah, P.: Activity recognition in residential spaces with internet of things devices and thermal imaging. Sensors **21**(3), 988 (2021)

18. Jiajun, X., Wang, G., Yufan, W., Ren, X., Gao, G.: Ultrastretchable wearable strain and pressure sensors based on adhesive, tough, and self-healing hydrogels for human motion monitoring. ACS Appl. Mater. Interfaces **11**(28), 25613–25623 (2019)

19. Saeed, U., et al.: Wireless channel modelling for identifying six types of respiratory patterns with SDR sensing and deep multilayer perceptron. IEEE Sens. J. **21**(18), 20833–20840 (2021)

20. Dong, B., et al.: Monitoring of atopic dermatitis using leaky coaxial cable. Healthc. Technol. Lett. **4**(6), 244–248 (2017)

21. Yang, X., et al.: s-band sensing-based motion assessment framework for cerebellar dysfunction patients. IEEE Sens. J. **19**(19), 8460–8467 (2018)

22. Haider, D., et al.: An efficient monitoring of eclamptic seizures in wireless sensors networks. Comput. Electr. Eng. **75**, 16–30 (2019)

23. Khan, S.A., et al.: An experimental channel capacity analysis of cooperative networks using universal software radio peripheral (USRP). Sustainability **10**(6), 1983 (2018)

24. Yang, X., et al.: Diagnosis of the hypopnea syndrome in the early stage. Neural Comput. Appl. **32**(3), 855–866 (2020). https://doi.org/10.1007/s00521-019-04037-8

25. Shah, S.A., Fioranelli, F.: Human activity recognition: preliminary results for dataset portability using FMCW RADAR. In 2019 International Radar Conference (RADAR), pp. 1–4. IEEE (2019)

26. Shah, S.A., Li, H., Shrestha, A., Yang, S., Fioranelli, F., Kernec, L.: Intelligent RF sensing for falls and health prediction - inshep – dataset (2019)

27. Amin, M.G., Zhang, Y.D., Ahmad, F., Dominic Ho, K.C.: Radar signal processing for elderly fall detection: the future for in-home monitoring. IEEE Signal Process. Mag. **33**(2), 71–80 (2016)

28. Fioranelli, F., Kernec, J.L., Shah, S.A.: Radar for health care: recognizing human activities and monitoring vital signs. IEEE Potentials **38**(4), 16–23 (2019)

29. Shah, S.A., Abbas, H., Imran, M.A., Abbasi, Q.H.: RF sensing for healthcare applications. Backscattering RF Sens. Future Wirel. Commun. 157–177 (2021)

30. Saeed, U., Jan, S.U., Lee, Y.-D., Koo, I.: Fault diagnosis based on extremely randomized trees in wireless sensor networks. Reliab. Eng. Syst. Saf. **205**, 107284 (2021)

31. Ashleibta, A.M., Abbasi, Q.H., Shah, S.A., Khalid, A., AbuAli, N.A., Imran, M.A.: Non-invasive RF sensing for detecting breathing abnormalities using software defined radios. IEEE Sens. J. **21**, 5111–5118 (2020)

32. Jan, S.U., Lee, Y.-D., Shin, J., Koo, I.: Sensor fault classification based on support vector machine and statistical time-domain features. IEEE Access **5**, 8682–8690 (2017)

33. Saeed, U., Lee, Y.-D., Jan, S.U., Koo, I.: CAFD: context-aware fault diagnostic scheme towards sensor faults utilizing machine learning. Sensors **21**(2), 617 (2021)

34. Huma, Z.E., et al.: A hybrid deep random neural network for cyberattack detection in the industrial internet of things. IEEE Access **9**, 55595–55605 (2021)

35. Churcher, A., et al.: An experimental analysis of attack classification using machine learning in IoT networks. Sensors **21**(2), 446 (2021)

36. He, K., Zhang, X., Ren, S., Sun, J.: Deep residual learning for image recognition. In: Proceedings of the IEEE Conference on Computer Vision and Pattern Recognition, pp. 770–778 (2016)

37. Géron, A.: Hands-on Machine Learning with Scikit-Learn, Keras, and TensorFlow: Concepts, Tools, and Techniques to Build Intelligent Systems. O'Reilly Media, Newton (2019)
38. Yin, M., Li, X., Zhang, Y., Wang, S.: On the mathematical understanding of ResNet with Feynman path integral. arXiv preprint arXiv:1904.07568 (2019)

Elderly Care - Human Activity Recognition Using Radar with an Open Dataset and Hybrid Maps

Xinyu Zhang[1,2], Qammer H. Abbasi[1] (iD), Francesco Fioranelli[3] (iD), Olivier Romain[4] (iD), and Julien Le Kernec[1,2(✉)] (iD)

[1] University of Glasgow, University Avenue, Glasgow G12 8QQ, UK
`julien.lekernec@glasgow.ac.uk`
[2] University of Electronic Science and Technology of China, Qingshuihe Campus: Chengdu High-tech Zone (West) 2006 West Avenue, Chengdu 611731, China
[3] TU Delft, Mekelweg 4, 2628 CD Delft, The Netherlands
[4] University Cergy-Pontoise, 6 Avenue du ponceau, 95000 Cergy-Pontoise, France

Abstract. Population ageing has become a severe problem worldwide. Human activity recognition (HAR) can play an important role to provide the elders with in-time healthcare. With the advantages of environmental insensitivity, contactless sensing and privacy protection, radar has been widely used for human activity detection. The micro-Doppler signatures (spectrograms) contain much information about human motion and are often applied in HAR. However, spectrograms only interpret magnitude information, resulting in suboptimal performances. We propose a radar-based HAR system using deep learning techniques. The data applied came from the open dataset "Radar signatures of human activities" created by the University of Glasgow. A new type of hybrid map was proposed, which concatenated the spectrograms amplitude and phase. After cropping the hybrid maps to focus on useful information, a convolutional neural network (CNN) based on LeNet-5 was designed for feature extraction and classification. In addition, the idea of transfer learning was applied for radar-based HAR to evaluate the classification performance of a pre-trained network. For this, GoogLeNet was taken and trained on the newly-produced hybrid maps. These initial results showed that the LeNet-5 CNN using only the spectrograms obtained an accuracy of 80.5%, while using the hybrid maps reached an accuracy of 84.3%, increasing by 3.8%. The classification result of transfer learning using GoogLeNet was 86.0% .

Keywords: Human activity recognition · Convolutional neural network · Transfer learning · Radar · Micro-Doppler · Hybrid maps

1 Introduction

1.1 Context

The development of public health and disease control has contributed much to increasing human life expectancy. However, along with the decreased average fertility rates, human

M. Ur Rehman and A. Zoha (Eds.): BODYNETS 2021, LNICST 420, pp. 39–51, 2022.
https://doi.org/10.1007/978-3-030-95593-9_4

longevity has resulted in the global issue of population ageing. World Population Ageing Report 2019 by the United Nations [1] summarised the previous trend of the population distribution in the world for the past two decades and estimated the trend for the next 30 years, from 2019 to 2050. The result showed the proportion of the global population for the old (aged over 65) had experienced a continuous increase, from around 6% in 1990 to 9% in 2019. Following the growing trend, the projected ageing population in 2050 would account for nearly 16%.

Human Activity Recognition (HAR) aims at conducting classification tasks to accurately identify human activities for further promoting proactive and timely healthcare [2]. Up to now, the most common methods of human activity detection are vision-based detection like using cameras and sensor-based detection such as using wearable sensors, radar and smartphone sensors [3, 4]. Among all the methods, radar technology outperforms the other for the following aspects [5–8]. Environmental insensitivity: radar detection is not influenced by harsh light; Contactless Sensing: users do not need to wear or connect with any devices, which provides a high capability of comfort and convenience; Privacy Protection: radar technology collects human activity data without showing their actual images, ensuring the privacy of individuals.

Much of the research [3, 9–11] around radar-based human activity recognition revolves around micro-Doppler signatures (spectrograms) [12], which provide rich information for classification.

1.2 Current Research Progress

Feature Extraction
In the research on HAR, it is apparent that one essential part is to extract features from the spectrograms and identify the movements represented in them. It can be found in previous research works that the features commonly used can be divided into several categories:

Physical Characteristics
Physical characteristics are characteristics with physical meanings. For instance, Kim [13] selected six features from a micro-Doppler map. Six features were extracted from the spectrogram, including the torso frequency where the scattering is strongest, the total bandwidth, the overall frequency shift, the Doppler bandwidth without micro-Dopplers, the normalised standard deviation (STD) of the signal intensity and the activity period. These are then used for classification. Further examples can be found for healthcare and animal welfare applications with physical characteristic extraction [3–5, 14–21].

Micro-doppler Maps (Spectrograms)
One main inconvenience of the feature extraction method based on extracting handcrafted features is that it relies heavily on the know-how of the radar engineer. As machine learning developed, many researchers began to directly consider the grayscale of RGB images of spectrograms as features. Then, convolutional neural networks derived from vision-based classification were applied to those images for classification [3–7, 10, 22]. Compared with the conventional hand-crafted feature extraction approaches, the use of

deep learning technology can increase the accuracy in classification. Through training and testing of a large number of data samples, deep learning seeks out the mapping relationship between data features and labels [23].

Classification Approaches

There have been numerous research works in solving HAR tasks. Because the movements of the human body are complex and each micro-motion can produce a unique micro-Doppler signature, many researchers have delved into extracting specific features from the micro-Doppler spectrograms and using classifiers to perform specific classification tasks.

At the start, conventional machine learning techniques, such as random forest, support vector machine (SVM) and K-nearest neighbour classifiers, were commonly researched. In 2009, Kim's team firstly used a support vector machine to identify activities from human micro-Doppler features [13]. In the experiment, the volunteers were asked to perform seven different activities. Then, they designed a variety of empirical features for each movement and extracted parameters according to those features. Finally, the team classified those seven activities by training a support vector machine model and received an average classification accuracy of 91.4%. In [24], a random forest was performed to classify the data information in a real-time manner. As a result, the average gesture recognition precision reached over 90%.

In recent years, with the development of GPU and deep neural networks, they have been applied to the human activity classification based on micro-Doppler characteristics as a powerful classifier. Deep learning technology can implement feature extraction and activity classification simultaneously, with minimal input from the human operator. In [25], the authors detected the micro-motion information of drones and obtained the micro-Doppler maps. They then carried out frequency-domain transformation to the Doppler features and obtained the cadence-velocity diagram (CVD). The two feature maps were merged and classified by the deep convolutional neural network. As a result, the accuracy reached more than 90% in drone classification. Kim [26] directly applied a deep convolutional neural network to the raw radar micro-Doppler spectrograms for classifying seven human activities. An accuracy of 90.9% was achieved.

Compared with traditional machine learning techniques, neural networks can independently extract features from the input data and reach higher classification accuracy. Deep learning techniques do not depend on the prior knowledge of the input data and tend to obtain better classification performance in more complex situations, at the price of increased need of labelled data amount for proper training.

At present, most of the research on radar-based HAR utilise the micro-Doppler map for feature extraction and activity classification. However, for some activities with similar movements, one map can be easily identified as the other map, producing the wrong prediction. Therefore, research attention on alternative or complementary radar data representations such as hybrid 2D maps to reduce the rate of false alarms increases. In [27], the authors incorporate the three-domain maps, time-Doppler map (micro-Doppler), time-range map and range-Doppler map. Three stacked auto-encoders were used to extract features and then fed the features into three softmax classifiers. The results showed that the classification accuracy gained after combining the three classifiers reached 96%, increasing from 93.3% using the micro-Doppler map, 95.4% using the range map and

90% using the range-Doppler map. From the study, it can be observed that though the micro-Doppler spectrograms contain rich information of the raw radar data, the possibility of false alarms is a challenge in radar-based HAR. Therefore, it is necessary to combine more information with the micro-Doppler maps to improve the HAR system performance.

For a raw radar echo received, the data contain I and Q channels, which can be synthesised into a complex signal. After the radar signal processing, the result is still in the complex form [8, 28], through which the magnitude and phase information can both be extracted. However, the majority of the researches on radar-based HAR only investigate the effect of the magnitude information but ignore the effect of the phase information. In [29], the authors use Histogram Oriented Gradient features from range maps exploiting both the phase information showed superior classification performance compared to amplitude range maps.

Hence, the question arises on whether processing the phase of the data can bring any benefit for classification. In order to increase the activity classification performance and reduce confusion between activities, we propose a novel approach by jointly processing the amplitude and the phase information of micro-Doppler patterns for recognition.

The remainder of this article is organised as follows. Section 2 - Methodology and Implementation - introduces the implementation of the HAR system in detail. With the hybrid maps created after radar signal processing, the implementation procedures of the self-designed CNN and GoogLeNet are explained in detail. Section 3 - Results and Discussion - describes the hardware and software environments for the experiment and presented the classification results in three situations. Then, it discusses the classification performances, the results of the classification will be presented and analysed. Finally, Sect. 5 - Conclusions and Future Work - summarises the contents and major contributions. Then, based on the discussion section, it identifies possible directions for further research.

2   Methodology and Implementation

2.1   Dataset Information

The data used in this paper come from an open dataset recorded by the University of Glasgow, "Radar signatures of human activities" [30]. The team used an FMCW radar, SDR-KIT-580B, produced by Ancortek with waveform generation and transmission modules, transmitting and receiving antennas, RF cables and other accessories, as shown in Fig. 1. The radar was operated at C-band (5.8 GHz), and the bandwidth was set as 400 MHz [22]. During the experiment, ten activities were performed by volunteers, as shown in Table 1. This is one of the largest dataset in radar-based HAR. The full details of the experiment are described in [22, 30].

2.2   Pre-processing

The chirps have a pulse repetition period of 1 ms with 128 samples per sweep. A fast Fourier transform is applied on the collected I&Q signal to extract the range information

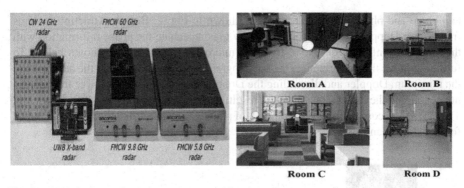

Fig. 1. The left shows the radar systems used by the radar team at the University of Glasgow. They used the rightmost radar, SDR-KIT-580B of Ancortek, to create the open dataset. The right shows four examples of the experiment environments for data collection adapted from [3, 22].

Table 1. 10 Activities recorded in the open dataset with their according duration. Note that the class "Not interested" includes four different tasks that the software should classify as not of interest for the classification to emulate an open dataset containing a multitude of classes and the detection of the classes of interest from all the activities that could be performed in front of the radar.

Number of samples	Activity Name		Duration [s]
250	Walking		10
316	Sitting on a chair		5
313	Standing up from a chair		5
314	Bending down and pick up a pen		5
314	Drinking couple of sips		5
226	Falling down		5
284	Not interested	Checking under the bed	10
		Moving objects	10
		Answering a phone call	5
		Bending and tying shoelaces	5

for each sweep (fast time) to obtain a range profile. A moving target indicator is used to suppress static targets from the radar returns. After collecting enough range profiles, a short-time Fourier transform is applied over each range bin (slow time). The window size is set to 200 ms, the overlap factor to 95% for a smooth spectrogram, and the zero-padding factor to 4 for a finer Doppler resolution. After this pre-processing, the spectrogram amplitude and phase can be extracted, as shown in Fig. 2. Before extracting features from micro-Doppler patterns, it is necessary to concatenate the phase information with the amplitude information. Also, from the micro-Doppler signature shown below. To further improve the performance, the spectrogram is cropped to contain the actions with the maximum Doppler and discarding the Doppler bins at higher and lower frequencies not containing the target signature. The resulting concatenated image is $120 \times 340 \times 3$. The 120×340 corresponds to the number of pixels per channel, and there are 3 channels for Red, Green and Blue.

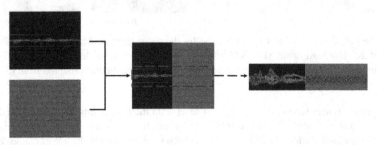

Fig. 2. The processing chain of micro-Doppler signatures and phase plots. Firstly, combine the two plots into one. Then, extract the main information inside the red dashed box by cropping the resulting image (Color figure online)

The hybrid maps of the 10 activities are shown in Fig. 3. Some activities can be easily distinguished, like moving objects and falling, while others are more difficult to tell apart because of the similarity of the micro-Doppler amplitude patterns, like answering a phone and picking up a pen. In total, there were 2017 images used in this project, and the number of samples per class is shown in Table 1.

2.3 Feature Extraction and Classification

The processed data inputs are in the form of RGB images. Thus, convolutional networks (CNN) normally used for image recognition were selected to extract features automatically and classify the data.

CNN Based on LeNet-5
Derived from [31], the key parameters of the convolutional and pooling layers are summarised in Table 2, where all units are pixels, for the proposed CNN based on LeNet5. The dropout layer was put to prevent data overfitting during the training process. After each convolutional layer, batch normalisation is implemented to normalise the output produced. The purpose of this layer is to speed up the convergence of model performance. The drop rate was set to be 0.5 to avoid overfitting. In this implementation, ReLU was used as the activation function for all nodes except in the output layer, which uses Softmax.

Transfer Learning – Use Pre-trained Model GoogLeNet
Transfer learning utilises a pre-trained model of one task to accomplish another task.

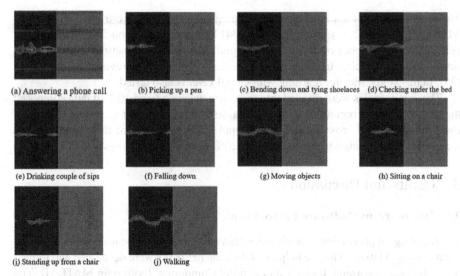

(a) Answering a phone call   (b) Picking up a pen   (c) Bending down and tying shoelaces   (d) Checking under the bed

(e) Drinking couple of sips   (f) Falling down   (g) Moving objects   (h) Sitting on a chair

(i) Standing up from a chair   (j) Walking

Fig. 3. Hybrid maps of the ten activities recorded in the open dataset, which concatenate micro-Doppler amplitude and phase.

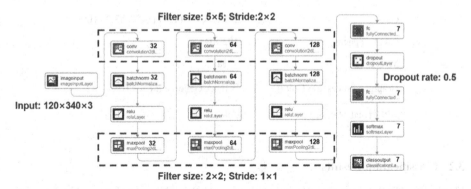

Fig. 4. Layout of the LeNet5-based CNN

Table 2. Parameters of the self-designed CNN about convolutional and pooling layers

Convolutional Layer	Filter Number	Filter Size	Stride	Pooling Layer	Pooling Area	Stride
Conv_1	32	5×5	1×1	maxpool_1	2×2	1×1
Conv_2	64	5×5	1×1	maxpool_2	2×2	1×1
Conv_3	128	5×5	1×1	maxpool_3	2×2	1×1

The main reasons for applying transfer learning are as follows. Pre-trained models like VGG [32], GoogLeNet [33] and ResNet [34] have been tested on large datasets and performances have been optimised. The second reason is that sometimes there is insufficient data to generalise from, so using a pre-trained model can prevent data overfitting [35]. In this study, transfer learning with GoogLeNet is also tested.

The data samples were divided into three sets, where a fixed 10% of data composed the test set. For the remaining dataset, because the dataset is not large and to prevent overfitting, five-fold cross-validation was applied. Hence, 80% of the remaining data were set as the training set, while the other 20% were the validation set.

3   Results and Discussion

3.1   Hardware and Software Environment

The radar signal processing, feature extraction and image classification were all implemented using Matlab. With the help of a GPU, the networks were developed and trained using the Deep Learning Toolbox and Parallel Computing Toolbox in MATLAB. The hardware and software environments are introduced in Table 3.

Table 3. Hardware parameters and software versions

CPU	Intel(R) Core (TM) i7-8700 3.2GHz
RAM Capacity	8192MB
MATLAB	2021a
Graphics Processing Unit (GPU)	NVIDIA GeForce RTX 3070
GPU Total Memory	8.59GB

3.2   Classification Results

Firstly, the HAR system was tested with training the CNN based on LeNet5. As for the hyperparameters, the initial learning rate for training was set as 0.0001, and the maximum epoch number was 20, as this was enough for convergence. There were 16 data samples in each mini-batch, and the training and validation data would be shuffled for every epoch. This guaranteed complete training with all data inputs. In terms of the validation process, one validation operation was performed every 20 iterations. The stochastic gradient descent with momentum (SGDM) optimiser was chosen to update the weights.

To evaluate the improvement over amplitude only classification, spectrograms (amplitude only size $120 \times 340 \times 3$) and the new hybrid images ($120 \times 340 \times 3$) were both trained using the CNN based on LeNet5. The confusion matrix for amplitude only is shown in Fig. 5 top left and for the hybrid maps in Fig. 5 top right.

For Transfer learning, the hybrid maps were resized to $224 \times 224 \times 3$. In addition, the last layers of GoogLeNet were replaced by new layers designed to fit the classification task. The confusion matrix is shown in Fig. 5, bottom left. A comparison of the overall performances of the 3 methods is shown in Fig. 5 bottom right.

3.3 Discussion

From Fig. 5, note that the hybrid maps which concatenate the magnitude and phase information produce higher accuracy than the spectrograms (amplitude only), with the classification accuracy increasing by 3.8%. The pre-trained GoogLeNet performed 1.7% better than the CNN based on LeNet5 at the cost of increased computational requirements. From the three confusion matrices, it is clear that compared with other activities, the activities labelled "Not interested" and "Picking up a pen" are confused for one another. After concatenating the spectrograms with phase plots, the average classification accuracy improved in these two categories by 20.9% and 0%, respectively, for the

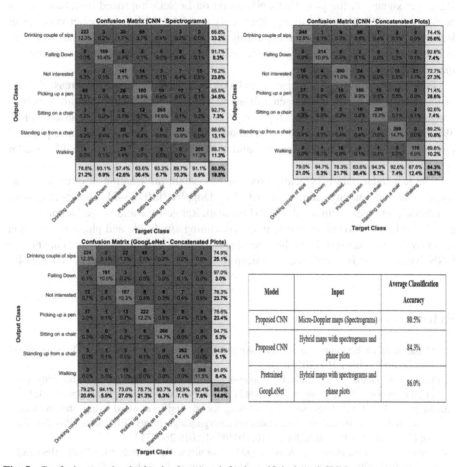

Fig. 5. Confusion matrix obtained using, (top left) the self-designed CNN on spectrograms, (top right) the self-designed CNN on hybrid maps, (bottom left) the pre-trained GoogLeNet, (bottom right) comparison of different methods for radar-based HAR.

CNN based on LeNet 5, and 15.6% and 15.1% for the GoogLeNet implementation. Thus, the proposed hybrid patterns can enhance the radar-based HAR performance.

Also, it is worth noting that through the training progress of GoogLeNet, though the mini-batch training accuracy converged to near 100% as the training went by, the validation accuracy was smaller than 100% (86–89% in the five folds), and so did the test accuracy. This may be caused by data overfitting. One possible reason is that the depth of GoogLeNet in MATLAB is 22, and the parameters are around 7 million [36] as opposed to 60k for LeNet5.

4 Conclusions and Future Work

In this study, the micro-Doppler amplitude and phase were combined to produce hybrid maps of radar signatures. After cropping the images onto the Doppler bins containing target signature, the proposed CNN based on LeNet5 improved the classification accuracy by 3.8% compared to amplitude only and 5.5% with GoogLeNet via transfer learning. These results show that exploiting the complex nature of the signals is essential in improving performances, as suggested in [37] calling to use complex numbers in machine learning architectures.

Future directions for this project would look at data augmentation to increase the size of the dataset for better model generalisation. Popular augmentation methods include image rotation, reflection and scaling along the x or y axis, cropping and translation [38, 39]. However, in radar, not all those techniques are valid as radar images have physical meaning. For example, rotation is not valid as this would never be produced by a radar system.

The raw radar data is typically processed to obtain information in three domains: range, time and velocity (can be described by Doppler shift) [3–5]. The spectrograms and phase plots were combined as a hybrid map. Range-time and range-Doppler maps could also be used to create hybrid maps containing amplitude and phase information either by concatenation or by adding the phase information as supplemental channels in CNN. These could be combined with deep fusion to further improve performance [40, 41].

References

1. Department of Economic and Social Affairs United Nations: Population Division World Population Ageing 2019 (2020)
2. Bulling, A., Blanke, U., Schiele, B.: A tutorial on human activity recognition using body-worn inertial sensors. ACM Comput. Surv. **46**(3), 33 (2014). https://doi.org/10.1145/2499621
3. Kernec, J.L., et al.: Radar signal processing for sensing in assisted living: the challenges associated with real-time implementation of emerging algorithms. IEEE Signal Process. Mag. **36**(4), 29–41 (2019). https://doi.org/10.1109/MSP.2019.2903715
4. Imran, M.A., Ghannam, R., Abbasi, Q.H., Fioranelli, F., Kernec, J.L.: Contactless radar sensing for health monitoring. In: Imran, M.A., Ghannam, R., Abbasi, Q.H. (eds.) Engineering and Technology for Healthcare (2021).. https://doi.org/10.1002/9781119644316.ch2

5. Fioranelli, F., Kernec, J.L., Shah, S.A.: Radar for Health care: recognizing human activities and monitoring vital signs. IEEE Potent. **38**(4), 16–23 (2019). https://doi.org/10.1109/MPOT. 2019.2906977

6. Jia, M., Li, S., Kernec, J.L., Yang, S., Fioranelli, F., Romain, O.: Human activity classification with radar signal processing and machine learning. International Conference on UK-China Emerging Technologies (UCET) **2020**, 1–5 (2020). https://doi.org/10.1109/UCET51 115.2020.9205461

7. Li, S., Jia, M., Kernec, J.L., Yang, S., Fioranelli, F., Romain, O.: Elderly Care: Using Deep Learning for Multi-Domain Activity Classification. International Conference on UK-China Emerging Technologies (UCET) **2020**, 1–4 (2020). https://doi.org/10.1109/UCET51 115.2020.9205464

8. Yang, S., Kernec, J.L., Fioranelli, F., Romain, O.: Human Activities Classification in a Complex Space Using Raw Radar Data. International Radar Conference (RADAR) **2019**, 1–4 (2019). https://doi.org/10.1109/RADAR41533.2019.171367

9. Li, X., He, Y., Jing, X.: A survey of deep learning-based human activity recognition in radar. Remote. Sens. **11**, 1068 (2019)

10. Gurbuz, S.Z., Amin, M.G.: Radar-based human-motion recognition with deep learning: promising applications for indoor monitoring. IEEE Sig. Process. Mag. **36**(4), 16–28 (2019). https://doi.org/10.1109/MSP.2018.2890128

11. Kernec, J.L., Fioranelli, F., Yang, S., Lorandel, J., Romain, O.: Radar for assisted living in the context of Internet of Things for Health and beyond. In: 2018 IFIP/IEEE International Conference on Very Large Scale Integration (VLSI-SoC), pp. 163–167 (2018), https://doi. org/10.1109/VLSI-SoC.2018.8644816

12. Chen, V.C.: The Micro-Doppler Effect in Radar. Artech House Publishers, Boston (2011)

13. Kim, Y., Ling, H.: Human activity classification based on micro-doppler signatures using a support vector machine. IEEE Trans. Geosci. Remote Sens. **47**(5), 1328–1337 (2009). https:// doi.org/10.1109/TGRS.2009.2012849

14. Fioranelli, F., et al.: Radar-based evaluation of lameness detection in ruminants: preliminary results. In: 2019 IEEE MTT-S International Microwave Biomedical Conference (IMBioC), pp. 1–4 (2019). https://doi.org/10.1109/IMBIOC.2019.8777830

15. Linardopoulou, K., Viora, L., Abbasi, Q.H., Fioranelli, F., Le Kernec, J., Jonsson, N.: Lameness detection in dairy cows: evaluation of the agreement and repeatability of mobility scoring. In: 74th Annual AVTRW Conference, 14–15 Septemper 2020 (2020)

16. Busin, V., et al.: Radar sensing as a novel tool to detect lameness in sheep. In: Ontario Small Ruminant Veterinary Conference, Ontario, Canada, 17–19 June 2019

17. Shrestha, A., et al.: Animal lameness detection with radar sensing. IEEE Geosci. Remote Sens. Lett. **15**(8), 1189–1193. https://doi.org/10.1109/LGRS.2018.2832650

18. Busin, V., et al.: Evaluation of lameness detection using radar sensing in ruminants. Vet. Record **185**(18), 572 (2019). https://doi.org/10.1136/vr.105407. PMID:31554712

19. Shrestha, A., Le Kernec, J., Fioranelli, F., Marshall, J.F., Voute, L.: Gait analysis of horses for lameness detection with radar sensors. In: RADAR 2017: International Conference on Radar Systems, Belfast, UK, 23–26 October 2017. ISBN:9781785616730. https://doi.org/10.1049/ cp.2017.0427

20. Li, H., et al.: Multisensor data fusion for human activities classification and fall detection. In: IEEE Sensors 2017, Glasgow, UK, 30 October–01 November 2017. ISBN: 9781509010127. https://doi.org/10.1109/ICSENS.2017.8234179

21. Li, X., Li, Z., Fioranelli, F., Yang, S., Romain, O., Kernec, J.L.: Hierarchical radar data analysis for activity and personnel recognition. Remote Sens. **12**(14), 2237 (2020)

22. Fioranelli, F., Shah, S.A., Li, H., Shrestha, A., Yang, S., Le Kernec, J.: Radar sensing for healthcare. Electr. Lett. **55**(19), 1022-1024 (2019). https://doi.org/10.1049/el.2019.2378

23. LeCun, Y., Bengio, Y., Hinton, G.: Deep learning. Nature **521**(7553), 436–444 (2015). https://doi.org/10.1038/nature14539

24. Smith, K.A., Csech, C., Murdoch, D., Shaker, G.: Gesture recognition using mm-wave sensor for human-car interface. IEEE Sens. Lett. **2**(2), 1–4 (2018). https://doi.org/10.1109/LSENS.2018.2810093

25. Kim, B.K., Kang, H., Park, S.: Drone classification using convolutional neural networks with merged doppler images. IEEE Geosci. Remote Sens. Lett. **14**(1), 38–42 (2017). https://doi.org/10.1109/LGRS.2016.2624820

26. Kim, Y., Moon, T.: Human detection and activity classification based on micro-doppler signatures using deep convolutional neural networks. IEEE Geosci. Remote Sens. Lett. **13**(1), 8–12 (2016). https://doi.org/10.1109/LGRS.2015.2491329

27. Jokanovic, B., Amin, M., Erol, B.: Multiple joint-variable domains recognition of human motion. In: 2017 IEEE Radar Conference (RadarConf), 8–12 May 2017. pp. 0948–0952 (2017). https://doi.org/10.1109/RADAR.2017.7944340

28. Loukas, C., Fioranelli, F., Le Kernec, J., Yang, S.: Activity classification using raw range and I & Q radar data with long short term memory layers. In: 2018 IEEE 16th Intl Conferenceon Dependable, Autonomic and Secure Computing, 16th Intl Conference on Pervasive Intelligence and Computing, 4th International Conference on Big Data Intelligence and Computing and Cyber Science and Technology Congress (DASC/PiCom/DataCom/CyberSciTech), pp. 441–445 (2018). https://doi.org/10.1109/DASC/PiCom/DataCom/CyberSciTec.2018.00088

29. Guendel, R.G., Fioranelli, F., Yarovoy, A.: Phase-based classification for arm gesture and gross-motor activities using histogram of oriented gradients. IEEE Sensors J. **21**(6), 7918–7927 (2021). https://doi.org/10.1109/JSEN.2020.3044675

30. Fioranelli, F., Shah, S.A., Li, H., Shrestha, A., Yang, S., Le Kernec, J.: Radar signatures of human activities. https://doi.org/10.5525/gla.researchdata.848

31. Lecun, Y., Bottou, L., Bengio, Y., Haffner, P.: Gradient-based learning applied to document recognition. Proc. IEEE **86**(11), 2278–2324 (1998). https://doi.org/10.1109/5.726791

32. Szegedy, C., et al.: Going deeper with convolutions. Proc. CVPR (2015). arXiv:1409.4842

33. Simonyan, K., Zisserman, A.: Very deep convolutional networks for large-scale image recognition. Proc. CVPR (2014). arXiv:1409.1556

34. He, K., Zhang, X., Ren, S., Sun, J.: Deep residual learning for image recognition. Proc. CVPR (2016). arXiv:1512.03385

35. Olivas, E.S., Guerrero, J.D.M., Sober, M.M., Benedito, J.R.M., Lopez, A.J.S.: Handbook of Research on Machine Learning Applications and Trends: Algorithms, Methods and Techniques - 2 Volumes. IGI Publishing (2009)

36. MATLAB: Pretrained Deep Neural Networks. The MathWorks Inc. https://www.mathworks.com/help/deeplearning/ug/pretrained-convolutional-neural-networks.html. Accessed 19 Apr 2021

37. Bruna, J., Chintala, S., LeCun, Y., Piantino, S., Szlam, A., Tygert, M.: A mathematical motivation for complex-valued convolutional networks (2015). arXiv:1503.03438v3

38. Gandhi, A.: Data augmentationǀhow to use deep learning when you have limited data — Part 2. Nanonets. https://nanonets.com/blog/data-augmentation-how-to-use-deep-learning-when-you-have-limited-data-part-2/. Accessed 19 Apr 2021

39. Li, J., Shrestha, A., Le Kernec, J., Fioranelli, F.: From Kinect skeleton data to hand gesture recognition with radar. J. Eng. **2019**(20), 6914–6919 (2019). https://doi.org/10.1049/joe.2019.0557

40. Li, H., le Kernec, J., Mehul, A., Gurbuz, S.Z., Fioranelli, F.: Distributed radar information fusion for gait recognition and fall detection. In: 2020 IEEE Radar Conference (RadarConf 2020), pp. 1–6 (2020). https://doi.org/10.1109/RadarConf2043947.2020.9266319
41. Li, H., Mehul, A., Le Kernec, J., Gurbuz, S.Z., Fioranelli, F.: Sequential human gait classification with distributed radar sensor fusion. In: IEEE Sensors J. **21**(6), 7590–7603 (2021). https://doi.org/10.1109/JSEN.2020.3046991

Wireless Sensing for Human Activity Recognition Using USRP

William Taylor[1]([✉])[iD], Syed Aziz Shah[2][iD], Kia Dashtipour[1][iD],
Julien Le Kernec[1][iD], Qammer H. Abbasi[1][iD], Khaled Assaleh[3],
Kamran Arshad[3], and Muhammad Ali Imran[1,4][iD]

[1] James Watt School of Engineering, University of Glasgow, Glasgow G12 8QQ, UK
`w.taylor.2@research.gla.ac.uk`
[2] Centre for Intelligent Healthcare, Coventry University, Coventry CV1 5RW, UK
[3] Faculty of Engineering and IT, Ajman University, 346, Ajman, UAE
[4] Artificial Intelligence Research Center (AIRC), Ajman University, Ajman, UAE

Abstract. Artificial Intelligence (AI) in tandem wireless technologies is providing state-of-the-art techniques human motion detection for various applications including intrusion detection, healthcare and so on. Radio Frequency (RF) signal when propagating through the wireless medium encounters reflection and this information is stored when signals reach the receiver side as Channel State information (CSI). This paper develops an intelligent wireless sensing prototype for healthcare that can provide quasi-real time classification of CSI carrying various human activities obtained using USRP wireless devices. The dataset is collected from the CSI of USRP devices when a volunteer sits down or stands up as a test case. A model is created from this dataset for making predictions on unknown data. Random forest was able to provide the best results with an accuracy result to 96.70% and used for the model. A wearable device dataset was used as a benchmark to provide a comparison in performance of the USRP dataset.

Keywords: Wireless sensing · Healthcare · RF sensing

1 Introduction

In recent years, healthcare monitoring technologies are becoming more common for improving the lives of vulnerable people [1,2]. Elderly people can be considered vulnerable people [3]. As the elderly population increases, the strain on nursing homes increase [4]. The United Nations (UN) estimates the global elderly population is likely to be around 2.1 billion in 2050 [5]. Healthcare monitoring can be used to provide real-time notifications to caregivers when care is required [6]. Monitoring can be achieved by observing the features of human movement obtained from technology [7]. The detection of elderly people falling is an example of how technology can be used to assist elderly people. Falling can cause serious injuries to people and in some cases cause death [8]. Fall detection

M. Ur Rehman and A. Zoha (Eds.): BODYNETS 2021, LNICST 420, pp. 52–62, 2022.
https://doi.org/10.1007/978-3-030-95593-9_5

systems used to alert care givers in real time so that care can be given when required. This relieves pressure from care givers and provides elderly people with more independence. The current methods of fall detection can be achieved using wearable devices such as mobile or smartwatches. The features of a human falling can then be passed to carers [9]. The main issue with wearable devices is when users do not wear the device for reasons of comfort or forgetfulness. Wearable devices are considered invasive as the wearable device is an instrument introduced onto the body. Non-invasive methods do not introduce instruments to the body. Recently, non-invasive and non-contact RF sensing based system is widely used to estimate human activity recognition. This is achieved by observing the Channel State information (CSI) that is represented in terms of amplitudes of the RF signals while humans move within the RF communication [10]. The wi-fi systems feature CSI to provide a description of how the RF signals propagate between transmitting and receiving nodes [11]. This research focus to exploit this CSI information. Therefore, the machine learning can be applied to detect patterns in the CSI and it can predict what human motion is taking place. This paper presents a machine learning model which can differentiate between a human standing up and sitting down using CSI with a real time application. Finally, the results are compared to a benchmark dataset which is collected using wearable devices.

The paper is organized as follows. Section 2 discusses related work on human activity recognition; Sect. 3 presents the proposed methodology; Sect. 4 provides the results and discussion and finally Sect. 5 concludes the paper.

2   Related Work

The following section lists some related works in the field of non-invasive RF sensing. Most of the current studies [12] used frequency-modulated continuous-wave (FMCW) radar systems. The human movements caused the radar signals to display a doppler shift. The doppler shifts is collected as samples of various human movements. The datasets are collected from multiple samples and machine learning is applied. The experimental results showed that the machine learning could distinguish differences in the doppler shifts for different human movements. The work of [13] used Wi-Fi signals to classify five different arm movements. The Wi-Fi router was used to communicate remotely to a laptop. In between the devices a human test subject made various arm movements. The CSI of the Wi-Fi signals was used as a data set for Long Short-Term Memory (LSTM) deep learning classification. Deep learning results achieved 96% accuracy. Other examples of work done on healthcare is present in [14]. Nipu et al. [15] exploited the CSI of RF signals for the identification of specific individuals. Experimentation used different volunteers to walk through the line of sight of two communication devices. The CSI was used as a dataset and machine learning was applied to try and extract the physical features of each volunteer. Random forest and decision tree algorithms were used and the results proved to have higher accuracy when the classification was only between two individuals. As the test subjects increased the accuracy decreased. Other work done using this dataset used four machine learning algorithms and ensemble learning of all four algorithms. The ensemble learning achieved an accuracy score of 93.83% [16].

3   Methodology

This section will discuss the experimental setup used in this research.

3.1   Data Collection

This research uses Universal Software Radio Peripheral (USRP) devices as the transmission and receiver of RF signals. The transmission device used is the USRP X300 model and the receiving device is the X310 USRP device. Each device is directly connected to its own a PC. On the PCs, the simulation software used is MatLab/Simulink. This simulation software enables the configuration of the devices to allow for the communication and capture of the CSI of the wireless exchange. Each USRP device is equipped with VERT2450 omni directional antennas. The devices were then setup in an office environment with 4 m between the communicating devices. The volunteers then performed the action of standing up and sitting down while USRP devices were communicating with each other. Each action was completed multiple times while the CSI for each instance was stored. multiple samples collected ensured that any error in performance could be filtered out in the data processing stage. The samples were collected while in a 7 × 8 m office which contained common furniture such as chairs and desks. The RF signals reflect on the volunteer as the sitting or standing motion occurs. The CSI data then stores the features of the movement in the form of signal propagation. There are many variations of how the signals will propagate, which is dependent on many factors just as posture, position of chair and different shapes and sizes of volunteers. However the general pattern of how the signals reflect from two different positions remains. Some ambient movement can cause the patterns to no longer be present in the CSI. These samples are not considered clear samples as the movement cannot be detected hence the reasoning behind taking a large range of samples for building a dataset. The complete dataset contains 60 samples. 30 samples for sitting and 30 samples for standing. Figures 1 and 2 show the 64 subcarrier CSI of the USRP transmissions. The time of transmission is shown along the X axis and the frequency change caused by the RF signals reflecting off the volunteer is shown in the Y axis. Figure 1 displays the CSI pattern of sitting down and Fig. 2 displays the CSI pattern of standing up. Figure 3 details the process used in this experimentation.

3.2   Machine Learning

Specifically, the dataset is used for various techniques of machine learning approaches. The machine learning algorithms are implemented using the Scikit

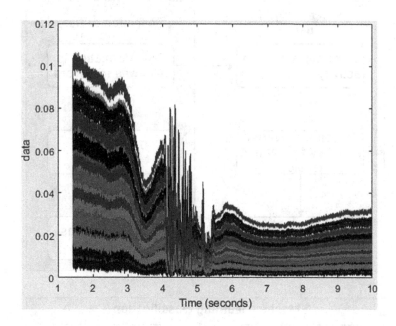

Fig. 1. Sitting down CSI

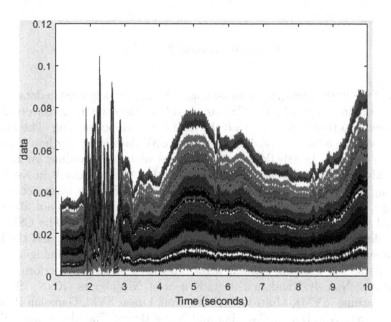

Fig. 2. Standing up CSI

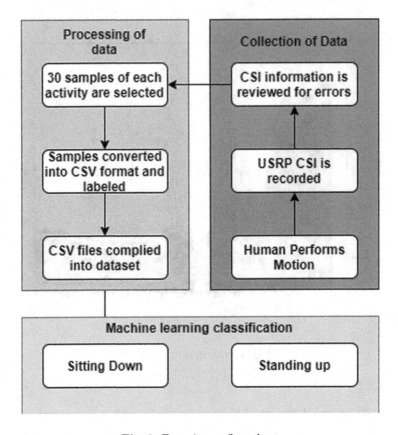

Fig. 3. Experiment flow chart

library of the Python programming language. Scikit is widely used in data science research and industry [17]. The CSI obtained from the samples is converted into CSV format so that Scikit can read the data for machine learning. The Pandas Python package is used to read and store the CSV data into a Python Variable. The data can then be labelled appropriately as sitting or standing. As the CSI data is always differentiating in each sample taken this can result in NAN values being present when python reads the CSV files. In order to overcome this challenge, the NAN values are replaced with 0 values. This does not affect the observed patterns when comparing different samples together. The CSV data is then divided between the actual CSI data of each sub carrier and the label for that sub carrier. The dataset is then divided between 70% training and 30% testing data. Ten machine learning algorithms used to test the performance of the dataset. Namely Random Forest, K nearest Neighbours (KNN), Support Vector Machine (SVM), Multi-layer Perceptron, Linear SVM, Gaussian Process, Decision Tree, Ada Boost, Gaussian and Naïve Bayes. The algorithms will be compared by considering the accuracy as evaluation metric. The comparative results will use the performance metrics of accuracy. Accuracy represents the

True positive (TP) classifications over the total classifications made. The other classifications made in machine learning are True Negative (TN), False Positive (FP) and False Negative (FN). The complete equation is shown in Eq. 1. It can be seen that the accuracy is the total number of correct classifications versus the total classifications made.

$$Accuracy = \frac{TP + TN}{TP + TN + FP + FN} \tag{1}$$

4   Results and Discussion

4.1   Machine Learning Algorithms Comparison

The first experiment used a range of machine learning algorithms to test the performance of the newly collected USRP dataset. The results compare the accuracy of each algorithm. Figure 4 shows the accuracy of each of the algorithms and how they compare to each other and Table 1 presents the actual percentage of accuracy of each algorithm.

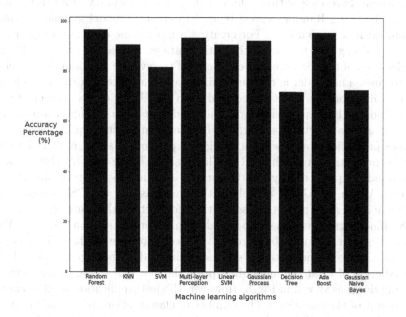

Fig. 4. Experiment flow chart

The machine learning experiments produced mostly high accuracy results with Random Forest, KNN, Multi layer Perception, Linear SVM, Gaussian Process and Ada Boost scoring over 90% accuracy. Random Forest had the best accuracy at 96.70% followed by Ada Boost with 95.48% accuracy. These results show that there are patterns in the CSI when volunteers stand up or sit down. These patterns can then be detected use machine learning techniques.

Table 1. Accuracy results of machine learning algorithms

Algorithm	Accuracy
Random Forest	96.70%
K nearest Neighbours	90.71%
Support Vector Machine	81.77%
Multi-layer Perception	93.40%
Linear SVM	90.71%
Gaussian Process	92.18%
Decision Tree	71.96%
Ada Boost	95.48%
Gaussian Naive Bayes	72.82%

4.2   Real Time Classification

The Random Forest algorithm achieved the highest accuracy of all tested algorithms. Therefore, Random Forest is used to create a model for making classifications on new unseen data. For creating a model, the data is no longer split between training and testing as the entire dataset is used for training. Python provides the Joblib library which can be used to save the Random Forest model for later use. The model is then used in an application which can provide real time classifications on new CSI received from the USRP devices. To create this application, the Flask web framework was used to create a web application. Flask was used as it is a python web framework and can execute the Python scripts to make predictions on new data using the previously saved model. The web interface presents users with a "Run Classification" button. This then allows a background script to use python to connect to MatLab and read the MatLab variables. When the USRP completes the transmission, the CSI is stored in a variable in MatLab. The Python script then connects to the MatLab session and the machine learning model can be used to make predictions on the CSI. While the script is running in the background, the web interface displays "Loading. . ." to the user. Once the prediction is generated the loading message is replaced with the prediction of what the model interprets the new CSI to be. Either standing or sitting down as shown in Fig. 5. However, the web application used to classify any amount of classifications. The number of classifications is dependent on the machine learning model used. The complete process of the web application is shown Fig. 6. For testing of this real time application, additional samples are taken. Six samples are taken for each sitting and standing. These samples are completely unseen to the training model. These samples are then used as the variable on MatLab and the real time application is used to make predictions on the samples. All 12 of these samples were correctly classified. This shows that the CSI for sitting and standing displays a specific pattern which can be detected by the created machine learning model.

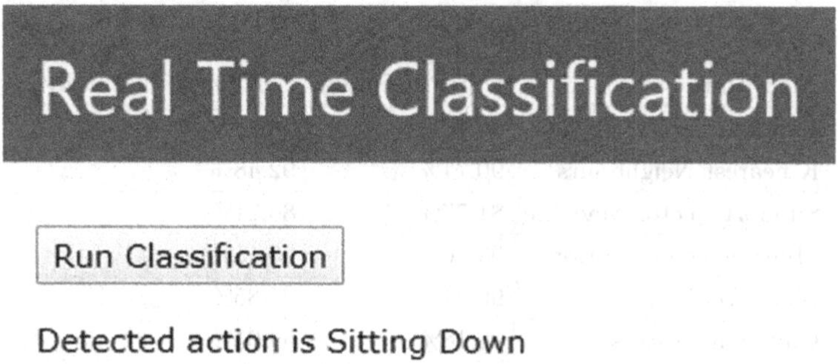

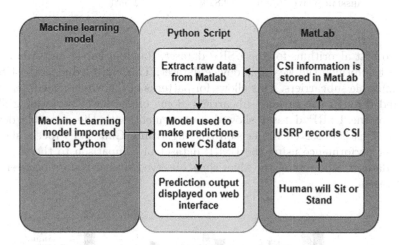

Fig. 5. Flask web interface displaying classification result

Fig. 6. Flask web interface process

4.3 Benchmark Dataset

The data collected from the USRP CSI has been shown to display patterns which can detected by most machine learning algorithms tested in this research. This shows that the Non-invasive CSI method is successful in motion detection. To provide a comparison between the performance of non-invasive techniques and invasive wearable devices, a publicly available dataset collected using wearable devices is used. D Anguita et al. [18] have publicly released a dataset detecting different human motions using accelerometers equipped on smartphones. The same machine learning techniques are applied to this dataset.

The results of the comparison show that the performance is similar with most of the algorithms between the two datasets. Random forest remained the highest performer between the two datasets with the results very similar around 96%. The accuracy for each algorithm between datasets is shown in Table 2 and the visual representation between the two datasets is shown in Fig. 7.

Table 2. Comparison of results

Algorithm	USRP accuracy	Benchmark accuracy
Random Forest	96.70%	96.49%
K nearest Neighbours	90.71%	92.48%
Support Vector Machine	81.77%	86.21%
Multi-layer Perception	93.40%	96.11%
Linear SVM	90.71%	91.85%
Gaussian Process	92.18%	54.01%
Decision Tree	71.96%	86.46%
Ada Boost	95.48%	92.23%
Gaussian Naive Bayes	72.82%	72.55%

The two best algorithms for the USRP dataset, Random Forest and Ada Boost both outperformed the wearable device dataset. This can be due to the USRP using multiple subcarriers. This allows for patterns in the wireless medium to be captured through the various subcarriers. Some of the lower performing algorithms of the USRP dataset showed improvement with the wearable device dataset. This is observed in decision tree algorithm. Gaussian Process showed a greater performance using the USRP dataset in comparison to the wearable device dataset. The rest of the algorithms observed similar results between the two datasets.

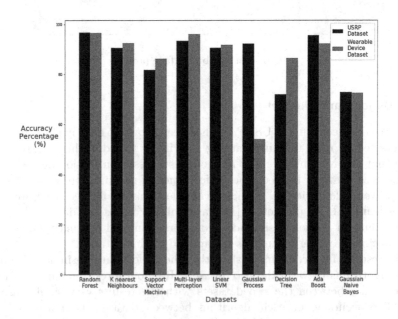

Fig. 7. Comparison of results

5   Conclusion

In this research paper, we have proposed a novel intelligent wireless sensing system using AI and USRP dataset and different algorithms that can detect the human motions of standing and sitting up. The dataset provides binary observations of CSI collected from USRPs as a volunteer stands and sits from a chair. The machine learning algorithms show good performance with the Random Forest algorithm producing the best performance with 96.70% accuracy. These results show that there is a distinctive pattern between the CSI of a volunteer sitting and standing. The web application designed was able to make predictions of new data based on a model build from training data. A comparison was also made between the newly created URSP dataset and a publicly available dataset, where data was collected using wearable devices. The same machine learning techniques were used, and results showed that performance was similar thus providing evidence that USRPs can detect motion at the same level as wearable devices.

Acknowledgement. William Taylor's studentship is funded by CENSIS UK through Scottish funding council in collaboration with British Telecom. This work is supported in parts by EPSRC EP/T021020/1 and EP/T021063/1. This work is supported in part by the Ajman University Internal Research Grant.

References

1. Dong, B., et al.: Monitoring of atopic dermatitis using leaky coaxial cable. Healthc. Technol. Lett. **4**(6), 244–248 (2017)
2. Abbasi, Q.H., et al.: Advances in body-centric wireless communication: Applications and state-of-the-art. Institution of Engineering and Technology (2016)
3. Yang, X., et al.: Diagnosis of the hypopnea syndrome in the early stage. Neural Comput. Appl. **32**(3), 855–866 (2019). https://doi.org/10.1007/s00521-019-04037-8
4. Mercuri, M., et al.: Healthcare system for non-invasive fall detection in indoor environment. In: De Gloria, A. (ed.) Applications in Electronics Pervading Industry, Environment and Society. LNEE, vol. 351, pp. 145–152. Springer, Cham (2016). https://doi.org/10.1007/978-3-319-20227-3_19
5. Liu, Y., et al.: A novel cloud-based framework for the elderly healthcare services using digital twin. IEEE Access **7**, 49088–49101 (2019)
6. Yang, X., et al.: Monitoring of patients suffering from REM sleep behavior disorder. IEEE J. Electromagn. RF Microwav. Med. Biol. **2**(2), 138–143 (2018)
7. Zhang, T., et al.: WiGrus: a Wifi-based gesture recognition system using software-defined radio. IEEE Access **7**, 131102–131113 (2019)
8. Santos, G.L., et al.: Accelerometer-based human fall detection using convolutional neural networks. Sensors **19**(7), 1644 (2019)
9. Yao, X., Khan, A., Jin, Y.: Energy efficient communication among wearable devices using optimized motion detection. In: 2019 IEEE Symposium on Computers and Communications (ISCC), pp. 1–6. IEEE (2019)
10. Zhao, J., et al.: R-DEHM: CSI-based robust duration estimation of human motion with WiFi. Sensors **19**(6), 1421 (2019)

11. Lolla, S., Zhao, A.: WiFi motion detection: a study into efficacy and classification. In: 2019 IEEE Integrated STEM Education Conference (ISEC), pp. 375–378. IEEE (2019)
12. Ding, C.: Fall detection with multi-domain features by a portable FMCW radar. In: 2019 IEEE MTT-S International Wireless Symposium (IWS), pp. 1–3. IEEE (2019)
13. Zhang, P.: Complex motion detection based on channel state information and LSTM-RNN. In: 2020 10th Annual Computing and Communication Workshop and Conference (CCWC), pp. 0756–0760. IEEE (2020)
14. Shah, S.A., Yang, X., Abbasi, Q.H.: Cognitive health care system and its application in pill-rolling assessment. Int. J. Numer. Model. Electron. Netw. Devices Fields **32**(6), e2632 (2019)
15. Nafiul Alam Nipu, Md., et al.: Human identification using WiFi signal. In: 2018 Joint 7th International Conference on Informatics, Electronics and Vision (ICIEV) and 2018 2nd International Conference on Imaging, Vision & Pattern Recognition (icIVPR), pp. 300–304. IEEE (2018)
16. Taylor, W., et al.: An intelligent non-invasive real-time human activity recognition system for next-generation healthcare. Sensors **20**(9), 2653 (2020)
17. Hao, J., Ho, T.K.: Machine learning made easy: a review of Scikit-learn package in python programming language. J. Educ. Behav. Stat. **44**(3), 348–361 (2019)
18. Anguita, D., et al.: A public domain dataset for human activity recognition using smartphones. In: Esann (2013)

Real-Time People Counting Using IR-UWB Radar

Kareeb Hasan[✉], Malikeh Pour Ebrahim, and Mehmet Rasit Yuce

Department of Electrical and Computer Systems Engineering, Monash University,
Melbourne, Australia
{kareeb.hasan2,melika.pour.ebrahim,Mehmet.Yuce}@monash.edu

Abstract. COVID-19 pandemic has introduced social distance regulations which are crucial to be followed by. In order to maintain proper social distancing, it is critical to regulate the number of people in a closed space. In this paper, we propose a people counting system based on Impulse Radio Ultra-Wideband radars for counting people walking through a doorway. The system uses two IR-UWB radars placed horizontally apart to create a lag effect when someone walks by the radars. This enables detection of movement's direction and subsequently, determination of the number of people in a room. The system proposed can be used for people counting in real-time and also on saved data which offers flexibility for real world applications. Several tests were conducted which shows the accuracy rate of system to be around 90%, validating the system. Contrary to conventional vision based people counting system, the proposed system is not limited by environmental factors such as light and also is privacy oriented.

Keywords: People counting · Occupancy counter · COVID-19

1 Introduction

Real-time people counting is an important feature that is useful in many circumstances. Situations such as monitoring congestion of railway or bus station, building or room occupancy is an increasingly important feature especially in current pandemic condition. Due to the COVID-19 pandemic, it is essential to regulate the number of people in a closed space, in order to adhere to the social distancing rules. Compliance of such rules is challenging for essential service providers such as pharmacies and supermarkets, where physical visits are essential. Therefore, an automatic monitoring system is required which can output the number of people in an enclosed area and allow the administrators to regulate the number of people as per the requirements.

Many research works have been conducted in people counting systems, with heavy emphasis in using vision sensors as the technology [1]. Typically, closed-circuit television(CCTV) footage is used to train neural network which can detect people using features such as head, shoulders, etc., and after training, the network is deployed to count the number of people on live footage [1]. However,

© ICST Institute for Computer Sciences, Social Informatics and Telecommunications Engineering 2022
Published by Springer Nature Switzerland AG 2022. All Rights Reserved
M. Ur Rehman and A. Zoha (Eds.): BODYNETS 2021, LNICST 420, pp. 63–70, 2022.
https://doi.org/10.1007/978-3-030-95593-9_6

vision based technology have several disadvantages, in that it is heavily dependent on the input video quality. Therefore, changes in illumination, haziness might affect the detection accuracy. In addition, the appearance of a person is also important for such technology e.g., a person covering their body while holding an umbrella might not be detected. However, a key disadvantage of vision based people counting system is the lack of privacy. Video monitoring is an aspect that make many people uncomfortable due to perceived privacy invasion. Since a people counting system is going to be reliant on Internet of Things (IoT) platform for processing, there are risk of video data compromise. Vision sensor based people counting systems are also usually reliant on heavy image processing, therefore high performance hardware are another component which might be required.

Other types of sensors have also been used for people counting research. In [2], passive infrared sensors were used, which although has the advantage of being illumination invariant, has poor resolution for large number of people. Thermal cameras, which offers privacy advantage compared to traditional cameras have also been used for people counting using a Convolutional Neural Network [3]. However thermal imaging based people counting system have difficulties in crowded situations where, due to high density, people block each other in the camera field-of-view. Furthermore, training a Convolutional Neural Network on thermal images, to achieve good accuracy rate, would involve collecting large amount of data, which is expensive in terms of both time and resource.

With high resolution, low power requirement and excellent penetration [4], Impulse Radio Ultra-Wideband (IR-UWB) is a trending technology for many applications such as vital sign detection [5], indoor positioning system [6], Time Of Arrival (TOA) [7], and also detection of people in disaster sites [8]. IR-UWB radar transmits a very short duration impulse signal, which occupies a wideband in frequency domain [9]. The reflected signal can then be analysed to extract useful information.

IR-UWB radar is a suitable technology for people counting and several research have been already conducted in this domain. In [10], Maximum Likelihood approach was used for people counting using IR-UWB radar. Similarly in [11], Convolutional Neural Network was used to count people using IR-UWB radar. However, both of these approaches were limited in the amount of people it can count, which is a critical drawback for a scalable people counting system in real world for application such as COVID-19 regulation monitoring. In [12], the count capacity limit was avoided by developing an in/out bound people counter.

In this study, a real-time people counting system using commercial IR-UWB radar has been developed, which can be used to count people in an enclosed space e.g., a room.

2   Methodology

The system developed uses the principle, that if a person entering and exiting a room can be detected, then the number of people inside a room can be counted using the expression:

Number of people in a room = Number of people entry - Number of people exit.

The basic overview of the system is illustrated in Fig. 1. By placing the proposed system beside a room entrance, any person going in or out can be detected, obtaining the total count of the number of people in the room. If there are multiple entrances to a room, then one system can be placed beside each entrance, and the result from each system can be integrated to output the total people count in the room as illustrated in Fig. 1.

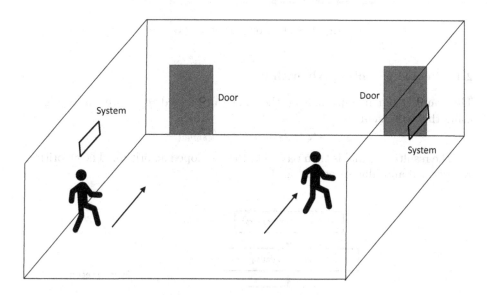

Fig. 1. System placement position in a room for people counting.

For this study, two commercial IR-UWB Radars, Xethru X4M200 by Novelda, were utilised. Both the radars have a centre frequency of 7.29 GHz. The radars were placed horizontally apart at distance d, to create a lag response when a person is walking in front of the radars, as shown in Fig. 2. This allows the direction of movement to be recognized and therefore, determine whether a person has moved in or out of a room. The separation distance d is a vital parameter, as too large distance d will output a clearer lag effect, enabling easier direction identification. But a person can walk in between the radars, distorting the return radar waveform. On the other hand, a small distance d will reduce the time taken by a person to walk across the two radars and thereby, reducing the accuracy in direction determination. Therefore, a value was chosen after trial and error. The algorithm was developed and run on Matlab platform using a laptop.

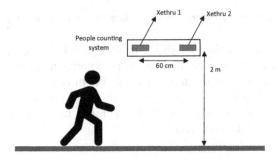

Fig. 2. System placement side view.

2.1 People Counting Algorithm

The I and Q signals output from the radars are mixed to create the IQ signal using the expression:

$$IQ = I_{signal} + i \times Q_{signal} \tag{1}$$

The resultant signal is then passed to the developed algorithm. The algorithm is described and illustrated in Fig. 3.

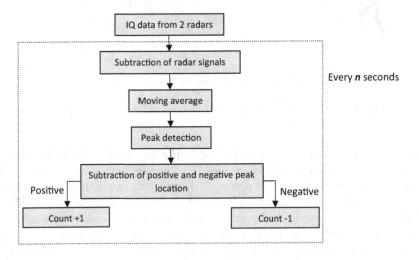

Fig. 3. Signal processing block diagram.

The algorithm is developed based on the principle of being able to run real-time. This is because, it will provide an opportunity for administrators to act in an instant, if the occupancy limit of a room is exceeded at any time. Each step of the algorithm is described as follows:

1. **Signal subtraction:** The IQ signal from the 2 Xethru radars are subtracted to ensure that the resultant output signal only contains the difference signal.
2. **Moving average:** To discard stray peaks and smoothen the signal.
3. **Peak detection:** Peak detection allows identifying positive and negative peak in the signal.
4. **Peak location subtraction:** The negative peak location is subtracted from the positive peak location. If the resultant number is positive, it indicates entrance to the room and vice versa for negative resultant number.

The algorithm takes the data and runs every specified n second e.g., every 3 s, 7 s, etc. After trial and error, n was set to 10 s. This value was chosen based on running the algorithm at real-time speed whilst keeping the computational cost low.

2.2   Experiment

The experiment was set up with the radars separation distance d set to 60 cm after trial and error. The vertical distance was set to 2 m. Two types of experiment were conducted: Controlled and Uncontrolled.

- **Controlled**: Specific number of people were instructed to walk up and down a corridor.
- **Uncontrolled**: Device was set up in a corridor and the experiment was conducted with free flowing crowd.

The main aim of the experiments were to monitor the accuracy of the algorithm, in determining the direction of movement (in to out, out to in) in real-time. Direct observation of people movements were used as reference.

3   Results

Figure 4 shows the ideal wave pattern for the algorithm, Fig. 5 illustrates each step of the signal processing blocks and Table 1 shows the experiment results.

Results in Table 1 validates the performance of the system as the results for both controlled and uncontrolled tests have an accuracy rate around 90%. Majority of the error during controlled test were due to the laptop slowing down as a result of driving two Xethru radars at the same time. In addition to that, uncontrolled test also had cases where a person would stop in the path to look at the system, thereby corrupting the data. Also, for uncontrolled test there was 1 instance where two people walked in side by side, resulting in an error.

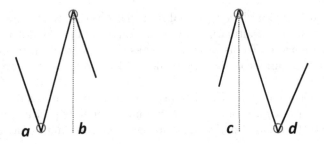

Fig. 4. *Left:* Ideal pattern for positive count where Positive peak **b** index minus Negative peak **a** index will give a positive number. *Right:* Ideal pattern for negative count where Positive peak **c** index minus Negative peak **d** index will give a negative number.

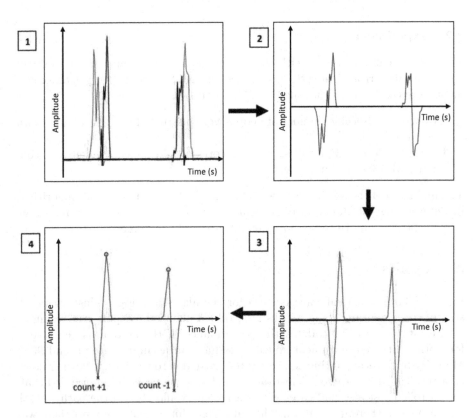

Fig. 5. Algorithm signal processing diagram. 1. IQ signal of both radars 2. Subtraction of the signals 3. Applying moving average 4. Peak detection and subtraction which enables determination of direction and hence, the count.

Table 1. Experimental results for the system in controlled and uncontrolled tests.

Test type	Controlled	Uncontrolled
Reference In	30	25
Reference Out	30	19
Predicted In	28	22
Predicted Out	27	17
Reference total	60	44
Predicted total	55	39
In accuracy rate (%)	93	88
Out accuracy rate (%)	90	89
Total accuracy rate (%)	92	89

4   Conclusion

In this paper, a real-time people counting system using IR-UWB radar has been proposed. Compared to conventional people counting technologies, which are predominantly camera based, the proposed technology does not have drawbacks of being light variant and privacy invasive. In addition, due to low algorithmic complexity, the system can be adapted to run on Raspberry Pi, and the IQ radar signal can be further utilised for additional functionalities such as posture classification. Two types of tests were conducted to validate the accuracy of the system developed. Overall, the high accuracy rate of the system demonstrate a feasible technology for robust people counting applications. In the future, further work will be done to improve the accuracy and also develop additional functionality for multiple people walking side by side.

References

1. Cruz, M., Keh, J.J., Deticio, R., Tan, C.V., Jose, J.A., Dadios, E.: A people counting system for use in CCTV cameras in retail. In: 2020 IEEE 12th International Conference on Humanoid, Nanotechnology, Information Technology, Communication and Control, Environment, and Management (HNICEM), pp. 1–6, (2020)
2. Wahl, F., Milenkovic, M., Amft, O.: A distributed PIR-based approach for estimating people count in office environments. In: 2012 IEEE 15th International Conference on Computational Science and Engineering, pp. 640–647 (2012)
3. Xu, M.: An efficient crowd estimation method using convolutional neural network with thermal images. In: 2019 IEEE International Conference on Signal, Information and Data Processing (ICSIDP), pp. 1–6 (2019)
4. Quan, X., Choi, J.W., Cho, S.H.: In-bound/out-bound detection of people's movements using an IR-UWB radar system. In: 2014 International Conference on Electronics, Information and Communications (ICEIC), pp. 1–2 (2014)
5. Hu, X., Jin, T.: Short-range vital signs sensing based on EEMD and CWT using IR-UWB radar. Sensors **16**, 2025 (2016)

6. Alarifi, A., et al.: Ultra wideband indoor positioning technologies: analysis and recent advances. Sensors **16**, 1–36 (2016)
7. Navarro, M., Najar, M.: TOA and DOA estimation for positioning and tracking in IR-UWB, pp. 574–579, October 2007
8. Yao, S.Q. Wu, S.Y., Tan, K., Ye, S.B., Fang, G.Y.: A vital sign feature detection and search strategy based on multiple UWB life-detection-radars. In: 2016 16th International Conference on Ground Penetrating Radar (GPR), pp. 1–6 (2016)
9. Advanced ultrawideband radar: signals, targets, and applications. CRC Press, Taylor & Francis Group, Boca Raton (2017)
10. Choi, J.W., Yim, D.H., Cho, S.H.: People counting based on an IR-UWB radar sensor. IEEE Sens. J. **17**(17), 5717–5727 (2017)
11. Yang, X., Yin, W., Zhang, L.: People counting based on CNN using IR-UWB radar. In: 2017 IEEE/CIC International Conference on Communications in China (ICCC), pp. 1–5 (2017)
12. Choi, J.W., Cho, S.H., Kim, Y.S., Kim, N.J., Kwon, S.S., Shim, J.S.: A counting sensor for inbound and outbound people using IR-UWB radar sensors. In: 2016 IEEE Sensors Applications Symposium (SAS), pp. 1–5 (2016)

Bespoke Simulator for Human Activity Classification with Bistatic Radar

Kai Yang[1,2], Qammer H. Abbasi[1] (iD), Francesco Fioranelli[3] (iD), Olivier Romain[4] (iD), and Julien Le Kernec[1,2(✉)] (iD)

[1] University of Glasgow, University Avenue, Glasgow G12 8QQ, UK
`julien.lekernec@glasgow.ac.uk`
[2] University of Electronic Science and Technology of China, Qingshuihe Campus: Chengdu High-tech Zone (West) 2006 West Avenue, Chengdu 611731, China
[3] TU Delft, Mekelweg 4, 2628 CD Delft, The Netherlands
[4] University Cergy-Pontoise, 6 Avenue du ponceau, 95000 Cergy-Pontoise, France

Abstract. Radar is now widely used in human activity classification because of its contactless sensing capabilities, robustness to light conditions and privacy preservation compared to plain optical images. It has great value in elderly care, monitoring accidental falls and abnormal behaviours. Monostatic radar suffers from degradation in performance with varying aspect angles with respect to the target. Bistatic radar may offer a solution to this problem but finding the right geometry can be quite resource-intensive. We propose a bespoke simulation framework to test the radar geometry for human activity recognition. First, the analysis focuses on the monostatic radar model based on the Doppler effect in radar. We analyse the spectrogram of different motions by Short-time Fourier analysis (STFT), and then the classification data set was built for feature extraction and classification. The results show that the monostatic radar system has the highest accuracy, up to 98.17%. So, a bistatic radar model with separate transmitter and receiver was established in the experiment, and results show that bistatic radar with specific geometry configuration (CB2.5) not only has higher classification accuracy than monostatic radar in each aspect angle but also can recognise the object in a wider angle range. After training and fusing the data of all angles, it is found that the accuracy, sensitivity, and specificities of CB2.5 have 2.2%, 7.7% and 1.5% improvement compared with monostatic radar.

Keywords: Radar · Micro-Doppler · Radar signature simulation · Human activity recognition

1 Introduction

Human activity recognition has become one of the current research hotspots. It can help to monitor different human behaviour states. Therefore, this technology has been widely used in security monitoring and medical health [1–3]. Nowadays, the most commonly used sensor in recognition is a camera, which can extract features by recording images

© ICST Institute for Computer Sciences, Social Informatics and Telecommunications Engineering 2022
Published by Springer Nature Switzerland AG 2022. All Rights Reserved
M. Ur Rehman and A. Zoha (Eds.): BODYNETS 2021, LNICST 420, pp. 71–85, 2022.
https://doi.org/10.1007/978-3-030-95593-9_7

of human motions, and then perform classification through machine learning or deep learning algorithms. However, the method of camera recording also has some drawbacks [4–7]. Images collected by the camera are easily affected by light conditions in the environment, and in addition, camera recording may infringe on personal privacy and may cause information leakage [6].

Because the use of a camera in private spaces is raising concerns with privacy and acceptance by users, radar is becoming an attractive sensing modality [8, 9]. Radar can see through walls and maintain good performance in any lighting conditions. Radar can penetrate obstacles to detect hidden targets. Finally, radar is a non-contact device. These benefits mean that radar technology has great application value in human activity recognition.

The world's ageing problem is getting worse, e.g., the proportion of the world's elderly population reached 9% in 2019. China is also facing a serious ageing problem. China Development Report [10] predicts that China's population over 65 will account for 14% in 2022, and the population over 60 years old will reach 500 million by 2015. Therefore, how to ensure the quality of life of the elderly and establish a complete medical and elderly care system will be a great challenge in China and in the world. In the daily life of the elderly, there are often unexpected falls or abnormal behaviours caused by diseases, which can be life-threatening in the case of unattended [11]. Thus, it is necessary to monitor Activities of Daily Living (ADL) of the elderly through equipment.

There have been much research works on the use of radar for human activity recognition. Chen proposed to use the micro-Doppler effect [12, 13] to obtain information on human motions. By using joint time-frequency analysis of radar signals, a time-dependent spectrum (spectrogram) description can be obtained. The motion of different body parts on the spectrum has different Doppler frequency shift trajectories. Therefore different motions will have different micro-Doppler signatures. There are short-time Fourier transform (STFT), continuous wavelet transform (CWT), Wigner Ville distribution (WVD) [14] for time-frequency transformation, while STFT is the most commonly used technology. Spectrogram data will be further processed to extract features. One method is physical component-based decomposition [15], which decomposes the spectrogram into components corresponding to different physical parts of the human body. However, how to track and decompose these signatures effectively is still complex, so it is challenging to implement this method. Another method is statistics-based decomposition, which is a feature decomposition method using Principal Component Analysis (PCA) or Singular Value Decomposition (SVD) [16, 17]. Through this method, the information with a small correlation is removed, and the main information is retained, which has the effect of data dimension reduction and noise reduction. In [18], PCA is used to extract the feature of the spectrogram. For classification, machine learning [16, 17] is a powerful tool to automate the task with algorithms such as K-Nearest Neighbor (KNN) is used in [19], Decision Tree and Naive Bayesian are used in [20], their final classification accuracy is greater than 90%. Most of the research on radar recognition for human activities are based on monostatic radar. However, the transmitter and receiver of monostatic radar are in the same position, so the observation angle is limited, and significant Doppler shift for classification purposes can be obtained only when the subject moves towards or away from the radar (when the aspect angle of the subject to the radar line of sight is 0° or 180°). The Doppler shift will be greatly reduced when the aspect angle is 90°, resulting in a significant decline in the classification performance of the spectrogram [21].

The transmitter and receiver of bistatic radar are separated and located in different positions, which can offer more freedom of acquiring complementary target's information, avoiding aspect angles with poor velocity measurements. Recording bistatic information is, however, demanding in terms of hardware resources to synchronise the radar nodes [22]. Researchers, therefore, turn to bespoke simulations to generate radar signatures that can complement experimental radar data [23–28]. The problem of aspect angle in [21, 29–31] and its effect on radar activity classification is seldom analysed in its entirety, as many studies consider target classification with subjects mostly moving in the radial direction in constrained trajectories. A person cannot be expected to always be facing a radar node. This would be impractical in daily life.

Because the aspect angle of the target influences the radar signatures, this has an influence on the micro-Doppler signatures and, therefore, the classification accuracy. Exploiting different radar geometry may help to counter the degradation with aspect angle. This paper proposes a parametric analysis of bistatic radar geometries to maintain performance with varying aspect angles from −90° to 90° using a bespoke simulation framework. It first analyses the suitability of the classification algorithm for practical implementation using the monostatic model. Secondly, the classification performances are tested when one algorithm is trained for signatures produced at each aspect as well as when one model is trained with the data from all angles.

The remainder of this paper is organised as follows. Section 2 will present the simulation framework. Section 3 will discuss the classification methods. Section 4 will provide the result of the classification of human activities. Section 5 will offer some insight in the results obtained from classification. Finally, Sect. 6 will conclude and provide future research directions.

2   Radar Simulation

The simulated radar operating frequency was set to 15 GHz, the range resolution is 0.01 m, and the monostatic radar model is based on [12], which uses canonical shapes to emulate the radar cross-section (RCS) of the human body, such as spheres and ellipsoids. Whereas in [12] the Boulic-Thalmann model [32] was used, this paper combines human motion capture (MOCAP HDM05) data containing the motion information of the human skeleton in each frame, sampled at 120 Hz [33]. This allows for a wider variety of actions to be explored for classification as the MOCAP dataset is not limited to an average subject and walking gait, as the Boulic-Thalmann model.

In addition to monostatic radar, this paper also explores bistatic configurations, for which the bistatic RCS of spheres and ellipsoids can be found in [34, 35]. The transmitter and receiver of bistatic radar are located in different positions, and there can be multiple transmitters and receivers. This allows the bistatic radar to have more observations, which may improve classification with varying target aspect angles. However, bistatic radar also leads in practical implementations to a more complex system and to the synchronisation challenge between transmitter and receiver. Hence, the value of establishing a simulator to get some initial data.

The baseline between transmitter and receiver is L, r_T and r_R is the distance from the transmitter to target and receiver to target, respectively, α_T and β_T is the azimuth and elevation angle of the transmitter, α_R and β_R is the azimuth and elevation angle of the receiver. The angle between the transmitter-to-target line and the receiver-to-target line is the bistatic angle φ (the angle between the moving direction of the target and the direction of the bisector).

There are three main factors that affect the Doppler shift in the bistatic radar system: the velocity of target V, the angle φ and the angle δ, so the formula of Doppler frequency shift is shown in (1).

$$f_D = \frac{2f}{c}|V|\cos\left(\frac{\varphi}{2}\right)\cos\delta \tag{1}$$

The received signal can be expressed as (2)

$$S(t) = \rho(x, y, z)\exp\left\{\left\{2\pi f \frac{|\mathbf{r}_T(t)| + |\mathbf{r}_R(t)|}{c}\right\}\right. \tag{2}$$

Note that the sampling frequency of the HDM05 database is only 120 Hz, and the Doppler frequency shift generated by human motion is often larger. This will cause the aliasing of the spectrogram according to Shannon-Nyquist sampling theory. Therefore, the HDM05 data is interpolated to increase the sampling frequency to 2 kHz, which ensures that the spectrogram has a ± 1 kHz Doppler unambiguous range, which is sufficient for the activities being considered. The spectrogram is generated using a 150-point Gaussian window with 95% overlap and 600-point FFT.

Five motion classes are considered: Walk, Jumping Jack, Hop, Squat, and Rotate Arms with associated labels from 1 to 5, in the same order. The dataset contains 130 samples from the HDM05 database. To obtain more data for machine learning, it is necessary to expand the dataset. The spectrogram is therefore segmented in smaller chunks, and a sliding window will be used. The window size is set to be 1.5 s to make sure at least one complete cycle of walking can be covered. Besides, there is a 33% overlap between each window. After segmentation, 71 samples were obtained for each motion, a total of 355 samples, and the size of each spectrogram is 600 × 471. In addition, for a more realistic simulation, additive white Gaussian noise (AWGN) was added to the samples to develop robustness against varying signal-to-noise ratio (SNR) levels (-5 dB, 0 dB, 5 dB and 10 dB) in the classification algorithms. To further increase the dataset, flipping the radar signatures upside down to obtain Doppler for a motion performed in the opposite direction of the original one allows doubling the size of the dataset. Finally, there are a total of 2840 samples (568 per class). The radar signatures obtained with a simulated monostatic radar configuration are shown in Fig. 1. All the simulations were performed in Matlab.

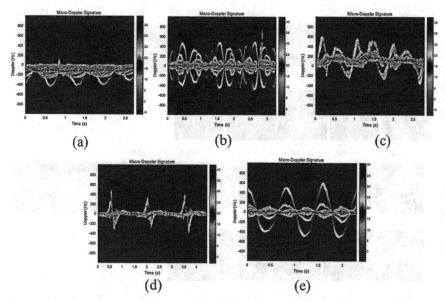

Fig. 1. Spectrograms of (a) Walking (b) Jump jack (c) Hop (d) Squat (e) Rotate arms in a monostatic radar environment.

In bistatic radar, the receiver, transmitter, and target are set, as shown in Fig. 2. Different geometries lead to different aspect angles, which alter the micro-Doppler signatures. Three circular bistatic radar (CB) geometries are considered with baselines of 10 m (CB10), 5 m (CB5) and 2.5 m (CB2.5), respectively. The distance to the centre of the scene is maintained at 7 m. The aspect angle θ is defined as the angle between the target heading and the radar line of sight when considering the transmitter. The effect of varying aspect angles (−90° to 90° with 15° steps) for different geometries for the walking activity is shown in Fig. 3.

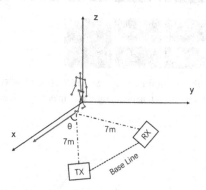

Fig. 2. The simulation geometry of a bistatic radar

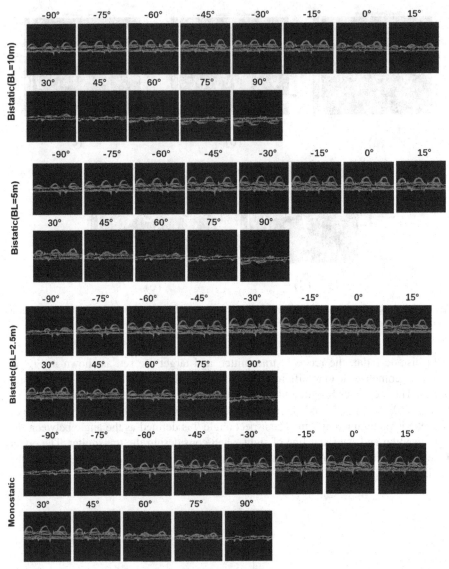

Fig. 3. Spectrograms for walking gait for configuration CB10, CB5, CB2.5 as bistatic geometries and for the monostatic radar case, when aspect angle changes from −90° to 90°

3   Classification

3.1   Feature Extraction

The spectrogram data can be used directly for classification. However, this increases computational complexity if the spectrogram is used as an image directly. Therefore, it is recommended to reduce the dimensionality of the data and extract the salient information for the given classification task. The traditional PCA will transform the spectrogram data into a one-dimensional vector, therefore, losing the spatial information. Hence, 2D-PCA [36] is used to extract features from the spectrograms. Compared with traditional PCA, 2D-PCA can evaluate the covariance matrix more accurately and compute the eigenvalues faster than PCA by at least 4 times but requires more components to describe the images. The comparison of reconstruction images for the varying numbers d of PCA is shown in Fig. 4. The quality of the image improves as d increases visually. However, through the KNN classifier (with the number of neighbours K = 5), it is found that the highest accuracy is obtained when $d = 15$, as shown in Fig. 5. Furthermore, a higher d value will result not just in a lower accuracy but also an increase in computational requirements resulting in a longer inference time.

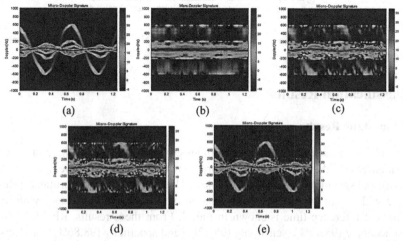

Fig. 4. (a) Original spectrogram (b) Reconstructed spectrogram ($d = 5$) (c) Reconstructed spectrogram ($d = 15$) (d) Reconstructed spectrogram ($d = 25$) (e) Reconstructed spectrogram ($d = 50$)

3.2 Classification Algorithm

Four classification algorithms are evaluated in this study, namely, KNN, Support Vector Machine (SVM) with a linear kernel, Decision Tree, and Random Forest (RF) [17]. These four algorithms have different advantages and disadvantages, so it is necessary to evaluate the classification effectiveness via various metrics, such as accuracy, specificity, sensitivity, training time and inference time.

To verify the classification performance, 10-fold cross-validation will be used. The data set is divided into ten parts: one is the test set and the rest the training set; this process is then repeated ten times until all parts are used as the test set. The following section presents the average results of the 10 folds.

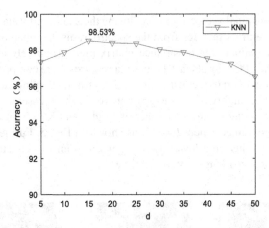

Fig. 5. Accuracy of classification of the 5 activities with KNN (K = 5) against the number of PCA values d

4   Classification Results

4.1   Monostatic Results

Some results are presented regarding performances with monostatic configuration. Confusion matrices of the different models are shown in Fig. 6. The average accuracy, sensitivity and specificity are shown in Table 1. The stability of the algorithms is shown in Fig. 7 with boxplots. Finally, the evaluation of classification efficiency with training time and inference time is shown in Fig. 8. From these results, RF achieves the highest accuracy (98.17%), sensitivity (95.42%) and specificity (98.86%); the decision tree has the worst classification performance. Furthermore, Fig. 7 shows that RF has a smaller deviation overall indicating better stability in performance, and KNN has the worst deviation. For the comparison of training time, SVM takes the longest time, while in inference time, it is faster than RF and KNN. Since training happens off-line, faster inference time and robust accuracy will be favoured for practical implementation. Hence, SVM is retained for further analysis.

4.2   Bistatic Results

To verify the classification performance of radars under different aspect angles ($-90°$ to $90°$), datasets are constructed for each rotation for the different radar geometries (monostatic, CB10, CB5, CB2.5). The accuracy for each aspect angle is shown in Fig. 9. Furthermore, the data from all the aspect angles are fused together to train a general model for each radar geometry, and the results are shown in Fig. 10.

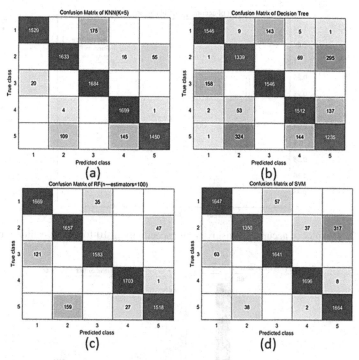

Fig. 6. Confusion matrices of (a) KNN (b) Decision Tree (c) Random Forest (d) SVM

The overall performance of CB2.5 is better since its accuracy in the range of $-75°$ to $75°$ is higher than that of the other radar geometries. Furthermore, the fusion data model in Fig. 10 shows that CB2.5 has higher accuracy, sensitivity and specificity than the other configurations as well.

Table 1. Average accuracy, sensitivity, specificity of 4 classifiers in monostatic radar system.

Classifier	KNN	Decision Tree	RF	SVM
Accuracy	0.9754	0.9370	0.9817	0.9755
Sensitivity	0.9384	0.8425	0.9542	0.9387
Specificity	0.9846	0.9606	0.9886	0.9847

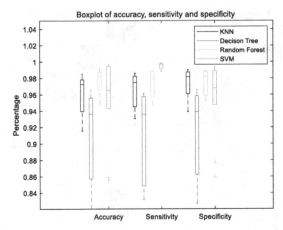

Fig. 7. Boxplot of accuracy, sensitivity and specificity in 10-fold cross-validation.

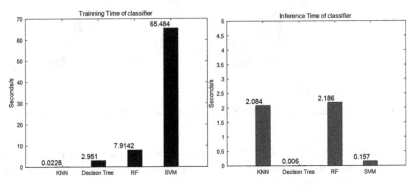

Fig. 8. Average (left) training time (right) inference time of 10-fold cross-validation.

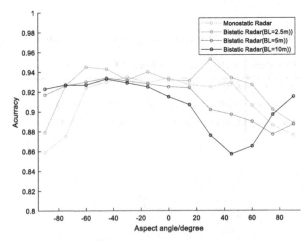

Fig. 9. Accuracy of CB10, CB5, CB2.5 and Monostatic Radar under different aspect angles with SVM.

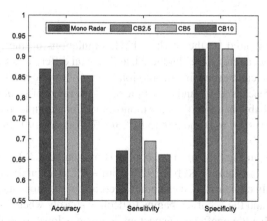

Fig. 10. Comparison of accuracy of different radar geometries after data fusion of all aspect angles with SVM

5 Discussion

5.1 Monostatic

We first completed the motion classification with a monostatic radar. Four machine learning algorithms are applied to compare which one will have better classification performance on the dataset. The classification results in Table 1 show that, except for the Decision Tree, the other three classifiers all achieve a good classification performance, their average accuracy all exceed 90%, and RF has the best accuracy (98.17%), sensitivity (95.42%) and specificity (98.86%), followed by SVM and KNN, while Decision Tree has the worst classification performance, its sensitivity is about 10% lower than the other three classifiers.

In Fig. 7, the width of the box reflects the fluctuation of the data. It illustrates that RF has the smallest fluctuations in accuracy, while SVM has a more obvious advantage in sensitivity. In specificity, KNN is slightly better than RF. RF is a relatively stable model in all three performance parameters. On the contrary, Decision tree shows the poorest performance in accuracy, sensitivity and specificity, so the stability of the model is the worst. In the comparison of time spent, Fig. 8 shows that the training time of SVM (65.48 s) is much longer than the others, followed by RF (7.91 s) and Decision Tree (2.95 s), KNN has the shortest training time (only 0.0228 s). While, for inference time, KNN and RF spend the longest time, which all exceed 2 s. KNN has a large number of calculations in the prediction stage. Therefore, inference takes more time. RF will produce multiple decision trees in model training, and it also depends on these decision trees for majority voting, resulting in a long time for model training and inference. For SVM, the model is complex, but its predictions only depend on the support vector, so the inference time is much shorter. In practical application, the inference time will have more influence on recognition efficiency, so Decision Tree and SVM seem to have more advantages, and since SVM is more accurate than Decision Tree, SVM was retained for further analysis.

5.2 Bistatic

For bistatic radar, inspired by the work in [21], simulations on the radar robustness against varying aspect angles were conducted, and several different radar geometries are tested. From Fig. 3, it can be seen that the motion from monostatic radar becomes hard to distinguish when θ reaches $\pm 90°$, and in bistatic radar, the range of aspect angles Doppler shifts are distinguishable is larger than for monostatic. For example, the spectrogram is clear for CB10 from $-90°$ to 0 and 75° to 90°; for CB5 from $-90°$ to 30°; for CB 2.5 from $-75°$ to 60°.

It can be seen from Fig. 9. that the overall performance of CB2.5 is better than the other three schemes. Its accuracy is above 92% from $-75°$ to 60° and reached the highest value (95%) at 30°. In comparison, the average accuracy of the monostatic radar is lower than that of CB2.5, and the accuracy begins to decline sharply when $\theta < -60°$ and $\theta > 60°$, which means that the unaffected aspect angle range is lower than that of CB2.5.

It is also found in Fig. 10 that the classification performance parameters of CB2.5 are higher than those of other geometries when all the aspect angles are fused together to train one model for all angles. For example, the accuracy, sensitivity and specificities of CB2.5 have 2.2%, 7.7% and 1.5% improvement compared with monostatic radar. Therefore, it is inferred from the above results that the CB2.5 bistatic radar has stronger robustness against aspect angle change than monostatic radar.

6 Conclusion

Human activity recognition based on radar has been one of the research hotspots in recent years. It has great application value in the field of healthcare and security. In this paper, the classification of human activity in the monostatic radar environment is simulated first and then upgraded into a bistatic radar environment with configurable radar geometries to explore the improvement of robustness against changes in aspect angle.

For feature extraction, 2D-PCA is applied, which can process images data more effectively compared with traditional PCA. It greatly reduces the data dimension, improving the efficiency of the algorithm. For classification, four machine learning algorithms are used, and it is concluded from the results that RF achieves the best results in classification accuracy, with a value up to 98.17%, and it also has better stability than the other three models. The accuracy and stability of SVM are second only to RF, but it has a shorter inference time, which means the classification efficiency is higher for embedded processing.

This paper also establishes bistatic radar models to test the classification performance of different radar geometry at different aspect angles. The results show that CB2.5 is more advantageous than monostatic radar in accuracy under each aspect angle. It is also found in fused data classification that the classification performance of CB2.5 is better than monostatic radar, so these results indicate that CB2.5 has better aspect angle robustness.

This paper explored the robustness against varying aspect angles with bistatic radar and monostatic radar. Other geometries with MIMO [37] and multi-static geometries [21] with more transmitters and receivers could be explored to improve robustness. Another aspect of the simulation to be considered is the incorporation of channel propagation and reflection from the clutter in indoor environments to increase the realism of the simulations.

Furthermore, for the operation of several radars in indoor spaces, the study of radar signals with software-defined radar to avoid interference should be considered and their associated performance [38–41].

Last but not least, this simulator considered discrete activities, whereas, in reality, people perform actions in a continuum. So, the simulator should work to generate continuous data for further improvement of the techniques for automatic segmentation [7, 42, 43].

References

1. Kernec, J.L., et al.: Radar signal processing for sensing in assisted living: the challenges associated with real-time implementation of emerging algorithms. IEEE Signal Process. Mag. **36**(4), 29–41 (2019). https://doi.org/10.1109/MSP.2019.2903715
2. Gurbuz, S.Z., Amin, M.G.: Radar-based human-motion recognition with deep learning: promising applications for indoor monitoring. IEEE Signal Process. Mag. **36**(4), 16–28 (2019). https://doi.org/10.1109/MSP.2018.2890128
3. Abdur Rahman, M.: A secure occupational therapy framework for monitoring cancer patients' quality of life. Sensors **19**(23), 5258 (2019)
4. Li, H., Cui, G., Kong, L., Guo, S., Wang, M., Yang, H.: Human target tracking for small aperture through-wall imaging radar. IEEE Radar Conf. (RadarConf) **2019**, 1–4 (2019)
5. Cippitelli, E., Fioranelli, F., Gambi, E., Spinsante, S.: Radar and RGB-depth sensors for fall detection: a review. IEEE Sens. J. **17**(12), 3585–3604 (2017). https://doi.org/10.1109/JSEN. 2017.2697077
6. Widen, W.H.: Smart cameras and the right to privacy. Proc. IEEE **96**(10), 1688–1697 (2008). https://doi.org/10.1109/JPROC.2008.928764
7. Shrestha, A., Li, H., Le Kernec, J., Fioranelli, F.: Continuous human activity classification from FMCW radar with Bi-LSTM networks. IEEE Sens. J. **20**(22), 13607–13619 (2020)
8. Li, X., Li, Z., Fioranelli, F., Yang, S., Romain, O., Kernec, J.L.: Hierarchical radar data analysis for activity and personnel recognition. Remote Sens. **12**(14), 2237 (2020)
9. Shrestha, A., et al.: Cross-frequency classification of indoor activities with DNN transfer learning. IEEE Radar Conf. (RadarConf) **2019**, 1–6 (2019). https://doi.org/10.1109/RADAR. 2019.8835844
10. Rapoza, K.: China's Aging Population Becoming More Of A Problem. Forbes (2017). https:// www.forbes.com/sites/kenrapoza/2017/02/21/chinas-aging-population-becoming-more-of-a-problem/#68537251140f
11. Shrestha, A., et al.: Elderly care: activities of daily living classification with an S band radar. The Journal of Engineering **2019**(21), 7601–7606 (2019)
12. Chen, V.C.: The Micro-Doppler Effect in Radar. Artech House Publishers (2011)
13. Chen, V.C., Ling, H.: Time-frequency transforms for radar imaging and signal analysis (2002)
14. Imran, M.A., Ghannam, R., Abbasi, Q.H., Fioranelli, F., Kernec, J.L.: Contactless radar sensing for health monitoring. In Engineering and Technology for Healthcare (2021)
15. Li, H., Shrestha, A., Heidari, H., Kernec, J.L., Fioranelli, F.: A multisensory approach for remote health monitoring of older people. IEEE J.Electromag., RF Micro. Med. Biol. **2**(2), 102–108 (2018)
16. Klaine, P.V., Imran, M.A., Onireti, O., Souza, R.D.: A survey of machine learning techniques applied to self-organizing cellular networks. Commun. Surveys Tuts. **19**(4), 2392–2431 (2017)

17. Goodfellow, I., Bengio, Y., Courville, A.: Deep Learning. MIT Press, Cambridge, MA (2016)
18. Erol, B., Amin, M.G.: Radar data cube processing for human activity recognition using multisubspace learning. IEEE Trans. Aerospace Electron. Syst. **55**(6), 3617–3628 (2019)
19. Guendel, R.G.: Radar Classification of Contiguous Activities of Daily Living. Master Thesis (2019). http://arxiv.org/abs/2001.01556
20. Baird, Z.J.: Human Activity and Posture Classification Using Single Non-Contact Radar Sensor by Affairs in partial fulfillment of the requirements for the degree of Master of Applied Science, pp. 55–87 (2017)
21. Zhou, B., et al.: Simulation framework for activity recognition and benchmarking in different radar geometries. IET Radar, Sonar Navig. **15**(4), 390–401 (2021). https://doi.org/10.1049/rsn2.12049
22. Fioranelli, F., Ritchie, M., Griffiths, H.: Bistatic human micro-doppler signatures for classification of indoor activities. IEEE Radar Conf. (RadarConf) **2017**, 0610–0615 (2017)
23. Manfredi, G., Russo, P., De Leo, A., Cerri, G.: Efficient simulation tool to characterize the radar cross section of a pedestrian in near field. Progress Electromag. Res. C **100**, 145–159 (2020). https://doi.org/10.2528/PIERC19112701
24. Du, H., He, Y., Jin, T.: Transfer learning for human activities classification using micro-doppler spectrograms. IEEE Int. Conf. Comput. Electromag. (ICCEM) **2018**, 1–3 (2018)
25. Du, H., Ge, B., Dai, Y., Jin, T.: Knowing the uncertainty in human behavior classification via variational inference and autoencoder. Int. Radar Conf. (RADAR) **2019**, 1–4 (2019)
26. Lin, Y., Le Kernec, J.: Performance analysis of classification algorithms for activity recognition using micro-doppler feature. In: 2017 13th International Conference on Computational Intelligence and Security (CIS), pp. 480–483 (2017)
27. Lin, Y., Le Kernec, J., Yang, S., Fioranelli, F., Romain, O., Zhao, Z.: Human activity classification with radar: optimization and noise robustness with iterative convolutional neural networks followed with random forests. IEEE Sens. J. **18**(23), 9669–9968 (2018)
28. Vishwakarma, S., Li, W., Tang, C., Woodbridge, K., Adve, R., Chetty, K.: SimHumalator: an open source wifi based passive radar human simulator for activity recognition arXiv:2103.01677 (2021)
29. Kim, Y., Toomajian, B.: Hand gesture recognition using micro-doppler signatures with convolutional neural network. IEEE Access **4**, 7125–7130 (2016)
30. Fioranelli, F., Ritchie, M., Griffiths, H.: Aspect angle dependence and multistatic data fusion for micro-doppler classification of armed/unarmed personnel. IET Radar Sonar Navig. **9**(9), 1231–1239 (2015)
31. Çağlıyan, B., Gürbüz, S.Z.: Micro-doppler-based human activity classification using the mote-scale bumblebee radar. IEEE Geosci. Remote Sens. Lett. **12**(10), 2135–2139 (2015)
32. Boulic, R., Thalmann, N.M., Thalmann, D.: A global human walking model with real-time kinematic personification. Vis. Comput. **6**(6), 344–358 (1990)
33. Müller, T., Röder, M., Clausen, B., Eberhardt, B., Krüger, A.: Weber, Documentation Mocap Database HDM05, Technical report, No. CG-2007–2, ISSN 1610–8892, Universität Bonn, June 2007
34. Crispin, J.W., Maffett, A.L.: Radar cross-section estimation for simple shapes. Proc. IEEE **53**(8), 833–848 (1965)
35. Trott, K.D.: Stationary phase derivation for RCS of an ellipsoid. IEEE Antennas Wirel. Propag. Lett. **6**, 240–243 (2007)
36. Yang, J., Zhang, D., Frangi, A.F., Yang, J.Y.: Two-dimensional PCA: a new approach to appearance-based face representation and recognition. IEEE Trans. Pattern Anal. Mach. Intell. **26**(1), 131–137 (2004)
37. Yang, F., Xu, F., Fioranelli, F., Le Kernec, J., Chang, S., Long, T.: Practical investigation of a MIMO radar system capabilities for small drones detection. IET Radar Sonar Navig. **15**(7), 760–774 (2021)

38. Le Kernec, J., Gray, D., Romain, O.: Empirical analysis of chirp and multitones performances with a UWB software defined radar: Range, distance and doppler. In: Proceedings of 2014 3rd Asia-Pacific Conference on Antennas and Propagation, pp. 1061–1064 (2014)
39. Le Kernec, J., Romain, O.: Empirical performance analysis of linear frequency modulated pulse and multitones on UWB software defined radar prototype. IET Int. Radar Conf. **2013**, 1–6 (2013)
40. Le Kernec, J.: Inter-range-cell interference free compression algorithm: performance in operational conditions. CIE Int. Conf. Radar (RADAR) **2016**, 1–5 (2016)
41. Le Kernec, J., Romain, O.: Performances of multitones for ultra-wideband software-defined radar. IEEE Access **5**, 6570–6588 (2017)
42. Li, H., Mehul, A., Le Kernec, J., Gurbuz, S.Z., Fioranelli, F.: Sequential human gait classification with distributed radar sensor fusion. IEEE Sens. J. **21**(6), 7590–7603 (2021)
43. Li, H., Shrestha, A., Heidari, H., Le Kernec, J., Fioranelli, F.: Bi-LSTM network for multimodal continuous human activity recognition and fall detection. IEEE Sens. J. **20**(3), 1191–1201 (2020)

Sensing for Healthcare

Detecting Alzheimer's Disease Using Machine Learning Methods

Kia Dashtipour[1,3]([⊠]), William Taylor[1], Shuja Ansari[1], Adnan Zahid[2],
Mandar Gogate[3], Jawad Ahmad[3], Khaled Assaleh[4], Kamran Arshad[4],
Muhammad Ali Imran[1,5], and Qammer Abbasi[1]

[1] James Watt School of Engineering, University of Glasgow, Glasgow, UK
kia.dashtipour@glasgow.ac.uk
[2] School of Engineering and Physical Science, Heriot-Watt University,
Edinburgh EH144AS, UK
[3] School of Computing, Edinburgh Napier University, Edinburgh, UK
[4] Faculty of Engineering and IT, Ajman University, Ajman 346, UAE
[5] Artificial Intelligence Research Center (AIRC), Ajman University, Ajman, UAE

Abstract. As the world is experiencing population growth, the portion of the older people, aged 65 and above, is also growing at a faster rate. As a result, the dementia with Alzheimer's disease is expected to increase rapidly in the next few years. Currently, healthcare systems require an accurate detection of the disease for its treatment and prevention. Therefore, it has become essential to develop a framework for early detection of Alzheimer's disease to avoid complications. To this end, a novel framework, based on machine-learning (ML) and deep-learning (DL) methods, is proposed to detect Alzheimer's disease. In particular, the performance of different ML and DL algorithms has been evaluated against their detection accuracy. The experimental results state that bidirectional long short-term memory (BiLSTM) outperforms the ML methods with a detection accuracy of 91.28%. Furthermore, the comparison with the state-of-the-art indicates the superiority of the our framework over the other proposed approaches in the literature.

Keywords: Machine learning · Deep learning · Detecting Alzheimer

1 Introduction

Alzheimer is from a family of diseases that can develop dementia, specially in elderly people. Dementia is a loss of memory and/or other mental disability that can cause physical damaged to the brain. Although Alzheimer is the most common type of dementia but there are different types of dementia [35,49], such as vascular dementia, Lewy Body disease, frontotemporal dementia, alcohol related dementia and HIV associated dementia, *etc.*. The most common type of dementia after Alzheimer's disease is vascular dementia which can happens after stroke. In addition, some of the causes of dementia are reversible such as thyroid problem and vitamin deficiencies. The dementia is not just a disease but its

M. Ur Rehman and A. Zoha (Eds.): BODYNETS 2021, LNICST 420, pp. 89–100, 2022.
https://doi.org/10.1007/978-3-030-95593-9_8

associated risks such as decline in the memory significantly reduces a person's ability to perform daily tasks. It is expected that the number of people affected from dementia will increase over the time. The early detection can not only help doctors to precisely make decision on the treatment but also help preventing the complications [21]. It is important to develop a system that can help in early detection of dementia.

The Alzheimer's disease has number of symptoms, especially in the elderly people that can cause problems to perform daily tasks due to memory loss. Although the Alzheimer is not normal due to aging, its risk factor increases with the aging. Most of the people who suffer from Alzheimer are aged 65 or above. However, it not uncommon to have this disease in the people younger than 65. For instance, more than two hundred thousand American aged less than 65 suffers from Alzheimer disease. Figure 1 shows the difference between the normal brain and Alzheimer's brain [47].

It can be noticed that the brain of the Alzheimer's disease in not only significantly smaller than the normal brain but is affected severely from neurological disorder and dysfunction. Additionally, Fig. 2 presents some of the common symptoms of the Alzheimer's disease. The most common types of symptoms are loss of memory, changes in the behaviour, difficulty with everyday task and confusion in familiar environments.

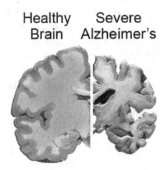

Healthy Severe
Brain   Alzheimer's

Fig. 1. Difference between a normal brain and a severe Alzheimer's brain [47].

Practically, no effective cure to treat Alzheimer's disease exist to date. However, there exist ways that can temporarily slow down the process of Alzheimer's symptoms and improve the quality of the life of the patient. To this end, significant research efforts are dedicated to find the effective ways of treating the Alzheimer's disease with a focus on preventing the disease from progressing over the time [39].

It is suggested that ML and DL algorithms, which have proven their significance in various fields, can help solve the problem of early detection of Alzheimer's disease clearly, ML and DL methods have their applications in

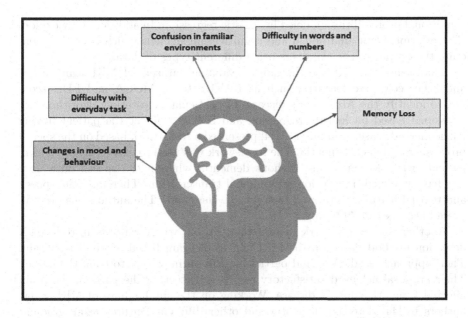

Fig. 2. Alzheimer symptoms

various domains, including but not limited to sentiment analysis [2,9–11,13–19,30,32,33], speech enhancement [27,28], cyber-security [31,34], image classification [36], energy efficiency [51], travel detection [5,6], posture detection [48], and atrial fibrillation [37,38], *etc.*. Therefore, the ML techniques including support vector machine (SVM), logistic regression, multi-layered perceptron and deep learning classifiers. In particular, feature selection is an important element of traditional ML classifiers which is inherently incorporated in DL classifiers. Generally, DL classifiers achieve better results on large datasets.

In this paper, we proposed a novel approach, based on ML and DL methods, to detect Alzheimer's disease. The obtained results from DL algorithm are compared against traditional ML algorithms [1,24–26]. In particular, bidirectional long short-term memory (BiLSTM) outperforms all the considered ML and DL methods, with a detection accuracy of 91.28%.

The rest of the paper is structured as follows. Section 2 provides the state-of-the-art in Alzheimer detection. Section 3 presents the proposed methodology. Section 4 provides the experimental results of the proposed Alzheimer detection and discussion, and finally Sect. 5 concludes the paper.

2 Related Work

In this section, we discuss the current state-of-the-art to detect dementia and Alzheimer's disease using DL and ML algorithms.

The work in [7] propose novel metrics to identify the Alzheimer's disease using pattern similarity score. The authors characterize the metrics in terms of conditional probabilities modeled by logistic regression. In addition, they explore the performance of anatomical and cognitive impairment which is used to generate the output of the classifiers using different types of data.

The authors in [41] use the online available datasets of MRI scan images and other cognitive features, such as RAVLT tests, MOCA and FDG score *etc.* to identify the Alzheimer's disease. In particular, clustering algorithms are developed based on logistic regression and SVM to detect the patient having Alzheimer's disease. Ammar et al. [4] presented a framework based on the speech processing to detect dementia. The framework was used to extract features from patients with dementia and without dementia wherein the speech data used was having verbal description and manual transcription. Therefore, the speech and textual features were used to train ML classifiers. The authors achieved an overall accuracy of 79% only.

Another interesting work in presented in [52] where authors introduced a detection method based on the MRI images of brain based on the Eigenbrain. Their approach used SVM and particle swarm optimization to train the model. Their proposal achieved satisfactory results in detecting the parts of the brain affected from Alzheimer's disease. Working on the similar lines of MRI scans, authors in [44] detected dementia and other different features using gradient boost and Artificial Neural Network (ANN) models. The authors achieved comparable results with the ones presented in [52]. The authors in [45] proposed a hybrid multimodal method based on the cognitive and linguistic features. The authors used ANN to train the model detect Alzheimer's disease and its severity. Their scheme achieved good results as compared to the state-of-the-art.

3   Methodology

This work proposes a novel Alzheimer's detection system using different ML and DL algorithms. In particular, the raw data coming from MRI scans is preprocessed before applying various ML and DL methods. Figure 3 presents an overall picture of the proposed Alzheimer detection system.

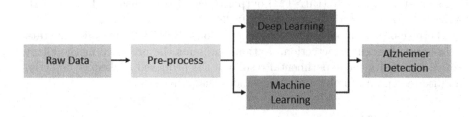

Fig. 3. Overview of Alzheimer detection framework

3.1 Machine Learning Methods

This subsection highlights our simulation settings to train different ML models. Scikit-learn is used to train ML classifiers. More specifically, radial basis function (RBF) kernel is used to train support vector machine (SVM). Elasticnet is used as a penalty for logistic regression, two hidden layers are used for multilayer perceptron (MLP), number of neighbors are set to 5 for k-nearest neighbors (KNN), epsilon is set to *float* for Naïve Bayes, max features are set to *int* for decision tree and finally number of estimate is set to 100 for random forest. It is worth mentioning that the ML classifiers are trained based on standard deviation, average, square root, skew, maximum and minimum value.

3.2 Deep Learning Methods

This subsection highlights our simulation settings to train different DL models. Mainly, two different DL models are used in this work, namely convolutional neural network (CNN) and LSTM The developed CNN architecture, inspired from [12, 29, 42], contains input, hidden and output layers where hidden layers are made up of convolutional, max pooling and fully connected layers. In particular, 10-layered CNN architecture is employed. On the other hand, LSTM architecture, inspired from [3, 8, 23, 43], contains two bidirectional LSMT along with 128 and 64 cells with dropout of 0.2. In addition, a dense layer with two neurons and softmax activation is used.

4   Experimental Results and Discussions

The dataset consists of 373 images from 150 subjects aged between 60 and 96. The MRI scan of each subject was taken for his one or two visits with a separation of at least one year between visits. All the subjects were right-handed with a mixture of men and women. Out of 150, 72 subjects were non-demented, with no mental disorder or dysfunction. On the other hand, 64 subjects were categorized as demented during their initial visit, including 51 with mild to moderate Alzheimer's disease. Importantly, the dataset is marked with five labels as normal, very mild dementia, mild dementia, moderate dementia, severe dementia.

In order to detect Alzheimer's disease, we compare the results of different ML classifiers including logistic regression, SVM, random forest, MLP, KNN, naïve bayes, decision tree and DL classifiers (1D-CNN, 2D-CNN, LSTM and BiLSTM). For ML classifiers, the features, such as skew, percentile, standard deviation, mean and square root are used to train the classifier. However, for DL classifiers raw data is used to train the models. It is important to that we used 5-fold and 10-fold cross-validation to perform the experiments. The considered evaluation parameters are precision, recall, f-measure and detection accuracy. It is evident from Tables 1 highlights are results of different ML and DL methods for a 5-fold cross validation settings. It can be noted that SVM provides the most promising results as compared to other ML methods such as logistic regression,

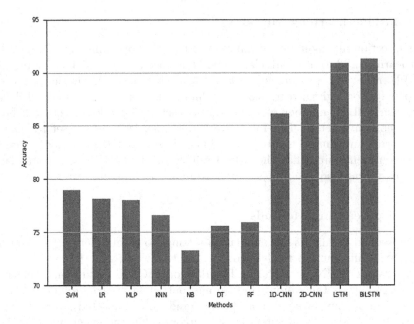

Fig. 4. 5-Fold summary of machine learning and deep learning results

MLP and *etc.* Overall, the experimental results show that the DL classifiers outperforms ML methods. However, the DL classifiers are expensive both in terms of computational resources and time.

Table 2 shows the summary of considered ML and DL results to the detect Alzheimer's disease for a 10-fold cross validation settings. Here again, SVM classifiers outperforms to other ML approaches such as logistic regression, MLP, KNN, Naive Bayes, decision tree and random forest. On the other hand, naive bayes gives the worst performance as compared to all ML and DL methods and also it took longer to train the model. Overall, DL methods perform better. In particular, BiLSTM achieved the best performance. However, BiLSTM took longer to train the model.

4.1   Discussion

It is important to note that the detection of Alzheimer's disease using ML methods is cost-effective (Computation and time) than DL algorithms. On the other hand, training deep learning classifiers is time and computationally expensive. Clearly, as shown in Figs. 4 and 5 the BiLSTM achieved better performance as compared to other methods in both 5-fold and 10-fold cross validation strategies. In addition to having such a promising results, our work has certain limitations as well (1) The dataset is very small with only 373 images in total. (2) The dataset considers people of aged 65 and above only (Table 3).

Table 1. Summary of machine learning and deep learning methods to detect Alzheimer using 5-fold cross-validation

Methods	Training accuracy	Testing accuracy	Precision	Recall	F-Score	Time
SVM	80.78	78.56	0.78	0.76	0.76	2 m 21 s
Logistic Regression	80.23	78.12	0.78	0.77	0.78	2 m 8 s
MLP	79.81	78	0.78	0.77	0.78	2 m 6 s
KNN	77.25	76.58	0.76	0.75	0.76	2 m 2 s
Naive Bayes	75.89	73.28	0.73	0.72	0.73	2 m 19 s
Decision Tree	76.98	75.59	0.75	0.74	0.75	2 m 11 s
Random Forest	76.85	75.89	0.75	0.75	0.75	2 m 31 s
1D-CNN	88.59	86.14	0.86	0.85	0.86	8 m 28 s
2D-CNN	89.45	87	0.87	0.86	0.87	9 m 1 s
LSTM	91.26	90.85	0.90	0.90	0.90	10 m 17 s
BiLSTM	93.21	91.28	0.91	0.91	0.91	10 m 12 s

Table 2. Summary of machine learning and deep learning methods to detect Alzheimer using 10-fold cross-validation

Methods	Training accuracy	Testing accuracy	Precision	Recall	F-Score	Time
SVM	82.24	80.75	0.80	0.79	0.80	2 m 33 s
Logisitc Regression	81.86	79.86	0.79	0.78	0.79	2 m 12 s
MLP	80.36	79.56	0.79	0.79	0.79	2 m 31 s
KNN	78.91	76.12	0.76	0.75	0.76	2 m 4 s
Naive Bayes	75.2	71.64	0.71	0.70	0.71	3 m
Decision Tree	78.69	75.9	0.75	0.74	0.75	2 m 19 s
Random Forest	75.97	73.29	0.73	0.72	0.73	2 m 8 s
1D-CNN	88.91	86.54	0.86	0.85	0.86	8 m 5 s
2D-CNN	89.43	87.01	0.87	0.86	0.87	8 m 29 s
LSTM	93.19	91.19	0.91	0.91	0.91	8 m 45 s
BiLSTM	95.59	93.19	0.93	0.93	0.93	9 m 16 s

Table 3. Comparison with state-of-the-art approach

Ref.	Accuracy	Precision	Recall	F-Score
Zhang et al. [52]	86.24	0.85	0.83	0.84
Dyrba et al. [20]	70.4	0.70	0.70	0.70
Escudero et al. [22]	79.1	0.78	0.76	0.75
Trambaiolli et al.[50]	75.56	0.75	0.73	0.71
Liu et al. [40]	84.40	0.84	0.82	0.82
Shankar et al. [46]	76.23	0.75	0.74	0.75
Our Approach	93.19	0.93	0.93	0.93

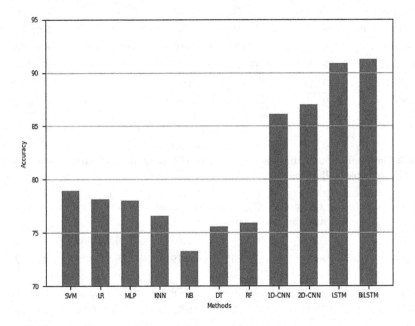

Fig. 5. 5-Fold summary of machine learning and deep learning results

5   Conclusion

The alzheimer's disease is the most challenging health problems scientists are facing since decades. In this paper, we present a novel framework based on the ML and DL algorithms including SVM, logistic regression, MLP, KNN, Naive Bayes, decision tree and random forest, 1D-CNN, 2D,CNN, LSTM and BiL-STM to automatically detect Alzheimer's disease. The extensive experimental results show that BiLSTM achieved better performance as compared to other ML and DL algorithms. As a future work, we intend to use transformers to detect Alzheimer's disease using images, visual and acoustic features.

Acknowledgement. This work is supported in part by the Ajman University Internal Research Grant.

References

1. Adeel, A., Gogate, M., Hussain, A.: Contextual deep learning-based audio-visual switching for speech enhancement in real-world environments. Inf. Fusion **59**, 163–170 (2020)
2. Ahmed, R., et al.: Deep neural network-based contextual recognition of Arabic handwritten scripts. Entropy **23**(3), 340 (2021)
3. Alqarafi, A.S., Adeel, A., Gogate, M., Dashitpour, K., Hussain, A., Durrani, T.: Toward's Arabic multi-modal sentiment analysis. In: Liang, Q., Mu, J., Jia, M., Wang, W., Feng, X., Zhang, B. (eds.) CSPS 2017. LNEE, vol. 463, pp. 2378–2386. Springer, Singapore (2019). https://doi.org/10.1007/978-981-10-6571-2_290
4. Ammar, R.B., Ayed, Y.B.: Speech processing for early alzheimer disease diagnosis: machine learning based approach. In: 2018 IEEE/ACS 15th International Conference on Computer Systems and Applications (AICCSA), pp. 1–8. IEEE (2018)
5. Asad, S.M., et al.: Mobility management-based autonomous energy-aware framework using machine learning approach in dense mobile networks. Signals **1**(2), 170–187 (2020)
6. Asad, S.M., Dashtipour, K., Hussain, S., Abbasi, Q.H., Imran, M.A.: Travelers-tracing and mobility profiling using machine learning in railway systems. In 2020 International Conference on UK-China Emerging Technologies (UCET), pp. 1–4. IEEE (2020)
7. Casanova, R., et al.: Alzheimer's disease risk assessment using large-scale machine learning methods. PloS One **8**(11), e77949 (2013)
8. Churcher, A., et al.: An experimental analysis of attack classification using machine learning in IoT networks. Sensors **21**(2), 446 (2021)
9. Dashtipour, K., Gogate, M., Adeel, A., Algarafi, A., Howard, N., Hussain, A.: Persian named entity recognition. In: 2017 IEEE 16th International Conference on Cognitive Informatics and Cognitive Computing (ICCI* CC), pp. 79–83. IEEE (2017)
10. Dashtipour, K., Gogate, M., Adeel, A., Hussain, A., Alqarafi, A., Durrani, T.: A comparative study of Persian sentiment analysis based on different feature combinations. In: Liang, Q., Mu, J., Jia, M., Wang, W., Feng, X., Zhang, B. (eds.) CSPS 2017. LNEE, vol. 463, pp. 2288–2294. Springer, Singapore (2019). https://doi.org/10.1007/978-981-10-6571-2_279
11. Dashtipour, K., Gogate, M., Adeel, A., Ieracitano, C., Larijani, H., Hussain, A.: Exploiting deep learning for Persian sentiment analysis. In: Ren, J., et al. (eds.) BICS 2018. LNCS (LNAI), vol. 10989, pp. 597–604. Springer, Cham (2018). https://doi.org/10.1007/978-3-030-00563-4_58
12. Dashtipour, K., Gogate, M., Adeel, A., Larijani, H., Hussain, A.: Sentiment analysis of Persian movie reviews using deep learning. Entropy **23**(5), 596 (2021)
13. Dashtipour, K., Gogate, M., Cambria, E., Hussain, A.: A novel context-aware multimodal framework for persian sentiment analysis. arXiv preprint arXiv:2103.02636 (2021)
14. Dashtipour, K., Gogate, M., Li, J., Jiang, F., Kong, B., Hussain, A.: A hybrid Persian sentiment analysis framework: integrating dependency grammar based rules and deep neural networks. Neurocomputing **380**, 1–10 (2020)

15. Dashtipour, K., Hussain, A., Gelbukh, A.: Adaptation of sentiment analysis techniques to Persian language. In: Gelbukh, A. (ed.) CICLing 2017, Part II. LNCS, vol. 10762, pp. 129–140. Springer, Cham (2018). https://doi.org/10.1007/978-3-319-77116-8_10

16. Dashtipour, K., Hussain, A., Zhou, Q., Gelbukh, A., Hawalah, A.Y.A., Cambria, E.: PerSent: a freely available Persian sentiment Lexicon. In: Liu, C.-L., Hussain, A., Luo, B., Tan, K.C., Zeng, Y., Zhang, Z. (eds.) BICS 2016. LNCS (LNAI), vol. 10023, pp. 310–320. Springer, Cham (2016). https://doi.org/10.1007/978-3-319-49685-6_28

17. Dashtipour, K., et al.: Multilingual sentiment analysis: state of the art and independent comparison of techniques. Cogn. Comput. 8(4), 757–771 (2016)

18. Dashtipour, K., Raza, A., Gelbukh, A., Zhang, R., Cambria, E., Hussain, A.: PerSent 2.0: Persian sentiment Lexicon enriched with domain-specific words. In: Ren, J., et al. (eds.) BICS 2019. LNCS (LNAI), vol. 11691, pp. 497–509. Springer, Cham (2020). https://doi.org/10.1007/978-3-030-39431-8_48

19. Dashtipour, K., et al.: Public perception towards fifth generation of cellular networks (5G) on social media. Frontiers in Big Data (2021)

20. Dyrba, M., et al.: Robust automated detection of microstructural white matter degeneration in Alzheimer's disease using machine learning classification of multicenter dti data. PloS One 8(5), e64925 (2013)

21. D'Andrea, M.R., Cole, G.M., Ard, M.D.: The microglial phagocytic role with specific plaque types in the alzheimer disease brain. Neurobiol. Aging 25(5), 675–683 (2004)

22. Escudero, J., et al.: Machine learning-based method for personalized and cost-effective detection of alzheimer's disease. IEEE Trans. Biomed. Eng. 6(1), 164–168 (2012)

23. Gepperth, A.R.T., Hecht, T., Gogate, M.: A generative learning approach to sensor fusion and change detection. Cogn. Comput. 8(5), 806–817 (2016). https://doi.org/10.1007/s12559-016-9390-z

24. Gogate, M., Adeel, A., Hussain, A.: Deep learning driven multimodal fusion for automated deception detection. In: 2017 IEEE Symposium Series on Computational Intelligence (SSCI), pp. 1–6. IEEE (2017)

25. Gogate, M., Adeel, A., Hussain, A.: A novel brain-inspired compression-based optimised multimodal fusion for emotion recognition. In: 2017 IEEE Symposium Series on Computational Intelligence (SSCI), pp. 1–7. IEEE (2017)

26. Gogate, M., Adeel, A., Marxer, R., Barker, J., Hussain, A.: DNN driven speaker independent audio-visual mask estimation for speech separation. arXiv preprint arXiv:1808.00060 (2018)

27. Gogate, M., Dashtipour, K., Adeel, A., Hussain, A.: CochleaNet: a robust language-independent audio-visual model for real-time speech enhancement. Inf. Fusion 63, 273–285 (2020)

28. Gogate, M., Dashtipour, K., Hussain, A.: Visual speech in real noisy environments (vision): a novel benchmark dataset and deep learning-based baseline system. In: Proceedings of the Interspeech 2020, pp. 4521–4525 (2020)

29. Gogate, M., Hussain, A., Huang, K.: Random features and random neurons for brain-inspired big data analytics. In: 2019 International Conference on Data Mining Workshops (ICDMW), pp. 522–529. IEEE (2019)

30. Guellil, I., et al.: A semi-supervised approach for sentiment analysis of Arab(ic+izi) messages: application to the Algerian dialect. SN Comput. Sci. 2(2), 1–18 (2021). https://doi.org/10.1007/s42979-021-00510-1

31. Huma, Z.E., et al.: A hybrid deep random neural network for cyberattack detection in the industrial internet of things. IEEE Access **9**, 55595–55605 (2021)
32. Hussain, A., et al.: Artificial intelligence-enabled analysis of UK and us public attitudes on Facebook and twitter towards covid-19 vaccinations. medRxiv (2020)
33. Hussien, I.O., Dashtipour, K., Hussain, A.: Comparison of sentiment analysis approaches using modern Arabic and Sudanese dialect. In: Ren, J., et al. (eds.) BICS 2018. LNCS (LNAI), vol. 10989, pp. 615–624. Springer, Cham (2018). https://doi.org/10.1007/978-3-030-00563-4_60
34. Ieracitano, C., et al.: Statistical analysis driven optimized deep learning system for intrusion detection. In: Ren, J., et al. (eds.) BICS 2018. LNCS (LNAI), vol. 10989, pp. 759–769. Springer, Cham (2018). https://doi.org/10.1007/978-3-030-00563-4_74
35. Ieracitano, C., Paviglianiti, A., Mammone, N., Versaci, M., Pasero, E., Morabito, F.C.: SoCNNet: an optimized sobel filter based convolutional neural network for SEM images classification of nanomaterials. In: Esposito, A., Faundez-Zanuy, M., Morabito, F.C., Pasero, E. (eds.) Progresses in Artificial Intelligence and Neural Systems. SIST, vol. 184, pp. 103–113. Springer, Singapore (2021). https://doi.org/10.1007/978-981-15-5093-5_10
36. Jiang, F., Kong, B., Li, J., Dashtipour, K., Gogate, M.: Robust visual saliency optimization based on bidirectional Markov chains. Cogn. Comput. **13**(1), 69–80 (2020). https://doi.org/10.1007/s12559-020-09724-6
37. Liaqat, S., Dashtipour, K., Arshad, K., Ramzan, N.: Non invasive skin hydration level detection using machine learning. Electronics **9**(7), 1086 (2020)
38. Liaqat, S., Dashtipour, K., Zahid, A., Assaleh, K., Arshad, K., Ramzan, N.: Detection of atrial fibrillation using a machine learning approach. Information **11**(12), 549 (2020)
39. Lindeboom, J., Schmand, B., Tulner, L., Walstra, G., Jonker, C.: Visual association test to detect early dementia of the alzheimer type. J. Neurol. Neurosurg. Psychiatry **73**(2), 126–133 (2002)
40. Liu, S., Liu, S., Cai, W., Pujol, S., Kikinis, R., Feng, D.: Early diagnosis of alzheimer's disease with deep learning. In: 2014 IEEE 11th International Symposium on Biomedical Imaging (ISBI), pp. 1015–1018. IEEE (2014)
41. Lodha, P., Talele, A., Degaonkar, K.: Diagnosis of Alzheimer's disease using machine learning. In: 2018 Fourth International Conference on Computing Communication Control and Automation (ICCUBEA), pp. 1–4. IEEE (2018)
42. Nisar, S., Tariq, M., Adeel, A., Gogate, M., Hussain, A.: Cognitively inspired feature extraction and speech recognition for automated hearing loss testing. Cogn. Comput. **11**(4), 489–502 (2019). https://doi.org/10.1007/s12559-018-9607-4
43. Ozturk, M., Gogate, M., Onireti, O., Adeel, A., Hussain, A., Imran, M.A.: A novel deep learning driven, low-cost mobility prediction approach for 5G cellular networks: the case of the control/data separation architecture (CDSA). Neurocomputing **358**, 479–489 (2019)
44. Rawat, R.M., Akram, M., Pradeep, S.S., et al.: Dementia detection using machine learning by stacking models. In: 2020 5th International Conference on Communication and Electronics Systems (ICCES), pp. 849–854. IEEE (2020)
45. Sarawgi, U., Zulfikar, W., Soliman, N., Maes, P.: Multimodal inductive transfer learning for detection of alzheimer's dementia and its severity. arXiv preprint arXiv:2009.00700 (2020)
46. Shankar, K., Lakshmanaprabu, S.K., Khanna, A., Tanwar, S., Rodrigues, J.J.P.C., Roy, N.R.: Alzheimer detection using group grey wolf optimization based features with convolutional classifier. Comput. Electr.l Eng. **77**, 230–243 (2019)

47. Taylor, K.: Dementia: A Very Short Introduction. Oxford University Press, Oxford (2020)
48. Taylor, W., Shah, S.A., Dashtipour, K., Zahid, A., Abbasi, Q.H., Imran, M.A.: An intelligent non-invasive real-time human activity recognition system for next-generation healthcare. Sensors **20**(9), 2653 (2020)
49. Tohgi, H., Abe, T., Kimura, M., Saheki, M., Takahashi, S.: Cerebrospinal fluid acetylcholine and choline in vascular dementia of Binswanger and multiple small infarct types as compared with alzheimer-type dementia. J. Neural Transm. **103**(10), 1211–1220 (1996). https://doi.org/10.1007/BF01271206
50. Trambaiolli, L.R., Lorena, A.C., Fraga, F.J., Kanda, P.A.M., Anghinah, R., Nitrini, R.: Improving Alzheimer's disease diagnosis with machine learning techniques. Clin. EEG Neurosci. **42**(3), 160–165 (2011)
51. Yu, Z., et al.: Energy and performance trade-off optimization in heterogeneous computing via reinforcement learning. Electronics **9**(11), 1812 (2020)
52. Zhang, Y., et al.: Detection of subjects and brain regions related to Alzheimer's disease using 3D MRI scans based on eigenbrain and machine learning. Front. Comput. Neurosci. **9**, 66 (2015)

FPGA-Based Realtime Detection of Freezing of Gait of Parkinson Patients

Patrick Langer[1], Ali Haddadi Esfahani[1], Zoya Dyka[1],
and Peter Langendörfer[1,2(✉)]

[1] IHP GmbH, 15326 Frankfurt (Oder), Germany
[2] BTU Cottbus-Senftenberg, 03046 Cottbus, Germany
langendoerfer@ihp-microelectronics.com

Abstract. In this paper we report on our implementation of a temporal convolutional network trained to detect Freezing of Gait on an FPGA. In order to be able to compare our results with state of the art solutions we used the well-known open dataset Daphnet. Our most important findings are even though we used a tool to map the trained model to the FPGA we can detect FoG in less than a millisecond which will give us sufficient time to trigger cueing and by that prevent the patient from falling. In addition, the average sensitivity achieved by our implementation is comparable to solutions running on high end devices.

Keywords: Freezing of Gait · Temporal convolution models FPGA based implementation · Tool assisted implementation · Body worn sensor nodes

1 Introduction

Detecting Freezing of Gait (FoG) and triggering countermeasures like cueing is an important issue with respect of quality of life of Parkinson patients. Parkinson patients are often so afraid of falling due to FoG, that their social life seriously suffers as they do no longer leave their flats. A proper device for detecting FoG needs to be wearable and, to avoid stigmatization, as unobtrusive as possible. The time for detecting FoG and triggering the cueing is limited by the normal time for taking a step which is about 300 ms. As the device needs to get some sensor data to do the assessment and then to trigger the cueing, the whole process should be limited to about 50 ms. This leads to strict hard real time requirements and extremely short processing time. In addition, cueing may not be triggered too often to avoid that the patient becomes too familiar and it is no longer helping if FoG really occurs. The occurrence of such habituation effects needs to be investigated in further research and long-term tests with patients.

Contributions of This Paper. We report on our FPGA implementation that provides extremely good parameters with its quite good average sensitivity well above 78, comparable to what is reported in literature for high end devices

© ICST Institute for Computer Sciences, Social Informatics and Telecommunications Engineering 2022
Published by Springer Nature Switzerland AG 2022. All Rights Reserved
M. Ur Rehman and A. Zoha (Eds.): BODYNETS 2021, LNICST 420, pp. 101–111, 2022.
https://doi.org/10.1007/978-3-030-95593-9_9

and a detection time of far less than 1 ms. The paper is structured as follows. Section 2 presents an overview of current research for FoG detection and its requirements. Furthermore, recent methods for the implementation of neural networks on FPGAs are discussed. Section 3 gives details about our own implementations and methods. Our experimental results are discussed in Sect. 4. Section 5 provides our conclusion and presents an outlook for our further research.

2   Related Work

2.1   Overview of Recent Methods of Detecting FoG

When it comes to Freezing of Gait (FoG), different algorithms have been used to identify an FoG event from sensor data (usually acceleration sensors). For example, in [8,17,18,30], threshold analysis methods are used, normally by applying those methods on extracted statistical features. Based on that, [3,24] employ Support Vector Machines (SVM) for FoG detection on sensor data. With the breakthrough of Machine Learning (ML) and Deep Learning (DL) methods, more recent research applied those technologies on FoG datasets to achieve new state of the art results. [15] tested different machine learning techniques for FoG detection. In [29], a Convolutional Neural Network (CNN) was trained on the raw sensor data and was used as an end-to-end classifier for FoG detection. As FoG detection is based on time series data usually from accelerometers, [31] claims that better results for FoG detection can be achieved when neural network architectures are used that are especially targeted at time series data. Historically this is associated with Recurrent Neural Networks (RNNs) [4], [14]. Especially Long short-term memory (LSTM) Units have achieved state of the art results on time series problems, such as speech recognition [10] or Human Activity Recognition (HAR) [19]. As such, [31] propose a combined CNN-LSTM architecture for FoG detection. The CNN is intended to learn the necessary feature extraction from the raw sensor data, whereas the LSTM shall learn the time-based dependencies in order to classify a time series and decide whether an FoG event occurred. A similar architecture was proposed by [26]. They evaluated a CNN combined with fully connected layers (Multilayer Perceptron, MLP) and a CNN combined with LSTM. They evaluated their models by means of sensitivity, specificity, area under the curve (AUC), geometric mean (GM) and equal error rate (EER). The CNN-LSTM achieved slightly better results (e.g. 0.849 vs. 0.844 sensitivity and the same for specificity). Thus, the authors state that the CNN-LSTM is the better architecture and should be used for future experiments.

Recently, it has been shown that CNNs in fact are able to learn (long-term) dependencies on time series data, contradicting common convictions that RNNs are the logical choice for such data sets. In [20], a special 1D convolutional model was developed for raw audio generation. Recent research suggests that similar convolutional models are able to learn long-term dependencies, possibly better than recurrent models and LSTMs [6]. Those models form a new group of CNNs, called Temporal Convolutional Models (TCNs), which achieved state of the art results on different datasets [6], yet inherently being a lot more straightforward by having a simpler architecture. In [13] it was proposed to combine TCNs and LSTMs in order to achieve better results in FoG detection (additionally, they also introduced an attentional mechanism). However, the TCN here was only used for the feature extraction, as in previous papers, not explicitly for learning dependencies in the time series data.

2.2 Requirements of FoG Detection Methods for Wearable Devices

Most of those publications especially focus on achieving better detection results and the applied methods have been trained and tested on modern GPUs. For example the mentioned TCN-LSTM architecture of [13] can be run in 0.52 ms but has only been evaluated on modern GPU (NVIDIA RTX 2060). From our understanding, there seems to be a gap in research between increasing accuracy and achieving real time capability for deployment in real world applications. While focusing on achieving better detection results, it is important to keep in mind that the proposed methods shall be deployed in wearable devices to aid parkinson patients. It is necessary that they can be run in real time efficiently. A freezing must be detected within at least 300 ms, so that an appropriate cueing signal can be issued fast enough in order to prevent patients from falling. As those wearable devices are powered by battery, the used hardware to run the neural network needs to be efficient, having an overall low power consumption.

2.3 Field Programmable Gate Arrays (FPGAs) for Inference of Neural Networks

Field Programmable Gate Arrays (FPGA) are often used as algorithm-specific hardware accelerator [5,21]. They can eventually be more efficient than generic computing units like CPUs or GPUs [7,22]. Recently, approaches to run neural networks on FPGAs are conducted, aiming for use cases in embedded applications or wearable devices. FoG detection was implemented with a specific neural network for those matters on an FPGA [16]. This architecture even has online learning capabilities, which means that the model on the FPGA can be trained continuously in action. However, the architecture itself is hardwired, it is not easily possible to switch to a more modern or sophisticated neural network. In order to speed up the development process and gain more flexibility means, to convert a neural network, trained in a common machine learning framework like TensorFlow or PyTorch, to some format applicable for the FPGAs would be needed. High Level Synthesis for machine Learning (HLS4ML) [12] is a project addressing this issues. Another approach was taken by Xilinx. They developed the so-called Deep Learning Processing Unit (DPU) [2] for their FPGAs. This is a programmable computation engine enabling FPGAs to run neural networks. Different types of DPUs with different supported layers are available, e.g. there is one for convolutional neural networks and one for recurrent neural networks. To the best of our knowledge, this technology represents the current state of the art of a generic method to deploy neural networks on FPGAs.

3 Methods

3.1 VitisAI to Run Neural Networks on FPGA

Methods of FoG detection should be executable in real-time on wearable devices and preferably only require a minimum amount of power. Therefore, we choose an FPGA as our targeted hardware and first explain how to use it to run neural networks. Xilinx provides a development environment for execution of neural networks on FPGAs. Currently, the machine learning frameworks Caffe, PyTorch and TensorFlow are supported. For this, the FPGA is configured (programmed) with Xilinx DPU. The DPU running inside the FPGA then is able to load a neural network from a file in a specific binary format (called xmodel). To generate this file from a certain model, it needs to be converted, which is a process containing two steps [1]:

1. Quantization: The trained model needs to be quantized. Currently, the DPU only supports 8-bit integer quantization. Thus, if the model was trained using 32-bit-floating-point values, those are converted to 8-bit integer values. This results in a loss of precision, possibly decreasing the accuracy of the neural network. This problem can partially be alleviated by so-called finetuning, which is also supported by the development tools.
2. Compilation: The quantized model is compiled into a binary file, which contains instructions to be run on Xilinx DPU.

Figure 1 shows the used hardware for our experiments, namely the UltraZED-EG hardware platform. It is a credit-card-sized FPGA platform based on a Xilinx XZCU3EG with some additional hardware. Additionally, a carrier card is available, which features peripheral connections, like USB or ethernet ports. The reason to use this platform is its small size and energy efficiency, but it currently does not support to execute recurrent layers and LSTM. We report on how we solved this issue in the following section.

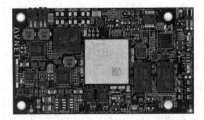

Fig. 1. UltraZED-EG. The used hardware platform for our experiments, which can used for embedded applications.

3.2   Hardware-Aware Implementation of a Temporal Convolutional Network for FoG Detection

As mentioned, usually RNNs are chosen for dealing with time series data. However, recently it has been shown that TCNs might achieve comparable or even better results [6]. When it comes to deciding which type of neural network shall be used for the implementation, a thorough analysis of benefits and drawbacks is essential. For the case of FoG detection, we especially consider the advantages of TCNs shown in Table 1 to be very important. In addition, it needs to be taken into account that TCNs potentially have a higher memory requirement during inference. When it comes to FPGA-based neural network accelerators, often memory bandwidth is the main limitation [25]. Thus, a recurrent neural network might have benefits when it comes to long input sequences or more complex problems, as the memory requirement during inference is potentially lower [6]. However, in the case of FoG detection, memory of modern FPGA systems is sufficient to run our proposed architecture very well.

Table 1. Advantages of TCNs compared to RNNs according to [6].

	TCN	RNN
Parallelism	Input sequence can be processed as a whole, convolution operations and filters are parallelizable. Especially important for FPGAs or other hardware accelerators	Each sample in the input sequence is processed one at a time (only sequential processing)
Stable gradients	Backpropagation path different from temporal direction of sequence, avoids vanishing/exploding gradient problem. Plus strategies like skip connections etc. can be used to build deep networks just as for conventional neural networks	LSTMs reduce risk of vanishing gradient problems, exploding gradients might still be a problem [27]
Receptive field size	Flexible, can be easily expanded, e.g. by increasing filter size or dilation factor. Might lead to better possibilities to learn long term dependencies.	Cannot be flexibly changed or influenced

So, from our point of view TCN are the better choice for an FPGA implementation. Another important aspect is that RNNs are not yet supported for our targeted FPGA platforms, neither by Xilinx VitisAI nor by other alternatives such as HLS4ML [12] etc. Xilinx provides a DPU able to execute RNNs only for Alveo platforms.

Implementation Details. For our implementations, which were done in Keras, we used [23] as a reference. After training, the model was converted to the binary file needed for the FPGA. For our tests, we used VitisAI version 1.3[1]. However, there were some restrictions for the conversion of the model in terms of supported layers and operations.

- First, the mentioned version of VitisAI only supports models built with Keras functional API. Furthermore, custom layers as used in [23] cannot be used.
- Second, Conv1D operations are not supported.

The latter issue can be remedied as follows. It is possible to replace any Conv1D operation with a Conv2D operation equivalently. For example, if the Conv1D operation uses a kernel of size 3, the Conv2D operation can use kernel of size 1×3, where 1 represents the height and 3 the width. However, while Conv1D operation in Keras supports causal (asymmetric) and non-causal (symmetric) padding, Conv2D operations only support the latter. However, as Keras is based on TensorFlow, a tf.pad layer can be used to do asymmetrical padding manually. But standard TensorFlow layers are currently only supported by VitisAI for TensorFlow 1, not for TensorFlow 2.

We realized causal padding with manual padding using tf.pad layer. The conversion for the FPGA worked well, however the used tools indicated that some of the layers of the converted model might not be run on the FPGA but on the CPU of the SoC automatically. This is not the case if non-causal padding is used.

To solve these issues, we came up with our own implementation of TCN which is convertible with VitisAI to be run on the FPGA (or FPGA + CPU accordingly). The desired form of padding can be chosen as desired. Training and conversion can be done end-to-end, no manual steps are required.

4   Experiments

4.1   Dataset Description

We trained our model using the Daphnet dataset [9,11] in order to compare our own results with the state-of-the-art publications using the same data set (such as [13] or [15]). It is a publicly available dataset of movement data recordings from 10 Parkinson patients. The age of those patients ranged from 59 to 75 years (66.4 years $\pm$ 4.8 years), whereas 3 patients were females. The patients were asked to perform three walking tasks as described in [9]. Three sensor nodes placed at different locations of the body, i.e. shank, thigh, and on the lower back of the patients, were used to record the data. Each sensor acquired data at a frequency 64 Hz. A physiotherapist marked FoG events through recorded videos of the experiments. In total, 8 h 20 min of acceleration signals were recorded, during which 237 FoG events occurred. Two of the ten patients did not show any freezing, their gait appeared as normal walking.

---

[1] https://github.com/Xilinx/Vitis-AI/tree/v1.3.

4.2 Performance Evaluation

Training Details. For evaluation, we used a patient dependent approach. This means that for each patient, a separate model was trained. As mentioned, two patients (patients four and ten) did not experience any FoG episodes during the recordings. Those patients were excluded from the training. The training dataset for each patient was composed of 80% of the corresponding data for the patient including all data of all other patients (except patients four and ten). The remaining 20% of the patients' data were used as validation dataset. The split of 80/20 was chosen as a it is a common split for initial evaluations. We might test additional variants in future work and might also do a R10Fold evaluation as seen in recent literature regarding FoG detection [13].

The daphnet dataset, is highly imbalanced. Therefore, common indicators such as accuracy might not be suitable to evaluate the detection performance of a model. Thus, we use sensitivity (true positive rate) and specificity (true negative rate), as used in other publications as well. We configured our architecture to use three residual blocks as described in [6], using a kernel size of 3 and 64 kernels per layer overall. For each patient (except four and ten), our model was trained five times for 1000 epochs using a learning rate of 0.001 and batch size 1000. Among all trainings and epochs, the best model for each patient was saved. Afterwards, it was quantized using Vitis AI tools and converted for FPGA. The quantized model is a TensorFlow graph and can be run on GPU as well.

4.3 Hardware Platform Details

For our experiments, an UltraZED-EG was used. It features a Xilinx XCZU3EG multiprocessor system on a chip (MPSoC). It contains 154.350 system logic cells, 216 Block RAM blocks (7.6 MB BRAM memory in total) and 360 DSP slices. It features an ARM Cortex-A53 processor aswell. In our case, the processor runs an Ubuntu based operating system including PYNQ[2]. A program on the operating system is responsible for loading the test data, feeding it to the model running on the FPGA and interpret the results. The model only needs 0.7 ms = 700 μs for execution on the FPGA. This number was consistent during the whole evaluation. The FPGA does not need any scheduling like CPUs or GPUs, thus the inference time is almost exactly the same each time the model is run.

Results on Standard Daphnet Dataset. In Table 2 we present our results of the model for each patient. We evaluated sensitivity and specificity on the original model, the quantized model running on GPU and the converted quantized model running on the FPGA.

---

[2] http://www.pynq.io/board.html.

Table 2. Results for dataset without augmentation

Patient	Original		Quantized		FPGA	
	Sens.	Spec.	Sens.	Spec.	Sens.	Spec.
Patient 1	0.0833	0.9987	0.0833	0.9889	0.0833	1.0000
Patient 3	0.4615	0.9760	0.4615	0.9680	0.3846	0.9640
Patient 3	0.4603	0.9514	0.5238	0.9114	0.4127	0.9114
Patient 5	0.4216	0.9394	0.3627	0.9303	0.3725	0.9394
Patient 6	0.0714	0.9943	0.0357	0.9448	0.0357	0.9946
Patient 7	0.3158	0.9968	0.3684	0.9968	0.3158	0.9935
Patient 8	0.6905	0.9052	0.4286	0.9138	0.2857	0.9483
Patient 9	0.4035	0.9663	0.4211	0.8653	0.3158	0.8384
Average	0.3635	0.9669	0.3356	0.9482	0.2758	0.9487

As can be seen, the overall specificity is quite high, 0.9669 on the original model run on GPU and still 0.9487 on FPGA. However, with this naive approach, the average sensitivity is quite low. This is due to the fact that the dataset is highly imbalanced, and the positive class (FoG event) is underrepresented. This issue was addressed by recent research. Different publications suggest using augmentation or rebalancing strategies to improve the dataset, such as [13, 28].

Results on Rebalanced Daphnet Set. Due to the lack of more balanced datasets, we as well used a simple oversampling strategy to virtually rebalance the dataset in order to evaluate our model in accordance with the current state of the art, which used augmentations. The results of the augmented dataset are presented in Table 3. In further research, we aim to build our own, better balanced dataset.

Table 3. Results for dataset without augmentation

Patient	Original		Quantized		FPGA	
	Sens.	Spec.	Sens.	Spec.	Sens.	Spec.
Patient 1	0.9995	0.9558	0.8103	0.9088	0.8966	0.9171
Patient 2	0.9996	0.9880	0.9692	0.9480	0.9487	0.9480
Patient 3	0.9995	0.9257	0.9199	0.8371	0.8846	0.8886
Patient 5	0.9994	0.9394	0.8518	0.8848	0.7787	0.8394
Patient 6	0.9998	0.9517	0.7059	0.7158	0.6053	0.9196
Patient 7	0.9999	0.9643	0.8000	0.7695	0.7316	0.9123
Patient 8	0.9988	0.9483	0.7000	0.9224	0.6048	0.9569
Patient 9	0.9997	0.9798	0.9146	0.8889	0.8043	0.8923
Average	0.9953	0.9566	0.8340	0.8594	0.7818	0.9093

On this rebalanced dataset, the sensitivity is significantly higher than on the non-augmented dataset. We achieve an average sensitivity of 0.9953 and specificity of 0.9566 with our model run on GPU, which is comparable to current state of the art results. However, after quantization, sensitivity and specificity suffer a significant drop (0.8340 sensitivity and 0.8594 specificity for the quantized model run on GPU, 0.7818 sensitivity and 0.90932 specificity for converted quantized model run on FPGA). This can be explained by the loss of precision, as the quantization converts the 32-bit float model to an 8-bit integer model.

5   Conclusions

In this paper we reported on an FPGA based implementation for detecting freezing of gait of Parkinson patients. We would like to stress the following points. Our implementation achieves almost the same values for sensitivity and specificity as reported in the literature for high end devices. Even after quantization, the results are quite good. So, the use of FPGAs to allow real time detection of FoG in wearables is a feasible solution. In our discussion with clinicians, they reported that false positives, if they do not occur too often, are not an issue and that patients rather like to get a cueing more often to be reassured the system is still working. So, 100% sensitivity is not the ultimate goal. On the other hand, a very fast detection of FoG is key when it comes to trigger proper cueing to prevent the patient from falling due to FoG. Here our implementation provides extremely good parameters with its quite good sensitivity and a detection time of far less than 1 ms. The latter is the parameter that makes fall prevention by a body worn sensor node feasible. Please note that we achieved this extremely fast processing even though we used a tool to map the trained model onto the FPGA. In our future work we aim at integrating our FPGA based solution with a wireless sensor node and to run experiments with Parkinson patients together with a clinical partner. In order to improve user experience, we will also work on increasing sensitivity. The loss of precision because of quantization can possibly be alleviated by finetuning the model. Xilinx already provides support for finetuning the converted models using their development tools. We are also interested to further reduce the processing time on the FPGA.

References

1. Vitis AI user guide. https://www.xilinx.com/support/documentation/sw_manuals/vitis_ai/1_3/ug1414-vitis-ai.pdf. Accessed 21 June 2021
2. Convolutional neural network with INT4 optimization on Xilinx devices white paper (2014)
3. Ahlrichs, C., et al.: Detecting freezing of gait with a tri-axial accelerometer in Parkinson's disease patients. Med. Biol. Eng. Comput. **54**(1), 223–233 (2015). https://doi.org/10.1007/s11517-015-1395-3
4. Almqvist, O.: A comparative study between algorithms for time series forecasting on customer prediction: an investigation into the performance of ARIMA, RNN, LSTM, TCN and HMM. Ph.D. thesis, June 2019

5. Andrey, G., Thirer, N.: A FPGA implementation of hardware based accelerator for a generic algorithm, November 2010. https://doi.org/10.1109/EEEI.2010.5662152
6. Bai, S., Kolter, J., Koltun, V.: An empirical evaluation of generic convolutional and recurrent networks for sequence modeling, March 2018
7. Betkaoui, B., Thomas, D.B., Luk, W.: Comparing performance and energy efficiency of FPGAs and GPUs for high productivity computing. In: 2010 International Conference on Field-Programmable Technology, pp. 94–101 (2010)
8. Bächlin, M., Hausdorff, J., Roggen, D., Giladi, N., Plotnik, M., Tröster, G.: Online detection of freezing of gait in Parkinson's disease patients: a performance characterization. In: BODYNETS 2009–4th International ICST Conference on Body Area Networks, p. 11, April 2009. https://doi.org/10.4108/ICST.BODYNETS2009.5852
9. Bächlin, M., Plotnik, M., Roggen, D., Giladi, N., Hausdorff, J., Tröster, G.: A wearable system to assist walking of Parkinson's disease patients. Methods Inf. Med. **49**, 88–95 (2009). https://doi.org/10.3414/ME09-02-0003
10. Chiu, C.C., et al.: State-of-the-art speech recognition with sequence-to-sequence models, pp. 4774–4778, April 2018. https://doi.org/10.1109/ICASSP.2018.8462105
11. Bächlin, M., et al.: Wearable assistant for parkinson's disease patients with the freezing of gait symptom. IEEE Trans. Inf. Technol. Biomed. **14**(2), 436–446 (2010)
12. Duarte, J., et al.: Fast inference of deep neural networks in FPGAs for particle physics. ArXiv arXiv:1804.06913 (2018)
13. Li, B., Yao, Z., Wang, J., Wang, S., Yang, X., Sun, Y.: Improved deep learning technique to detect freezing of gait in Parkinson's disease based on wearable sensors. Electronics **9**, 1919 (2020). https://doi.org/10.3390/electronics9111919
14. Mahmoud, A., Mohammed, A.: A survey on deep learning for time-series forecasting. In: Hassanien, A.E., Darwish, A. (eds.) Machine Learning and Big Data Analytics Paradigms: Analysis, Applications and Challenges. SBD, vol. 77, pp. 365–392. Springer, Cham (2021). https://doi.org/10.1007/978-3-030-59338-4_19
15. Mazilu, S., et al.: Online detection of freezing of gait with smartphones and machine learning techniques (2012). https://doi.org/10.4108/icst.pervasivehealth.2012.248680
16. Mikos, V., et al.: A wearable, patient-adaptive freezing of gait detection system for biofeedback cueing in Parkinson's disease. IEEE Trans. Biomed. Circuits Syst. (2019). https://doi.org/10.1109/TBCAS.2019.2914253
17. Moore, S., MacDougall, H., Ondo, W.: Ambulatory monitoring of freezing of gait in Parkinson's disease. J. Neurosci. Methods **167**, 340–8 (2008). https://doi.org/10.1016/j.jneumeth.2007.08.023
18. Moore, S., et al.: Autonomous identification of freezing of gait in Parkinson's disease from lower-body segmental accelerometry. J. Neuroeng. Rehabil. **10**, 19 (2013). https://doi.org/10.1186/1743-0003-10-19
19. Murad, A., Pyun, J.Y.: Deep recurrent neural networks for human activity recognition. Sensors **17**, 2556 (2017). https://doi.org/10.3390/s17112556
20. Oord, A., et al.: Wavenet: A generative model for raw audio, September 2016
21. Possa, P., Schaillie, D., Valderrama, C.: FPGA-based hardware acceleration: a CPU/accelerator interface exploration. In: 2011 18th IEEE International Conference on Electronics, Circuits, and Systems, pp. 374–377 (2011). https://doi.org/10.1109/ICECS.2011.6122291
22. Qasaimeh, M., Denolf, K., Lo, J., Vissers, K., Zambreno, J., Jones, P.: Comparing energy efficiency of CPU, GPU and FPGA implementations for vision kernels, May 2019. https://doi.org/10.1109/ICESS.2019.8782524
23. Remy, P.: Temporal convolutional networks for Keras (2020). https://github.com/philipperemy/keras-tcn

24. Rodríguez-Martín, D., et al.: Home detection of freezing of gait using support vector machines through a single waist-worn triaxial accelerometer. PLoS One **12**, e0171764 (2017)
25. Shawahna, A., Sait, S.M., El-Maleh, A.: FPGA-based accelerators of deep learning networks for learning and classification: a review. IEEE Access **7**, 7823–7859 (2019)
26. Sigcha, L., et al.: Deep learning approaches for detecting freezing of gait in Parkinson's disease patients through on-body acceleration sensors. Sensors **20**, 1895 (2020). Basel, Switzerland
27. Sutskever, I., Vinyals, O., Le, Q.V.: Sequence to sequence learning with neural networks. In: NIPS (2014)
28. Um, T.T., et al.: Data augmentation of wearable sensor data for Parkinson's disease monitoring using convolutional neural networks. In: Proceedings of the 19th ACM International Conference on Multimodal Interaction (2017)
29. Wang, J., Liu, Q., Chen, H.: Detection of freezing of gait for Parkinson's disease patients based on deep convolutional neural networks. Chin. J. Biomed. Eng. **36**, 418–425 (2017). https://doi.org/10.3969/j.issn.0258-8021.2017.04.005
30. Zach, H., et al.: Identifying freezing of gait in parkinson's disease during freezing provoking tasks using waist-mounted accelerometry. Parkinsonism Relat. Disord. **21** (2015). https://doi.org/10.1016/j.parkreldis.2015.09.051
31. Zhang, Y., Gu, D.: A deep convolutional-recurrent neural network for freezing of gait detection in patients with Parkinson's disease, pp. 1–6, October 2019. https://doi.org/10.1109/CISP-BMEI48845.2019.8965723

Received WiFi Signal Strength Monitoring for Contactless Body Temperature Classification

Vincent Ha and Ani Nahapetian[✉]

California State University, Northridge, USA
vincent.ha.887@my.csun.edu, ani@csun.edu

Abstract. Currently, non-contact body temperature monitoring requires specialized thermometers, such as non-contact infrared thermometers (NCIT), to achieve a reading. This work explores an alternative way of classifying temperature using the ubiquitous WiFi waveform. By merely observing the change in the received signal strength indicator (RSSI), body temperature can be classified as below normal, normal, or warm. Using a smartphone as the receiver and a router or another phone as the transmitter, experimental results show that temperature is inversely correlated with RSSI. The findings also indicate that WiFi RSSI is less variable when the temperature is cooler. Our classification can correctly identify the temperature class from a single RSSI reading 56.86% of the time. It can correctly identify a cool reading 61.11% of the time, a normal reading 58.82% of the time, and a warm reading 50% of the time.

Keywords: Body temperature · WiFi · Smartphones

1 Introduction

As a result of the Covid-19 pandemic, there has been an explosive growth of body temperature monitoring in an expanded number of settings. Temperatures, which serve as a proxy for infection, are being taken daily to allow for entry into schools, workplaces, and retails settings.

Body temperature measurement can and has typically been carried out using physical contact with a mercury or digital thermometer. While this method has high accuracy, it requires prolonged contact and sanitation of the thermometer following each use. Commercially available contactless thermometers, known as non-contact infrared thermometers (NCIT), use technology that measures the reflected infrared radiation. They do not require contact but are not as accurate as the contact thermometers.

This paper examines the feasibility of using only smart phones and no other specialized hardware to make contactless body temperature readings. While infrared sensors are cheap and affordable, there are alternative waveforms that are more ubiquitous and universally available on smartphones. In this paper, we focus on WiFi as that waveform.

Due to the ubiquity of smart phones and other mobile devices, people universally have access to a WiFi transducer. In this work, WiFi received signal strength indicator

M. Ur Rehman and A. Zoha (Eds.): BODYNETS 2021, LNICST 420, pp. 112–125, 2022.
https://doi.org/10.1007/978-3-030-95593-9_10

(RSSI) and its relationship to temperature is explored, thus opening the potential for measuring temperature using only the WiFi hardware of a smart phone and an installed app.

In this work, a series of experiments were carried out that measured the RSSI of a WiFi access points as temperature was varied, thus quantifying the relationship between temperature and WiFi signal strength. The experiments showed that the accessibility of temperature monitoring can be improved by leveraging the nature of wireless signals and the infrastructure that comes with living in the digital age.

2 Related Work

2.1 WiFi for Localization

Although, the main functionality of WiFi is to provide wireless connectivity in a local area network, its ubiquity has enabled its expanded use for localization. There have been many studies that evaluate the use of WiFi signals for indoor localization and positioning monitoring [1, 3, 4, 6].

WiFi RSSI is heavily influenced by the environment [13] and so filtering has been shown to improve its effectiveness in localization. Researchers have looked at the improved accuracy of using Kalman [8], Gaussian [9, 10] and newer filters [11] on the smartphones RSSI readings.

2.2 RF Monitoring of Human Vital Signs and Activity

Researchers have previously explored monitoring human vital signs using wireless technology. One such study uses mmWave (60 GHz) RSSI to track human's heartbeat and breathing [2]. A more recent study uses a similar approach to analyzing sleeping posture using RF-reflection [5]. Both studies use reflection and orientation of the subject to determine their vital sign.

In 2016, a study demonstrated the use of radio waves and wearable devices to track a person's activity [12]. A more recent study in 2018 showed how Bluetooth signals can be used to track and classify a person's actions [7], by looking for specific patterns in the Bluetooth RSSI readings.

While WiFi channel state information (CSI) is not available yet for mobile phones, researchers have used CSI to count individuals in a crowd [14]. By leveraging the response of movement by the Channel Frequency Response and using CSI to extract useful information, their trained-once model has an accuracy of 74% to 52% [14].

2.3 Temperature Studies on Wireless Network

The impact of temperature on wireless connectivity has been explored before. Studies have shown that sensor nodes require less energy to transmit during cooler temperatures and are able to maintain a more stable link [19]. In 2013, a study demonstrated the effect of hot temperature on wireless network. It showed that RSSI can decrease up to 8 dBm when measured at 65 °C [17]. Another study in 2013 further explored how temperature can affect the communication protocol and its resulting data transmission rate [18].

2.4 Temperature Sensing Technology

Smartphones are equipped with temperature sensors to monitor internal hardware temperature. A study done in 2015 leveraged this technology to track skin temperature. The researchers were able to achieve 99% accuracy, but their method requires skin-contact and can only track the surface temperature of the skin [20].

Similarly, a study in 2018 used the CPU's temperature to estimate outdoor temperature in a field [22]. They achieved an average error of 1.5 °F.

Chen et al. developed bespoke hardware to monitor body temperature. They use an in-ear thermometer to monitor core temperature with a smart phone application [21]. The sensor is equipped with an infrared thermometer which transmits the temperature readings to a paired app.

As for contactless temperature monitoring, other than commercially available NCIT devices [15, 16], contactless temperature monitoring requires visual cues and an RGB-thermal camera [23].

3 Approach Overview

In this work, to measure an individual's body temperature, the person is positioned between a WiFi transmitter and a WiFi receiver; and the change in the WiFi reading is used to classify the person's body temperature as below normal, normal, or warm. As shown in Fig. 1, the person stands in front of any WiFi access point and a smartphone is used to examine the change in the WiFi received signal and determine if the person is warm.

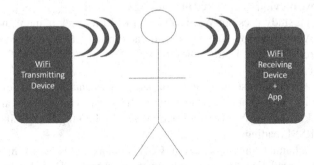

Fig. 1. System overview with the person stepping between a WiFi transmitter and a WiFi receiver to determine the person's body temperature, as observed in the changes with the WiFi received signal strength.

For the system prototype, a bespoke software app was developed that monitored the WiFi received signal strength. Both the signal strength and its change over time were used for classification.

The WiFi received signal strength indicator (RSSI) is reported in decibels in relation to milliwatts (dBm). The range of the reference typically falls between −30 dBm and −100 dBm but can approach 0. The stronger the signal, the larger and the less negative the reading.

4 Experimental Set-Up

A software app was developed that records the RSSI reading over time with a sample rate of approximately one scan per every 3 to 4 s. It carries out a WiFi scan for access points. Upon receipt of a result, the app records the strength and the time of the receipt for each access point that it has found.

The experimental setup utilizes two separate devices, with one designated as the WiFi wireless signal transmitter and the other as the WiFi wireless signal receiver. A Samsung Galaxy S10 was used as a receiving device. Depending on the experiment, either a SageCom Router as an access point or a Samsung Galaxy S10e smartphone was used as the transmitting device.

Downloading or uploading data can cause interference in the reading of RSSI. Therefore, both devices were disconnected from any mobile network. The phones were not connected to the internet during the experiments. The receiving phone is not paired with any wireless devices or networks. WiFi scan throttling is disabled to ensure continuous scan.

The model collects multiple RSSI readings for analysis. The collected RSSI in dBm is plotted onto a graph and the slope of the regression line is used to determine the overall trend of the dBm. Any spikes or oscillations within the reading is recorded, except for outliers that lie far beyond the clustered set of data.

5 Experiments

Three different types of experiments were carried out. In the first two experiments, changes in a bowl of water's temperature were used to simulate the human body. In the first experiment, the smart phone recording the WiFi RSSI was placed near the bowl of water, while in the second experiment the smartphone was submerged in the bowl. The third set of experiments measured the temperature of a human hand, after it was dipped in ice water and dipped in warm water.

5.1 Water Bowl Experiments

The first experiment involved changing the temperature of a bowl of water and observing changes in RSSI. A bowl of water is placed in between two mobile devices. The devices are placed equidistant from the foot of the bowl. The receiving phone simultaneously keeps track of the signal dBm from both the transmitting phone and the router. An aquarium thermometer is submerged in the water bowl to monitor the water of the temperature. Figure 2 illustrates the setup of the experiment.

The experiment was carried out three times using three different water temperatures: hot, cold, and room temperature. Cold is defined as having water temperature of 44.2 °F to 46.9 °F. Room temperature is defined as having water temperature of 73.5 °F. Hot is defined at having temperature of 131 °F to 149.5 °F.

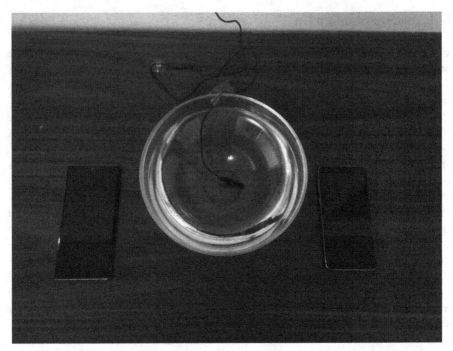

Fig. 2. Two smart phones are placed equidistant from the foot of the bowl. An aquarium thermometer is placed submerged in the water to monitor the water of the temperature.

The graph in Fig. 3 shows the RSSI under the effect of cooling hot water. A total of 65 samples were collected over the course of 4 min. The initial temperature of the water was 149.5 °F, which fell to 131 °F by the end of the observation period. The average dBm for this round was −23.1538.

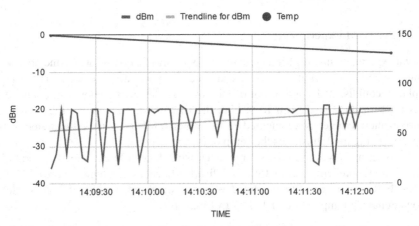

Fig. 3. Signal and temperature over time for hot water. Slope shows a positive slope in relation to the decrease in water temperature.

In Fig. 3, the overall trendline for the signal shows a positive slope. Despite the oscillation of signal, as temperature decreases, there is a slight increase in signal strength. Also, the RSSI variability decreases as the temperature decreases.

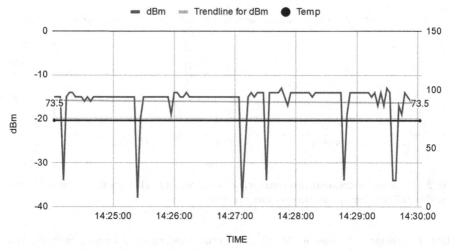

Fig. 4. Signal and temperature over time for room temperature water. Signal is relatively stable with room temperature water.

Figure 4 shows the RSSI readings for the room temperature water. The signal remains stable, which is in line with the water temperature which is also kept stable throughout the observation period, remaining at a constant 73.5 °F. A total of 75 samples were collected over the course of 6 min. The average dBm for this round was -16.0181.

Figure 5 shows the RSSI readings for the cold water. The RSSI is relatively constant. Although temperature increases by a small amount, this is not reflected in the slope of the trend line. A total of 75 samples were collected over the course of 4 min. The initial water temperature was 44.2 °F, which gradually increased to 46.9 °F. The average dBm for this round was -14.5811.

Table 1 gives the average and the standard deviation of the WiFi RSSI for the three different temperature tests. Comparing the results from the three different instances, an inverse relationship between temperature and WiFi RSSI is observed. The results show an inversely linear relationship between temperature and average signal strength. As temperature increases, not only does the signal strength decrease, but the variability also increases.

5.2 Submerged Water Bowl Experiments

To further isolate the key hypothesis, the smart phone was submerged into a bowl of water to record the change in RSSI. The water was boiled and left to cool naturally during the observation period. The phone is placed within 2 resealable plastic bags to prevent water from damaging the phone. It is then placed submerged into the bowl. There

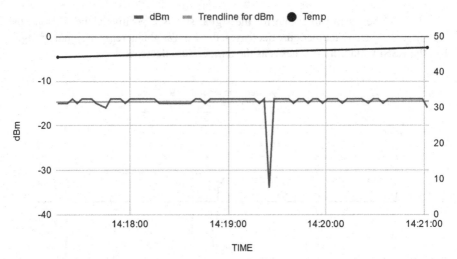

Fig. 5. Signal and temperature over time for cold water. Signal is relatively stable with cold water, despite small increase in water temperature over time.

Table 1. Average RSSI, standard deviation, small size, temperature, and time span for the three water temperatures.

Water temp	Average RSSI	RSSI STDEV	Sample size	Start temp	End temp	Time span
Cold	−14.58108108	2.330757909	75	44.2	46.9	4 min
Room temp	−16.08108108	4.869467292	75	73.5	73.5	6 min
Hot	−23.15384615	5.67403838	65	149.5	131	4 min

is ample space between the bottom of the bowl and the phone, as shown in Fig. 6. A temperature sensor is placed inside the bowl as before.

Figure 7 shows the RSSI as the water temperature changes. A total of 549 samples were collected. The initial temperature of the water was 108.1 °F, which fell to 92.9 °F by the end of the observation period. When the water temperature reaches 96.6 °F, there is a noticeable stabilization effect on the reading. The overall regression line follows a positive slope as temperature falls. Figures 8a,b show that when the water temperature remains constant, the RSSI signal remains constant as well. These results match with the finding from the previous experiments and confirms the hypothesis that temperature does affect RSSI of the WiFi signal. The experiment also shows that signal strength's variability decreases in cooler temperatures. As temperature decreases, the WiFi signal increases.

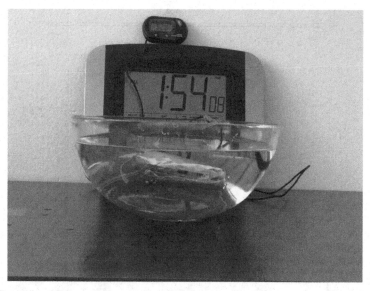

Fig. 6. Smartphone submerged in water bowl with an aquarium thermometer to monitor the water of the temperature.

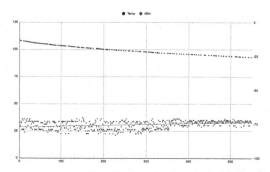

Fig. 7. Signal and temperature over time for bowl of water. RSSI increases and its standard deviation decreases as the temperature increases.

5.3 Hand Experiments

In the next series of experiments, the presence and the temperature of a person is measured using changes in WiFi RSSI. The person's hand is used for the experiment, as it can be cooled or warmed by dipping the hand into cold and warm water.

The setup, as show in Fig. 9, includes two phones facing away from each other. Due to the location of the WiFi adapter on the devices, this orientation has the strongest baseline signal. In the experiment, the person places the hand in between the two phones equidistant from both phones for a period of seconds before removing the hand.

There are three classes of temperature. There is the hand at normal temperature. There is the hand dipped in ice water which has a cool temperature. There is the hand dipped in warm water, which results in the hand having a warm temperature. Following

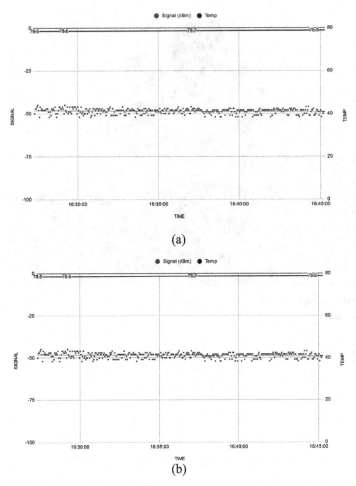

Fig. 8. Signal and temperature over time for bowl of room temperature water. Signal is relatively stable with room temperature water.

the dipping into water, the hand is quickly dried and then placed exactly between the two phones. The placement is kept for at least 4 s due to the limitation of WiFi Scanning of the hardware.

Due to heat loss or heat gain, the exact temperature of the hand at the time of detection is not possible to isolate. Instead, the reading of the hand is taken just before and after the detection to ensure the closest temperature estimation. There are three temperature group for each of the test run, cold, normal, and warm. The respective temperature range for them are, 82 °F to 84° for cold, 98 °F for normal, and 103 °F to 104 °F for warm. A total of 4 separate trials were run.

As shown in Fig. 10, a person standing in between the two smartphones can be detected. This indicates the need to isolate change in RSSI caused by obstruction from the change in RSSI caused by temperature changes.

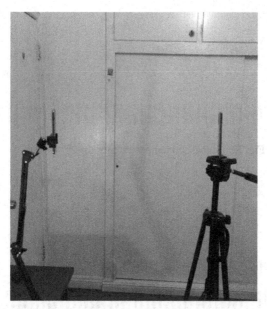

Fig. 9. Two smart phones are setup to face one another so that the WiFi adapter have direct access. This orientation is found to have the clearest signal reception.

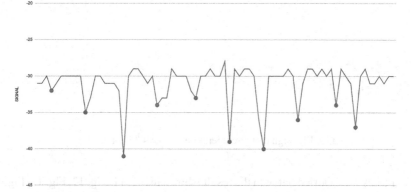

Fig. 10. The RSSI reading over time, as a person steps between the two devices. The dots indicated the moment of detection of the person. All 10 instances of the human obstruction are successfully detected.

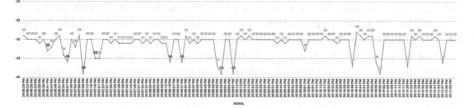

Fig. 11. Signal and temperature for the 1st hand trial.

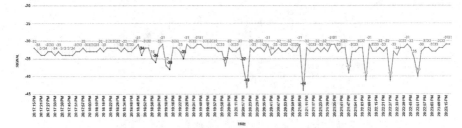

Fig. 12. Signal and temperature for the 2nd hand trial.

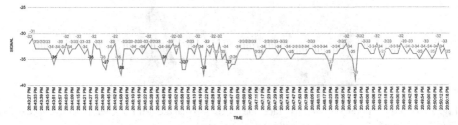

Fig. 13. Signal and temperature for the 3rd hand trial.

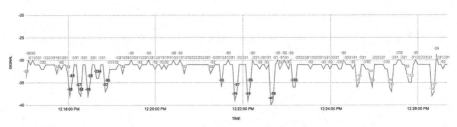

Fig. 14. Signal and temperature for the 4th hand trial.

Four trials were carried out with the results shown in Fig. 11, Fig. 12, Fig. 13, Fig. 14. In the figures, each color-coded entry indicates the detection of the hand. Green signifies normal temperature, which is 98 °F. Red signifies a temperature reading of 103 °F to 104 °F. Cyan signifies a reading of 82 °F to 84 °F.

For the first trial, there were 4 instances for each temperature class and all twelve instances were detected. For the remaining trials, there were 5 instances for each temperature classes, and an average of 80% of the instances were detected. Table 2 gives the average and standard deviation of the readings for the four trials.

In all the trials, WiFi RSSI is larger under cool temperature than warm temperature. Additionally, there is a smaller standard deviation at cooler temperatures. These experiments are therefore successful in isolating the obstruction element from the temperature element.

Table 2. RSSI reading average and standard deviation for the cool, normal, and warm hand experiments across the four trials.

	Trial #1	Trial #2	Trial #3	Trial #4
Average cool temp	−36.875	−40.25	−36	−35.9
STDEV cool temp	0.6291528696	0.9574271078	2	1.197219
Average normal temp	−35.5	−35.25	−36.375	−36.2
STDEV normal temp	2.516611478	1.658312395	0.4787135539	1.619327707
Average warm temp	−37.25	−40.33333333	−36.83333333	−37.55555556
STDEV warm temp	1.5	3.511884584	0.8819171037	1.666666667

5.4 Hand Temperature Classification

To classify an RSSI reading as either cool, normal, or warm temperature, a baseline range for normal temperature is determined. The readings are classified as warm, if the RSSI is less than the baseline's minimum value. The readings are classified as cool, if the RSSI is more than the baseline's maximum value. The readings are classified as normal if they are within the baseline's range.

Table 3 shows the confusion matrix for the total 51 samples across the four trials. A cool reading has a 61.11% chance of being correctly identified. The chance of being misclassified as normal is 5.56% and the chance of it being misclassified as warm is 33.33%. A normal reading has a 58.82% of being correctly identified. The chance of being misclassified as cool is 29.41% and being misclassified as warm is 11.76%. The A warm reading has a 50% chance of being correctly identified. There is a 43.75% chance of it being misclassified as cool and 6.25% chance as normal. Overall, there a 56.86% chance of a reading being correctly identify. This is an improvement from the 33% chance of randomly guessing from among three temperature group.

Table 3. Classification confusion matrix

Predicted	Cool	Actual normal	Warm
Cool	**61.11%**	29.41%	43.75%
Normal	5.56%	**58.82%**	6.25%
Warm	33.33%	11.76%	**50.00%**
Overall accuracy		**56.86%**	

6 Conclusion

We explored the impact of temperature on WiFi signals, as measured with commercial smartphones. The experimental results confirm that temperature does influence received WiFi signal strength and signal variability and thus can be used to classify temperature. A classification accuracy of 56.86% was achieved on a single reading across a three-class library of cool, normal, and warm.

References

1. Chen, Y., Lymberopoulos, D., Liu, J., Priyantha, B.: FM-based indoor localization. In: Proceedings of the 10th International Conference on Mobile systems, Applications, and Services (MobiSys 2012), pp. 169–182. Association for Computing Machinery, New York (2012). https://doi.org/10.1145/2307636.2307653
2. Yang, Z., Pathak, P.H., Zeng, Y., Liran, X., Mohapatra, P.: vital sign and sleep monitoring using millimeter wave. ACM Trans. Sen. Netw. **13**(2), 14, 32 (2017), https://doi.org/10.1145/3051124
3. Chintalapudi, K., Padmanabha Iyer, A., Padmanabhan, V.N.: Indoor localization without the pain. In: Proceedings of the Sixteenth Annual International Conference on Mobile Computing and Networking (MobiCom 2010), pp. 173–184. Association for Computing Machinery, New York (2010), https://doi.org/10.1145/1859995.1860016
4. Zeng, Y., Pathak, P.H., Mohapatra, P.: Analyzing Shopper's Behavior through WiFi Signals. In: Proceedings of the 2nd Workshop on Workshop on Physical Analytics (WPA 2015), pp. 13–18. Association for Computing Machinery, New York (2015). https://doi.org/10.1145/2753497.2753508
5. Yue, S., Yang, Y., Wang, H., Rahul, H., Katabi, D.: BodyCompass: monitoring sleep posture with wireless signals. Proc. ACM Interact. Mob. Wearable Ubiquitous Technol. **4**(2), Article 66 (2020), 25 p (2020). https://doi.org/10.1145/3397311
6. Liu, H.-H., Liu, C.: Implementation of Wi-Fi signal sampling on an android smartphone for indoor positioning systems. Sensors **18**(2) 3 (2017). https://doi.org/10.3390/s18010003
7. Vance, E., Nahapetian, A.: Bluetooth-based context modeling. In: Proceedings of the 4th ACM MobiHoc Workshop on Experiences with the Design and Implementation of Smart Objects (SMARTOBJECTS 2018). Article 1, pp. 1–6. Association for Computing Machinery, New York (2018). https://doi.org/10.1145/3213299.3213300
8. Sung, Y.: RSSI-based distance estimation framework using a Kalman filter for sustainable indoor computing environments. Sustainability **8**, 11 (2016). https://doi.org/10.3390/su8111136
9. Ito, K., Xiong, K.: Gaussian filters for nonlinear filtering problems. IEEE Trans. Autom. Control **45**(5), 910–927 (2000). https://doi.org/10.1109/9.855552
10. Luo, J., Zhan, X.: Characterization of smart phone received signal strength indication for WLAN indoor positioning accuracy improvement. J. Netw. **9**, 3 (2014). https://doi.org/10.4304/jnw.9.3.739-746
11. Shi, Y., Shi, W., Liu, X., Xiao, X.: An RSSI classification and tracing algorithm to improve trilateration-based positioning. Sensors **20**(15), 4244 (2020). https://doi.org/10.3390/s20154244
12. Fang, B., Lane, N.D., Zhang, M., Boran, A., Kawsar, F.: BodyScan: enabling radio-based sensing on wearable devices for contactless activity and vital sign monitoring. In: Proceedings of the 14th Annual International Conference on Mobile Systems, Applications, and Services (MobiSys 2016), pp. 97–110. Association for Computing Machinery, New York (2016), https://doi.org/10.1145/2906388.2906411

13. Tshiluna, N.B., et al.: Analysis of bluetooth and Wi-Fi interference in smart home. In: 2016 International Conference on Advances in Computing and Communication Engineering (ICACCE) (2016). https://doi.org/10.1109/icacce.2016.8073716

14. Domenico, S.D., De Sanctis, M., Cianca, E., Bianchi, G.: A Trained-once Crowd Counting Method Using Differential WiFi channel state information. In: Proceedings of the 3rd International on Workshop on Physical Analytics (WPA 2016), pp. 37–42. Association for Computing Machinery, New York (2016). https://doi.org/10.1145/2935651.2935657

15. Khan, S., et al.: Comparative accuracy testing of non-contact infrared thermometers and temporal artery thermometers in an adult hospital setting. Am. J. Infect. Control 49(5), 597–602 (2021). https://doi.org/10.1016/j.ajic.2020.09.012

16. Teran, C.G., Torrez-Llanos, J., Teran-Miranda, T.E., Balderrama, C., Shah, N.S., Villarroel, P.: Clinical accuracy of a non-contact infrared skin thermometer in paediatric practice. Child Care Health Dev. 38(4), 471–476 (2011). https://doi.org/10.1111/j.1365-2214.2011.01264.x

17. Boano, C., et al.: Hot Packets: a systematic evaluation of the effect of temperature on low power wireless transceivers. In: Proceedings of the 5th Extreme Conference on Communication (ExtremeCom 2013). Þórsmörk, Iceland (2013)

18. Keppitiyagama, C., Tsiftes, N., Alberto Boano, C., Voigt, T.: Temperature hints for sensornet routing. In: Proceedings of the 11th ACM Conference on Embedded Networked Sensor Systems (SenSys 2013), Article 25, pp. 1–2. Association for Computing Machinery, New York. https://doi.org/10.1145/2517351.2517441

19. Alberto Boano, C., Tsiftes, N., Voigt, T., Brown, J., Roedig, U.: The impact of temperature on outdoor industrial sensorNet applications. IEEE Trans. Ind. Inform. 6(3), 451–459 (2010), https://doi.org/10.1109/tii.2009.2035111

20. Egilmez, B., Memik, G., Ogrenci-Memik, S., Ergin, O.: User-specific skin temperature-aware DVFS for smartphones. In: Proceedings of the 2015 Design, Automation & Test in Europe Conference & Exhibition (DATE 2015), pp. 1217–1220. EDA Consortium, San Jose (2015)

21. Chen, X., Xu, C., Chen, B., Li, Z., Xu, W.: In-ear thermometer: wearable real-time core body temperature monitoring: poster abstract. In: Proceedings of the 18th Conference on Embedded Networked Sensor Systems (SenSys 2020), pp. 687–688. Association for Computing Machinery, New York (2020). https://doi.org/10.1145/3384419.3430442

22. Krintz, C., Wolski, R., Golubovic, N., Bakir, F.: Estimating outdoor temperature from CPU temperature for IoT applications in agriculture. In: Proceedings of the 8th International Conference on the Internet of Things (IOT 2018). Article 11, pp. 1–8. Association for Computing Machinery, New York (2018). https://doi.org/10.1145/3277593.3277607

23. Wei, P., Yang, C., Jiang, X.: Low-cost multi-person continuous skin temperature sensing system for fever detection: poster abstract. In: Proceedings of the 18th Conference on Embedded Networked Sensor Systems (SenSys 2020). pp. 705–706. Association for Computing Machinery, New York (2020). https://doi.org/10.1145/3384419.3430398

A Preliminary Study of RF Propagation for High Data Rate Brain Telemetry

Mariella Särestöniemi[1,2(✉)], Carlos Pomalaza-Raez[3], Kamran Sayrafian[4],
Teemu Myllylä[1,5], and Jari Iinatti[1]

[1] Centre for Wireless Communications, University of Oulu, Oulu, Finland
mariella.sarestoniemi@oulu.fi
[2] Research Unit of Medical Imaging, Physics and Technology, Faculty of Medicine,
University of Oulu, Oulu, Finland
[3] Purdue University of Technology, West Lafayette, USA
[4] National Institute of Standards and Technology, Gaithersburg, MD, USA
[5] Optoelectronics and Measurement Techniques Research Unit, Faculty of Information
Technology and Electrical Engineering, University of Oulu, Oulu, Finland

Abstract. This paper presents the preliminary results of a study on the radio frequency (RF) propagation inside the human skull at several Industrial, Scientific and Medical (ISM) and ultrawideband UWB frequencies. These frequency bands are considered as possible candidates for high data rate wireless brain telemetry. The study is conducted using a high-resolution 3D computational model of the human head. Power flow analysis is conducted to visualize propagation inside the brain for two different on-body antenna locations. Furthermore, channel attenuation between an on-body directional mini-horn antenna and an implant antenna at different depths inside the brain is evaluated. It is observed that radio frequency propagation at 914 MHz sufficiently covers the whole volume of the brain. The coverage reduces at higher frequencies, specially above 3.1 GHz. The objective of this comparative analysis is to provide some insight on the applicability of these frequencies for high data rate brain telemetry or various monitoring, and diagnostic tools.

Keywords: Brain computer interface · Brain monitoring · Frequency channel response · Implant communications · In-body propagation

1 Introduction

There has been a growing interest in the development of non-invasive acute brain injury detection and continuous monitoring systems in recent years [1–12]. Advances in microelectronics is also contributing to significant progress in invasive monitoring systems such as intra cranial pressure and brain oxygenation monitoring [5–8]. In addition, Brain Computer Interface (BCI) as a multidisciplinary research area has drawn considerable attention due to its attractive and transformative applications across many verticals in wireless communications including E-Health [1–3, 9]. Low-power, reliability, and security are essential requirements for wireless monitoring of the brain signals. Some BCI

© ICST Institute for Computer Sciences, Social Informatics and Telecommunications Engineering 2022
Published by Springer Nature Switzerland AG 2022. All Rights Reserved
M. Ur Rehman and A. Zoha (Eds.): BODYNETS 2021, LNICST 420, pp. 126–138, 2022.
https://doi.org/10.1007/978-3-030-95593-9_11

applications may require wireless links that can support high data rates reaching 100 Mbps [1, 2]. In order to meet these requirements, in-depth propagation studies at various frequency bands are essential in the design of a wireless brain telemetry system.

Wireless propagation inside the human body at different frequency bands including Industrial, Scientific and Medical (ISM), Wireless Medical Telemetry Service (WMTS), Ultra WideBand (UWB), and Medical Device Radio Communications Service (MedRadio) is an attractive and challenging topic of research in Body Area Networks [13–18]. However, there are only few such studies in the literature for brain implant communication [16–24]. Most of the existing studies are based on simple tissue-layer models. Those models are more relevant for applications where the brain implant is relatively close to the skull. For wireless monitoring applications where the implant could be located deeper inside the brain, it is important to study propagation using more realistic models of the human head. It is also necessary to identify which frequency bands would be suitable for different brain monitoring or implant communication applications. This identification should take into the account all desirable requirements for the wireless communication link. The main objective of this paper is to study radio waves propagation inside the human skull at several frequency bands. The novelty of this paper compared to other brain propagation studies in the literature is the use of a more accurate computational model of the human head, and a directional on-body antenna which allows for evaluation at several frequency bands appropriate for medical applications.

The rest of this paper is organized as follows: Sect. 2 presents the simulation environment and the antennas used in this study. Section 3 presents the simulation results for two different on-body antenna locations, including power flow analysis and channel characteristics evaluations. Conclusions and future work are provided in Sect. 4.

2 Simulation Environment and Antenna Models

2.1 Simulation Model

This study is conducted using Simulia CST studio suite[1] 3D electromagnetic simulation software [25] which is based on Finite Integration Technique (FIT). The anatomical 3D head model from the CST's Hugo voxel-based body model shown in Fig. 1a has been used for simulation purposes. Hugo voxel-based head model includes brain tissue structure with separate grey and white matters as depicted in the 2D cross section in Fig. 1b. The frequency-dependent dielectric properties of the voxel tissues are obtained using four-pole Cole-Cole modeling described in [26]. Relative permittivity ε_r and conductivity ρ of the most relevant tissues in the head are presented in Table 1 [27].

2.2 Mini-horn Antenna

A directional bio-matched mini-horn antenna, shown in Fig. 2, has been used for our evaluations in this paper. The mini-horn antenna originally presented in [28] has been

---

[1] Commercial products mentioned in this paper are merely intended to foster understanding. Their identification does not imply recommendation or endorsement by National Institute of Standards & Technology.

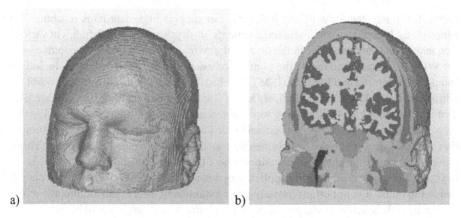

Fig. 1. a) Hugo voxel model b) Cross-section of the head model

Table 1. Dielectric properties of the head tissues at several frequencies

Tissue	0.914 GHz ε_r / p [S/m]	2.45 GHz ε_r / p [S/m]	3.1 GHz ε_r / p [S/m]	4.0 GHz ε_r / p [S/m]	5.8 GHz ε_r / p [S/m]
Skin	41.3 / 0.9	38.0 / 1.46	37.4 / 1.79	36.6 / 2.34	35.1/3.72
Fat	11.3 / 0.11	10.8 / 0.27	10.6 / 0.40	10.4 / 0.50	9.86/8.32
Muscle	55.0 / 0.95	52.7 / 1.74	51.8 / 3.02	50.8 / 3.02	48.5/4.96
Skull bone	20.8 / 0.34	18.5 / 0.81	17.8 / 1.04	16.9 / 1.40	15.4/2.15
Brain grey matter	52.7 / 0.95	48.9 / 1.81	47.9 / 2.30	46.6 / 3.09	44.0/4.99
Brain white matter	38.8 / 0.60	36.2 / 1.21	35.4 / 1.57	34.5 / 2.14	32.6/3.49

modified and updated for this study in order to obtain better matching with the voxel-based head model [11]. The modified structure has dimensions $h = 2.7$ cm and $d = 1.8$ cm (see Fig. 2). The antenna is composed of water-filled holes which mimics the frequency-dependent relative permittivity of the underlying tissue over its entire bandwidth. The bio-matched mini-horn antenna has been designed to operate while tightly attached to the skin surface. Although the resolution of the Hugo voxel model is high, pixelization on the head surface could lead to air gaps between the antenna and the skin as explained in [11]. This effects negatively on the antenna matching and hence the resulting channel simulations as shown in [11]. To alleviate this problem, the air gaps have been replaced by a thin layer of skin between the antenna and the surface of the head where the antenna is placed [11]. This "smoothing layer" creates a better and more realistic contact between the antenna and the scalp. Further details of the antenna structure can be found in [28].

For RF propagation evaluation, two antenna locations on the surface of the head have been considered: Location 1) on the side, and Location 2) on the top, see Fig. 3a–b. These locations are selected due to their different propagation environments. At location 1, there is a relatively thick muscle tissue below the mini-horn antenna; however, no such muscle exists at location 2. Figure 4. presents the antenna reflection coefficients, i.e., S_{11} parameter, of the mini-horn antenna after adjustment with the smoothing layers at locations 1 and 2.

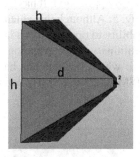

Fig. 2. Mini-horn on-body antenna designed for in-body communication.

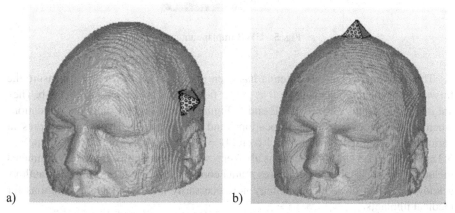

a)   b)

Fig. 3. On-body antenna locations: a) Location 1 (above the temporal bone on the left side), b) Location 2 (top of the head)

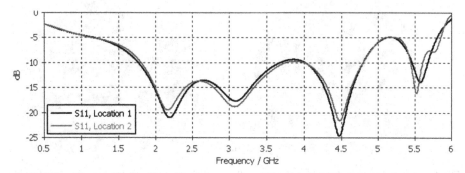

Fig. 4. Reflection coefficient of the mini-horn antenna placed on Hugo's scalp at locations 1 and 2

2.3   Implant Antenna

The implant antenna used in this study is a double-loop UWB antenna originally introduced in [29] for capsule endoscopy application. It has a cylindrical shape with a size of
11 mm by 15 mm as shown in Fig. 5. Although this antenna might not be applicable for
practical brain implants, its capability to operate over a large bandwidth (i.e., 1–6 GHz)
will allow us to carry out the preliminary RF propagation study in this paper. In addition
to the 1–6 GHz frequency range which this antenna has been designed for, it offers
reasonable performance at the ISM (902−928) MHz band as well.

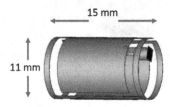

Fig. 5. UWB implant antenna

The locations where this antenna has been placed inside the brain to measure the
forward channel coefficients as well as power flow values are shown in Fig. 6a–b. They
are marked as points A, B, C, D, E and F. Figure 6a and Fig. 6b show these locations
when the mini-horn antenna is at location 1 and 2, respectively. These points represent
various propagation depths of A = 1.6 cm, B = 3.0 cm, C = 4.3 cm, D = 5.3 cm, E =
6.3 cm and F = 7.3 cm. The locations also represent different propagation environments
including muscle layers and white/grey matter compositions inside the brain. The authors
acknowledge that these locations may not necessarily indicate practical locations for
medical implants.

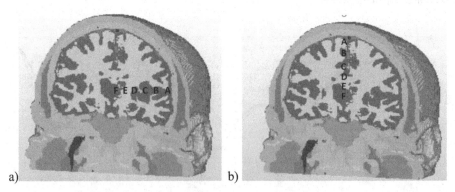

Fig. 6. Implant locations for which the power flow and channel attenuation have been evaluated
a) on-body antenna at location 1 and b) on-body antenna at location 2

The S11 parameter of this antenna while located at point A is presented in Fig. 7. Further details of the antenna structure, radiation pattern, as well as Specific Absorption Rate (SAR) have been studied in [29].

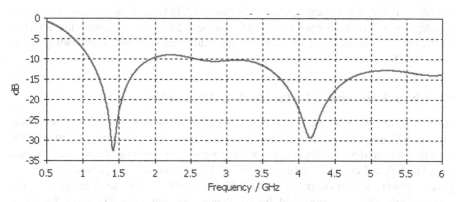

Fig. 7. Reflection coefficient of the implant antenna inside the brain tissue

3   Simulation Results

3.1   Power Flow Results for the On-Body Antenna Location 1

In-body propagation results at different frequencies using the notion of power flow is presented in this section. Power flow is the time-averaged magnitude of the Poynting vector [26]. The Poynting vector represents the directional energy flux (the energy transfer per unit area per unit time) of an electromagnetic field. The flux of the Poynting Vector through a certain surface represents the total electromagnetic power flowing through that surface. Here, the power flow values (expressed in decibels) have been normalized so that 0 dB represents the maximum. Figures 8a–e present the power flows (ranging from 0 to −65 dB) on the horizontal (left) and vertical (right) cross-sections of the brain at 915 MHz, 2.45 GHz, 3.1 GHz, 4.0 GHz, and 5.8 GHz, respectively. These figures correspond to location 1 of the mini-horn antenna. Power flow values at locations A, B, C, D, E and F are also provided in Table 2.

As observed in Fig. 8a, at 915 MHz, a good coverage is obtained throughout the whole volume of the head with power flow values well within the selected 65 dB range. At this frequency, the power flow values decrease gradually from −35 dB to −54 dB as the propagation depth increases from point A = 1.6 cm to point F = 7.3 cm. At 2.45 GHz, the power flow plots indicate coverage of only ¾ of the head volume (Fig. 8b). As expected, power loss in the brain tissue increases with higher frequencies and the size of the covered volume specially declines for UWB. The power flow plots at 3.1 GHz and 4 GHz indicate a coverage of half and almost 1/3 of the brain volume respectively (see Figs. 8c–d). Again, power flow values gradually decrease as the propagation distance increases (Table 2).

One might note that at point A, power flow at 914 MHz is smaller compared to its values at 2.45 GHz and 3.1 GHz. This is inconsistent with the fact that propagation loss is typically smaller at lower frequencies. However, as observed in Fig. 4, the reflection coefficient of the mini-horn antenna at 2.45 GHz is significantly better compared to 914 MHz. This results in larger power flow value at 2.45 GHz. However, as the propagation depth increases, higher power loss in the tissue at 2.45 GHz overcomes the reflection coefficients discrepancy and power flow values drop below their corresponding values for 914 MHz.

3.2   Channel Attenuation for the On-Body Antenna Location 1

In this section, we evaluate the channel frequency responses between the mini-horn antenna at location 1 and the implant antenna when placed at locations A through F. The objective is to understand the impact of the propagation depth on the channel attenuation. The forward channel coefficients (S21) at locations A–F are presented in Fig. 9. Assuming that a maximum pathloss of 65 dB is tolerable in order to maintain a reliable communication link, it is observed that the channel attenuations at 914 MHz, 2.45 GHz, and 3.1 GHz are within the acceptable threshold for all considered propagation depths. Maximum attenuations for these frequencies (which occurs at location F) are −54 dB, −58 dB, and −63 dB, respectively. However, at 4 GHz, the channel attenuation is manageable only at the implant locations A–D. At implant locations E and F, a receiver with higher sensitivity would be required as channel attenuation for these locations are over 70 dB. At 5.8 GHz, only locations A and B experience channel attenuation within the 65 dB margin. These results are aligned with the power flow observations discussed in Sect. 3.1.

3.3   Power Flow Results for the On-Body Antenna Location 2

In this subsection, a similar propagation study is conducted for the on-body antenna location 2 (see Fig. 3b). For brevity, only the power flow results have been provided. Figures 10a–d presents the power flows on the horizontal (left) and vertical (right) cross-sections of the brain at 915 MHz, 2.45 GHz, 3.1 GHz, and 5.8 GHz, respectively. The magnitude ranges from 0 to −65 dB similar to the on-body antenna location 1. Power flow values at locations A, B, C, D, E, and F are also provided in Table 3.

It is observed that the power flow values resulting from the on-body antenna location 2 are generally at higher levels compared to the antenna location 1. This is mostly due to the existence of the temporalis muscle which is a thick muscle layer on each side of the head filling the temporal fossa. This muscle directly sits on the propagation path from the antenna location 1. RF attenuation in the muscle tissue is typically high due to its dielectric properties [16]. Another reason for higher values of power flow from location 2 is the amount of grey matter that exist between the implant and the on-body antenna. Compared to the white matter in the brain tissue, the propagation loss in the grey matter is substantially higher due to its dielectric properties [16]. Since there is more grey matter on the propagation path between the implant and the on-body antenna location 1, the attenuation would be higher, resulting in relatively lower power flow values.

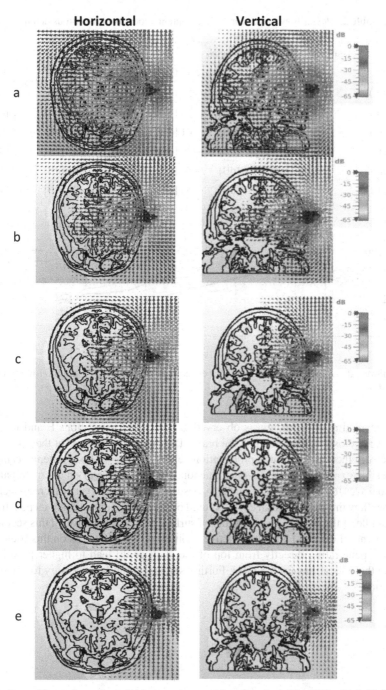

Fig. 8. Power flows from the mini-horn antenna at location 1 a) 914 MHz, b) 2.45 GHz, c) 3.1 GHz, d) 4.0 GHz, and e) 5.8 GHz

Table 2. Power flow values for on-body antenna location 1 at various depths

Location and distance from the surface	Frequencies				
	0.914 GHz	2.45 GHz	3.1 GHz	4.0 GHz	5.8 GHz
A (1.6 cm)	−35 [dB]	−32 [dB]	−33 [dB]	−35 [dB]	−48 [dB]
B (3.0 cm)	−38 [dB]	−38 [dB]	−41 [dB]	−45 [dB]	−62 [dB]
C (4.3 cm)	−43 [dB]	−41 [dB]	−51 [dB]	−57 [dB]	−81 [dB]
D (5.3 cm)	−45 [dB]	−49 [dB]	−54 [dB]	−63 [dB]	−93 [dB]
E (6.3 cm)	−48 [dB]	−53 [dB]	−59 [dB]	−71 [dB]	−101 [dB]
F (7.3 cm)	−54 [dB]	−58 [dB]	−63 [dB]	−78 [dB]	−110 [dB]

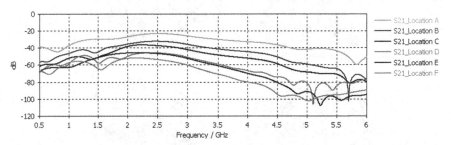

Fig. 9. Forward channel coefficient (S21) for different implant locations and mini-horn antenna location 1

An interesting phenomenon is observed at 5.8 GHz for locations E and F. These locations are closer to the center of the brain. The power flow values at these locations unexpectedly increase, although propagation depth from the on-body antenna is higher. One possible explanation for this phenomenon is the existence of an alternate path for the radio waves to arrive at these points. As observed in Fig. 10e (vertical cross-section), a stronger flow through the nasal cavities could be the reason for better signal penetration to the middle of the brain. The possibility of surface propagation through this secondary route (i.e., nasal cavities) and constructive addition of the RF waves on this route with the waves penetrating directly from top of the skull could lead to higher power flow values at these locations for 5.8 GHz. Further studies would be necessary to verify this justification.

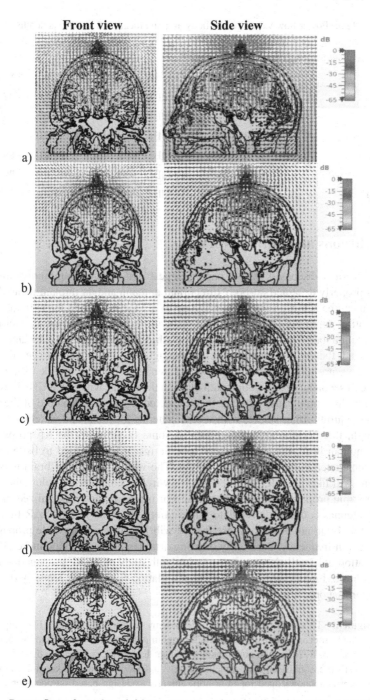

Fig. 10. Power flows from the mini-horn antenna at location 2 a) 914 MHz, b) 2.45 GHz, c) 3.1 GHz, d) 4.0 GHz, and e) 5.8 GHz

Table 3. Power flow values for on-body antenna location 2 at various depths

Location and distance from the surface	Frequencies				
	0.914 GHz	2.45 GHz	3.1 GHz	4.0 GHz	5.8 GHz
A (1.6 cm)	−32 [dB]	−30 [dB]	−28 [dB]	−29 [dB]	−37 [dB]
B (3.0 cm)	−35 [dB]	−35 [dB]	−38 [dB]	−39 [dB]	−59 [dB]
C (4.3 cm)	−38 [dB]	−40 [dB]	−44 [dB]	−49 [dB]	−73 [dB]
D (5.3 cm)	−40 [dB]	−42 [dB]	−48 [dB]	−57 [dB]	−84 [dB]
E (6.3 cm)	−42 [dB]	−47 [dB]	−53 [dB]	−61 [dB]	−79 [dB]
F (7.3 cm)	−44 [dB]	−54 [dB]	−60 [dB]	−70 [dB]	−70 [dB]

4   Conclusions and Future Work

Simulation results discussed in this paper suggest that reliable communication link between a properly designed on-body directional antenna and an implant located deep in the brain can be achieved from 914 MHz up to 3.1 GHz. Beyond those frequencies, communication depth may be limited. Our evaluations also point to the impact of the on-body antenna location on the propagation depth. When the antenna is located on the top of the head, the gap between the left and the right brain hemispheres (i.e., the great longitudinal fissure) could lead to better signal penetration to the middle of the brain. Existence of a secondary propagation path through the nasal cavity at 5.8 GHz is another phenomenon that could cause stronger than expected signal in the middle of the brain. This would require further studies with several antenna locations and voxel models.

Although, this preliminary study provided some insight into the RF propagation inside the human head, more application-specific research is needed to better understand and characterize the propagation media. The wide spectrum of brain telemetry applications will likely result in a diverse set of wireless connectivity solutions, necessitating multiple propagation channel studies. For brain implants, specialized custom-designed antennas considering regulatory and safety issues as well as SAR limitation for the human brain are needed. These factors will impact the achievable propagation depth at a given frequency. Possibility of using array antennas to create more efficient communication links will also require more in-depth study of the RF propagation inside the human brain. Finally, verification of the simulation results with properly designed head phantoms should also be conducted.

Acknowledgment. This work is supported by Academy of Finland 6Genesis Flagship (grant 318927) and the European Union's Horizon 2020 programme under the Marie Sklodowska-Curie grant agreement No. 872752. Mikko Linnanmäki from ExcellAnt is acknowledged for UWB capsule antenna's redesign based in documentation given in [29]. Mikko Parkkila and Uzman Ali from Radientum is acknowledged for mini-horn antenna re-design based on documentation in [28].

References

1. Chavarriaga, R., Cary, C., Contreras-Videl, J.L., McKinney, Z., Bianchi, L.: Standardization of neurotechnology for brain-machine interfacing: state of the art and recommendations. IEEE Open J. Eng. Med. Biol. **2**, 71–73 (2021)
2. Song, Z., et al.: Evaluation and diagnosis of brain diseases based on non-invasive BCI. In: 2021 9th International Winter Conference on Brain-Computer Interface (BCI) (2021)
3. Song, L., Rahmat-Samii, Y.: An end-to-end implanted brain-machine interface antenna system performance characterizations and development. IEEE Trans. Antennas Propag. **65**(7), 3399–3408 (2017). https://doi.org/10.1109/TAP.2017.2700163
4. Chen, W., Lee, C.W.L., Kiourti, A., Volakis, J.L.: A multi-channel passive brain implant for wireless neuropotential monitoring. IEEE J. Electromagnet. RF Microwaves Med. Biol. **2**(4), 262–269 (2018)
5. Roldan, M., et al.: Non-invasive techniques for multimodal monitoring in traumatic brain injury: systematic review and meta-analysis. J. Neurotrauma **37**(23), 2445–2453 (2020)
6. Manoufali, M., Bialkowski, K., Mobashsher, A.T., Mohammed, B., Abbosh, A.: In situ near-field path loss and data communication link for brain implantable medical devices using software-defined radio. IEEE Trans. Antennas Propag. **68**(9), 6787–6799 (2020)
7. Albert, B., Zhang, J., Noyvirt, A., Setchi, R., Sjaaheim, H., Velikova, S., et al.: Automatic EEG processing for the early diagnosis of traumatic brain injury. In: 2016 World Automation Congress (WAC), pp. 1–6, July 2016
8. Evensen, K.B., Eide, P.: Measuring intracranial pressure by invasive, less invasive and non-invasive means, limitations and avenues for improvement. Fluids Barrierd CNS **17**(1), 34 (2020)
9. Imaduddin, S.M., Fanelli, A., Vonberg, F., Tasker, R.C., Heldt, T.: Pseudo-Bayesian model-based noninvasive intracranial pressure estimation and tracking. IEEE Trans. Biomed. Eng. **67**(6), 1604–1615 (2019)
10. Barone, D.G., Czosnyka, M.: Brain monitoring: do we need a hole? An update on invasive and noninvasive brain monitoring modalities. Sci. World J. (2014)
11. Särestöniemi, M., et al.: Detection of brain hemorrhage in white matter using analysis of radio channel characteristics. In: Alam, M.M., Hämäläinen, M., Mucchi, L., Niazi, I.K., Le Moullec, Y. (eds.) BODYNETS 2020. LNICSSITE, vol. 330, pp. 34–45. Springer, Cham (2020). https://doi.org/10.1007/978-3-030-64991-3_3
12. Hakala, J., Kilpijärvi, J., Särestöniemi, M., Hämäläinen, M., Myllymäki, S., Myllylä, T.: Microwave sensing of brain water – a simulation and experimental study using human brain models. IEEE Access **8**, 111303–111315 (2020). https://doi.org/10.1109/ACCESS.2020.300 1867
13. Patel, P., Sarkar, M., Nagaraj, S.: Wireless channel model of ultra wideband radio signals for implantable biomedical devices. Health Technol. **8**(1–2), 97–110 (2017). https://doi.org/10.1007/s12553-017-0199-x
14. Särestöniemi, M., Pomalaza-Raez, C., Sayrafian, K., Iinatti, J.: In-body propagation at ISM and UWB frequencies for abdominal monitoring applications. In: IoT Health Workshop, ICC Conference, Montreal, Canada (2021)
15. Dove, I.: Analysis of radio propagation inside the human body for in-body localization purposes. Master thesis, Faculty of Electrical Engineering, Mathematics and Computer Science, University of Twente, Netherlands, August 2014
16. Teshome, A.K., Kibret, B., Lai, D.T.H.: A Review Of Implant Communication Technology In WBAN: progress and challenges. IEEE Rev. Biomed. Eng. **12**, 88–99 (2019)
17. Mohamed, M., Maiseli, B.J., Ai, Y., Mkocha, K., Al-Saman, A.: In-body sensor communication: trends and challenges. IEEE Electromagn. Compat. Mag. **10**(2), 47–52 (2021)

18. Aminzadeh, R., Thielens, A., Zhadobov, M., Martens, L., Joseph, W.: WBAN channel modeling for 900 MHz and 60 GHz communications. IEEE Trans. Antennas Propag. **69**(7), 4083–4092 (2021)
19. Hout, S., Chung, J.: Design and characterization of a miniaturized implantable antenna in a seven-layer brain phantom. IEEE Access **7**, 162062–162069 (2019)
20. Bahrami, H., Mirbozorgi, S.A., Ameli, R., Rusch, L.A., Gosselin, B.: Flexible, polarization-diverse UWB antennas for implantable neural recording systems. IEEE Trans. Biomed. Circ. Syst. **10**(1), 38–48 (2016)
21. Rana, B., Shim, J.-Y., Chung, J.-Y.: An implantable antenna with broadside radiation for a brain-machine interface. IEEE Sens. J. **19**(20), 9200–9205 (2019)
22. Nguyen, D., Seo, C.: An ultra-miniaturized antenna using loading circuit method for medical implant applications. IEEE Access **9**, 111890–111898 (2021)
23. Moradi, E., Björninen, T., Sydänheimo, L., Carmena, J.M., Rabaey, J.M., Ukkonen, L.: Measurement of wireless link for brain-machine interface systems using human-head equivalent liquid. IEEE Antennas Wirel. Propag. Lett. **12**, 1307–1310 (2013)
24. Bahrami, H., Mirbozorgi, S.A., Rusch, L.A., Gosselin, B.: Biological channel modeling and implantable UWB antenna design for neural recording systems. IEEE Trans. Biomed. Eng. **62**(1), 88–98 (2015). https://doi.org/10.1109/TBME.2014.2339837
25. Dassault Simulia CST Suite. https://www.3ds.com/
26. Orfanidis, J.: Electromagnetic Waves and Antennas (2002). Revised 2016. http://www.ece.rutgers.edu/~orfanidi/ewa/
27. https://www.itis.ethz.ch/virtual-population/tissue-properties/databaseM
28. Blauert, J., Kiourti, A.: Bio-matched horn: a novel 1–9 GHz on-body antenna for low-loss biomedical telemetry with implants. IEEE Trans. Antennas Propag. **67**(8), 5054–5062 (2019)
29. Shang, J., Yu, Y.: An ultrawideband capsule antenna for biomedical applications. IEEE Antennas Wirel. Propag. Lett. **18**(12), 2548–2551 (2019)

Anomalous Pattern Recognition in Vital Health Signals via Multimodal Fusion

Soumyadeep Bhattacharjee[1,3]($\boxtimes$), Huining Li[2], and Wenyao Xu[2]

[1] Transit Middle School, East Amherst, NY, USA
[2] State University of New York at Buffalo, Buffalo, NY, USA
[3] Gifted Math Program, State University of New York at Buffalo, Buffalo, NY, USA
{sbhattac,huiningl,wenyao.xu}@buffalo.edu

Abstract. Increasingly, caregiving to senior citizens and patients requires monitoring of vital signs like heartbeat, respiration, and blood pressure for an extended period. In this paper, we propose a multimodal synchronized biological signal analysis using a deep neural network-based model that may learn to classify different anomalous patterns. The proposed cepstral-based peak fusion technique is designed to model the robust characterization of each biological signal by combining the list of dominant peaks in the input signal and its corresponding cepstrum. This works as an input to the following multimodal anomaly detection process that not only enables accurate identification and localization of aberrant signal patterns but also facilitates the proposed model to adopt an individual's unique health characteristics over time. In this work, we use Electrocardiogram (ECG), Femoral Pulse, Photoplethysmogram (PPG), and Body Temperature to monitor an individual's health condition. In both publicly available datasets as well as our lab-based study with 10 participants, the proposed cepstral-based fusion module attains around 7 to 10% improvement over the baseline of time-domain analysis and the proposed deep learning classifier reports an average accuracy of 95.5% with 8 classes and 93% (improvement of 3%) with 17 classes.

Keywords: Vital signal · Peak fusion · Anomaly detection

1 Introduction

Vital biological Signals, such as heart and respiratory rate, are some of the first-level means to evaluate an individual's physical health scenario. For example, cardiac motion, which is a primary indicator of an individual's well-being, is often a unique identifier for each person as no two individuals have the same size, anatomy, or position of heart. While there are scientific tools to estimate basic health conditions from such biological signals, being bulky and hard to use in nature, they are primarily used within a clinical environment, under the supervision of a health professional. Hence, it is typical that these signs are only checked rarely at the annual doctor's visit or when the patient's physical health has already drastically deteriorated and symptoms are too prevalent to ignore.

© ICST Institute for Computer Sciences, Social Informatics and Telecommunications Engineering 2022
Published by Springer Nature Switzerland AG 2022. All Rights Reserved
M. Ur Rehman and A. Zoha (Eds.): BODYNETS 2021, LNICST 420, pp. 139–157, 2022.
https://doi.org/10.1007/978-3-030-95593-9_12

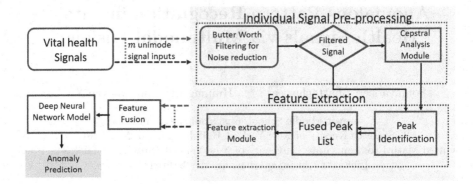

Fig. 1. The proposed multimodal anomalous pattern recognition framework

The situation becomes more complicated in a COVID-19 like pandemic scenario, where common people around the world, specifically the elderly patients, who are amongst the most vulnerable sections of the community, are trying hard to stay away from the hospitals and clinics to ensure safety. So, the probability of missing the regular health check process is now higher than ever. In fact, to address the criticality, an intensive and expensive medical procedure often turns out to be imperative or unavoidable. However, with early detection and regular monitoring processes in place, such exorbitant events may be circumvented.

Unconstrained means to monitor these vital body signals have rapidly emerged as a popular alternative to the conventional health check process in the last decade [1–6]. However, these appliances require frequent charging and are mostly wearable, making the patient uncomfortable (like causing skin irritation), specifically the elderly population. Many times, they also find it awkward due to the devices' external visibility often compromising the privacy of their personal health information. All these pose severe challenges in continual and accurate data collection. A set of works employ unobtrusive devices, which can be easily installed in frequently used furniture that often appears in closed body contact with the patients [7–12]. However, the quality of the signal recorded using such devices often may relies on the frequency of the direct contact between the device surface and the patient's body.

As such, an obvious way to inconspicuously monitor a person's physical health is to embed sensors into objects most frequented by an individual. Studies have shown that people usually spend most of their day doing activities that require the person to be seated such as sitting while attending meetings, sitting while eating, sitting in cars, sitting while watching television [13]. A set of recent works [14–20] which mainly focus on building a hardware system like a chair, often rely on measurements obtained from only one type of signal and thereby have an access to only a limited amount of user's health information. Additionally, frequently their prediction models derive aggregated decisions on the user's health condition without allowing enough personalization. On the other hand, works [21–25] focusing primarily on its recognition sub-task tend to fail in a real-life problem setting, where signals collected from the patients are often too noisy for these machine learning-based systems to make an accurate prediction. Toward this, we aim to develop a generic signal processing and anomaly detection framework that may be deployed both in obtrusive and unobtrusive environments to measure and analyze vital signals of humans in real-time. While the proposed algorithm is invariant to its deployment environment, the proposed system has been installed within a *SmartChair* for real-life evaluation, as such a chair-like setting is known to be a complex application setting in this problem scenario. The extensive set of experiments demonstrate the effectiveness of the proposed cepstral-based peak fusion module by reporting 7 to 10% improvement over the baseline of a time-domain analysis. Furthermore, the proposed deep anomaly detection reports an average accuracy of 95.3% with 8 classes and 93% (improvement of 3%) with 17 classes.

An overview of the proposed method is illustrated in Fig. 1. In our experiments, we have used three vital body signals: respiratory rate, heart rate, and femoral pulse [10, 18, 26–28]. The primary contributions of the proposed system include:

1. *Generic Machine Learning Based Framework* that may analyze both uni- and multi-modal signals within an integrated noise-tolerant framework. The proposed algorithm develops a robust peak detection module by fusing peaks in time and cepstral domain to identify an exhaustive and accurate peak list, which works as an input to the proposed deep learning-based prediction model to predict an individual's personalized health pattern in an automated manner.
2. *Deep Anomaly Detection Strategy*, which enables a continual deep learning-based monitoring process to precisely localize the anomalies in the time domain.
3. *Real-life Demonstration in an Unobtrusive Experiment Setting*, wherein the proposed multimodal signal processing and analysis framework is deployed with a *SmartChair* health monitoring system that may simultaneously capture different types of vital signals from different parts of the seat occupant's body (over a wide range of ages) without forcing an interruption in their daily work schedule.
4. *Extensive Evaluation and Comparative Study* demonstrates an improved performance both in the publicly available datasets as well as our real-life lab experimental settings.

The rest of the paper is organized as follows: Sect. 2 briefly describes related works. The proposed method is explained in Sect. 3. Section 4 and 5 respectively present the experimental results and conclusion.

2   Related Works

In this section, we will briefly describe a set of related research, which can be categorized in parts: (1) Methods focusing on building an intelligent software system, wherein authors assume that a good quality annotated data collection is always available for training a sophisticated machine learning model and the quality of the signals captured during test time may also be considered to be reasonably noise-free, and (2) Methods aiming to build a hardware system that will collect the streaming data for further analysis using machine learning-based methods.

2.1   Health Anomalous Pattern Recognition

Traditional machine learning methods, like Multi-Layer Perceptron (MLP) [29–31], Support Vector Machine (SVM) [32–35], and K nearest neighbors (KNN) [30,31,36,37] have already been used extensively to analyze vital health signals. A set of recent works introduce deep learning models [38–43] for improved performance. Deshmane and Madhe [44] have shown some impressive results on ECG Based biometric human identification using the Convolutional Neural Network model. In contrast to the traditional neural networks, Recurrent Neural Network (RNN) can be used for processing sequential data (e.g., cardiac signal) due to their internal state of memory and connection between the nodes. To explore the temporal granular details, RNN and its variant Long Short Term Memory (LSTM) [45–48] based models have also been introduced for the task. Given the prior knowledge of adjustment between input and output, it can map various sequences with sequences. However, in a practical scenario, specifically in a home-based computationally constrained setting, it is challenging to apply RNN-based methods for continual monitoring tasks, due to its scalability issues. In contrast to these methods, to ensure computational tractability, we use a small set of hand-crafted features to compute a compact feature descriptor that is passed as an input to the subsequent neural network-based prediction module. This not only helps attain a scalable prediction module but also ensures easy adaptability to an individual's personalized health signal patterns.

2.2   Vital Signal Sensing Modality

Vital signals like ECG have been widely used to determine the health condition in many works [42,49–51]. Kim et al. [52] studies of ECG measurement on the toilet seat for ubiquitous health care. Wu et al. [53] use a capacitive coupling ECG sensor to obtain the signal. While the signal capturing module for many of these methods is unobtrusive in nature, they may still demand the seat occupant's attention to ensure a perfect connection between the body and the sensor and accurate angular arrangement, which may cause interruption to the seat occupant's daily routine. A set of recent works have installed multi-channel ECG signals in a chair-based acquisition system to identify the motion artifacts [54]. Important to note that the system either requires the physiological activity in the same fashion as the enrollment stage or periodical resampling of the training dataset [55]. Therefore, the signal capturing process fails to be sustainable enough to ensure long-term usage.

Another set of works design the radio frequency (RF) methods [56] based on the signal reflection, require an off-body reader with the antenna in the far fields, while making the signal acquisition process for a single individual from multiple points, more challenging. A few research have utilized femoral pulse as a component of an active near-field coherent sensing (NCS) system [26,57–59].

However, the arterial blood pressure is dependent on individual's personal characteristics (e.g., age, height, gender), health conditions, and the administration of vasoactive drugs on the patient. Therefore, it is important to have a personalized prediction model that may effectively utilize the femoral pulse as a vital health signal to evaluate a patient's health condition. In this paper, we use the ECG, PPG, and SCG vital signals to evaluate the subject's physical condition. These specific vital signals are chosen as other possible signal resources such as Phonocardiography and Echocardiography are either obtrusive or require high expenses and are difficult to install on chairs.

3 Methodology

We design a generic machine learning-based classification model that performs a comprehensive and synchronized vital health signal analysis both in a uni-modal or multi-modal environment, wherein each mode may represent a signal generated from a unique body part of the participant and make a comprehensive prediction on the health condition of the individual. More specifically, given an annotated data collection $\mathcal{D} = \{(s^j, y^j)\}_j$, where each vital body signal s^j is described using a m-mode ($m \geq 1$) representation, i.e., $s^j = \{x_l^j\}_{l=1}^m$ and the corresponding label y^j is the label for the signal s^j. As shown in Fig. 1, each mode-specific signal is pre-processed via the proposed signal processing module in parallel and later may get combined through feature fusion. In this section, we will describe the process in detail.

3.1 Signal Preprocessing

Noise Filtering. In the real-life setting, the signals received via the sensors are often noisy, due to the individual's movements or shifts during measurements, dampening and noise from clothing, and noise introduced by the sensor itself. Therefore, any raw input signal is somewhat noisy. To address this challenge, we perform an initial noise filtering using Butterworth filter [60] to process each incoming signal to ensure an accurate prediction performance.

The Butterworth Filter is a filter that separates the high-frequency noise from the signal, such that frequency values within the range of the frequency boundaries are reflected in the signal without a significant amount of change. Also, the impact of higher frequencies is reduced by a significant factor, which is dependent on the filter order, in the filtered out signal. The sharpness of the transition from stopband to passband is controlled by the order, a predefined constant in our experiments. The low-pass Butterworth filter is designed as a rational function, defined as follows:

$$|H(j\omega)|^2 = \frac{H_0}{(1 + \omega/\omega_0)^{2n}}, \tag{1}$$

where $H_0 = 1$ the maximum passband gain and $\omega_0 = 1$ rad/sec. In our experiments, we have filtered the signal with a cutoff at 2.5 Hz and a fifth-order Butterworth filter, i.e. we have $n = 5$. The filtered signal x is treated as an input for further analysis. Unless mentioned otherwise, any reference of the signal x in the latter part of the paper will assume it as a filtered signal. We use the Scipy Python library [61] to implement the Butterworth filter.

Peak Identification. In order to analyze the signal characteristic, the first objective of this paper is to propose a robust peak detection scheme that may identify an exhaustive peak list within a signal against the different types of noise resources (e.g. non-stationary effects, low SNR, or several environmental settings of the patient like high heart rate exhibited after exercise) with minimum false positives. In this work, we compute a moving average based on a one-sided window proportional to the sampling frequency, where the proportionality constant is constant and user-defined. In all our experiments, we have chosen the proportionality factor as 0.75 and the sampling frequency as 100. Within each window, any heart rate lying above moving average (where the signal demonstrates a sharp change in gradient) is considered as a peak. While this approach works well in an ideal signal, in presence of a low SNR ratio, the precision performance may still deteriorate significantly resulting in the generation of some false peaks or end up losing some significant peaks in the input signal. An intuitive approach to mitigate the risk of false peak identification is to raise the moving average threshold. However, selecting a universal threshold that would work for all possible noisy signal settings, is difficult and may not be chosen automatically. Therefore, we employ an adaptive approach to dynamically set the threshold by computing the standard deviation of RR intervals [62,63]. In general, the standard deviation of RR intervals is not large. Marking an extra peak or misplacing a R peak may increase the standard deviation significantly, which indicates the possibility of some false peak identification. Therefore, minimizing RRSD will be key to finding a threshold that finds the most accurate number of peaks. However, if RRSD is zero, then there can be two possibilities: either we have a perfect signal or we are seeing the consequences of undetected noises. So, to provide for the best solution, we choose a threshold from a predefined range that would satisfy both $min(RRSD) > 1$ and $RRSD > 1$. We use Heartpy [64] Python library function for the implementation task.

Peak Identification in the Cepstral Domain. Note that the peak detection in the input signal x is similar to detecting pitch from an audio signal. However, identifying peaks from x directly may not be sufficient in isolation, due to having the chance of missing some important peaks. In fact, this may in turn impact on deteriorating the following feature extraction task. Toward this end, for an improved peak detection performance, we use Cepstrum of the signal x for a granular-level peak analysis. As such, Cepstrum analysis, which is a nonlinear signal processing technique, is typically used for pitch detection (similar in some aspects to peak detection) in audio and speech. The real cepstrum of a signal x [65] is calculated as follows:

$$c_x(t) = \frac{1}{2\pi} \int_{-\pi}^{\pi} ln|X(\omega)|e^{j\omega t}\, d\omega, \qquad (2)$$

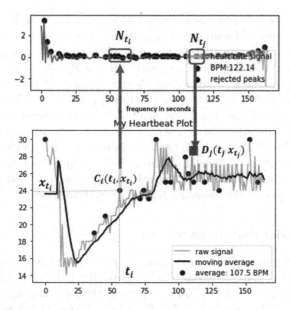

Fig. 2. Peak fusion process: an arrow displays the corresponding peak positions in the input signal (displayed in graph at the top), and the Cepstrum signal (displayed in graph at the bottom.

where $X(\omega)$ is the Fourier transform of the sequence $x(t)$. The proposed peak detection scheme (as described in Sect. 3.1) is employed to parallelly capture a set of peaks in the cepstral domain representation c_x of the input signal x.

Note that in order to ensure an accurate heart rate prediction, we aim to first identify the peaks in an input signal, which will later be used for identifying several key features like beats-per-minute (BPM), Inter-beat-interval (IBI), Root mean square of the successive differences (RMSSD), etc. We will discuss these features more in Sect. 3.2. As such in the cepstral domain, the magnitude of the cepstral coefficient is naturally related to the periodicity of the signal, which is the focus in heart rate estimation and higher values of the cepstrum coefficients reflect increased Signal to Noise Ratio (SNR). A fusion of signal peaks at the cepstrum domain is advantageous to produce a more exhaustive and accurate peak list, which forms the basis of the following feature fusion module (Fig. 2).

Peak Fusion Algorithm. The cepstrum signal c_x is used as a derived representative for the original unimode input signal x. The proposed method uses both c_x and x to identify sets of peaks which are fused to obtain a more exhaustive set of peaks in the signal x.

Given $\mathcal{P}$ as the set of identified peaks in x, as shown in Fig. 5, for every peak at $C_i \in \mathcal{P}$ with co-ordinate $(t_i, x_{(t_i)})$ in the signal x, there is a set of peaks in the corresponding time-domain neighborhood N_{t_i} around t_i for the cepstrum signal, c_x. Intuitively multiple such peaks in c_x within the close neighborhood N_{t_i} around t_i do not provide any new peak information. Therefore, while fusing we eliminate all such redundant peaks within N_{t_i} retaining only the common peak identified at C_i. This is the scenario, which we refer to as *Remove Upward*. This process is repeated for all peaks in $\mathcal{P}$, resulting in retaining only those peaks in c_x, which were not captured within any neighborhood N_{t_i} for any $C_i \in \mathcal{P}$. The set of these remaining peaks in c_x is denoted as $\mathcal{P}_{c_x}$. As illustrated in Fig. 5, to capture these missing peaks within the fused peak list for x, we analyze a close neighborhood N_{t_j} around every remaining peak in $\mathcal{P}_{c_x}$. The time instant t_j within N_{t_j} at which the signal magnitude $c_x[t_j]$ is maximum is mapped down to identify an additional peak D_j with magnitude $x[t_j]$ in x. This process is referred to as *Add Downward*. The process is repeated for all elements of $\mathcal{P}_{c_x}$. The combined peak list obtained at the end of a sequence of *Remove Upward* followed by a sequence of *Add Downward* is treated as the fused peak list that is used as the input to the following feature extraction module.

3.2 Multimodal Feature Extraction

Given the fused peak list obtained from the processed signal x, we derive several handcrafted signals including RRSD; RMSSD; BPM; IBI; SDNN; SDSD; NN20; NN50; PNN20; and PNN50 to represent the incoming signal in terms of a compact feature descriptor $f_x \in \mathbb{R}^d$. RRSD can be computed as the standard deviation between the RR intervals (difference in time between the R-peaks) of a heart signal. RRSD can be computed as the standard deviation between the RR intervals (difference in time between the R-peaks) of a heart signal. RMSSD is defined as the root mean square of successive RR-Intervals and calculated by squaring each RR-interval. Then, the resulting values are averaged before the square root of the total is obtained. BPM can be calculated as the total number of peaks divided by the amount of time passed. IBI, the inter beat interval, can be calculated as the overall average of the RR Intervals. SDNN reflects the changes in heart rate due to cycles longer than 5 min. SDNN can be measured by computing the standard deviation of the time between the consecutive R-peaks. SDSD can be computed as the standard deviation of the successive differences between adjacent RR intervals. NN20 and NN50 can be computed by measuring the number of successive RR intervals that differ by more than 20 and 50 milliseconds respectively. PNN20 and PNN50 can be obtained by dividing NN20 and NN50 by a total number of RR intervals respectively.

In a multimodal environment, feature descriptor collection $\{f_{x_l}^j\}_l^m$ representing multiple unimode signals $s^j = \{x_l^j\}_{l=1}^m$ is transformed into a fused feature $f = \phi(\{f_{x_l}^j\}_l^m)$. In this work, we use vector concatenation function [66] as ϕ to produce md dimensional fused feature f^j.

3.3 Anomalous Pattern Recognition

Given an input signal x, we feed the feature vector f_x (as defined above) into a Neural Network model consisting of 3 fully connected (FC) layers with rectified linear unit (ReLU) activation function. The activation of the last FC layer is fed into a softmax layer to obtain the probabilistic category membership scores for

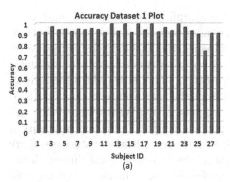 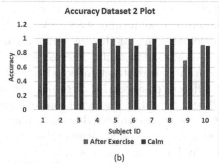

Fig. 3. Peak detection performance in the OHSU ECG signal dataset [67] (shown in (a)) and our in-house dataset with 13 participants (shown in (b)).

the incoming signal's anomaly score. While adding more layers makes the network more expressive, it simultaneously becomes harder to train due to increased computational complexity, vanishing gradients, and model over-fitting. The standard backpropagation algorithm is employed to update the fully connected layer weight parameters.[1] The loss function L is defined as follows:

$$L(\mathbf{W}) = -\frac{\sum_{y \in \mathcal{Y}} \sum_{j=1}^{|\mathcal{D}|} (\mathbf{1}(y^j = y)) log(p(y^j = y | s^j; \mathbf{W})}{|\mathcal{D}|}, \qquad (3)$$

where $\mathbf{1}.$ is the indicator function, $\mathbf{W}$ represents the neural network weight parameters and $log(p(y^j = y | s^j; \mathbf{W})$ computes the probabilistic score of the sample x_i for the class $y \in \mathcal{Y}$. The learning task is formulated as solving the minimization problem defined as: $\min_{\mathbf{W}} L(\mathbf{W})$.

4   Experiments

The proposed method is evaluated from two different perspectives: 1) accuracy evaluation of the peak detection module and 2) the effectiveness of its two-class neural network based prediction module, where the goal is to precisely identify the 'anomalous' signal characteristics of a participant in near real-time. Different datasets are used to evaluate the performance of the model.

4.1   Dataset

To evaluate the performance of our peak detection algorithm, which forms the core of the subsequent prediction module, we use two datasets: the publicly available Oregon Health and Science University (OHSU) ECG signal dataset with 28 participants [67] and our in-house dataset with 13 participants. The

---

[1] https://nrs.harvard.edu/URN-3:HUL.INSTREPOS:37364585.

OHSU dataset has recorded its signals at a sampling rate of 200 Hz and at an amplitude resolution of 4.88 muV. We have used only the health signals from 26 participants. As for the remaining 2 participants, the ECG signals were missing at several time instants. Therefore, we have not used these 2 participants' data. In our in-house dataset collected via the prototype *VitalChair* (which has sensors at different positions for recording signals from the seat occupant and details to follow in Sect. 4.2), the synchronized Femoral pulse (FP), Wrist Pulse (WP), and ECG signals are collected from 13 participants sitting at 7 different positions in a chair for 30 seconds. Among the participants, 4 are high school students, 6 are healthy functioning adults, and 3 are senior adults who have gone through heart surgeries in the past year. The system performs sensor fusion, analyzing the signal patterns to highlight potential anomalous patterns if any. Tests include two scenarios: 1) heart rate of a person at 'calm' state, 2) excited state after 30 min of 'after exercise'.

To evaluate the performance of the proposed neural network model that uses a compact feature descriptor derived from the identified fused peak list as input to predict the participant's health condition, we use Mendeley ECG 1000 Fragments Dataset [25] and our in-house dataset. The Mendeley ECG 1000 Fragments Dataset [25] is the publicly available dataset that we have used to evaluate our framework. This dataset has data from 45 different patients in different health conditions, which comprise of: 2 types of normal rhythms including a pace-maker rhythm and a normal sinus rhythm; 15 types of cardiac dysfunctions including Atrial premature beat, Atrial flutter, Atrial fibrillation, Supraventricular tachyarrhythmia, Pre-excitation (WPW), Premature ventricular contraction, Ventricular bigeminy, Ventricular trigeminy, and Ventricular tachycardia. All the recorded signals are documented at a sampling rate 360 Hz and a gain of 2200 [adu/mV]. In our experiments we have used the above-mentioned 2 types of normal rhythm signal collection as our 'normal' class, which combined together is referred to as *Class 8*, while all the other classes are treated as a specific type of 'anomalous' classes. The class population ratio between two types of classes (i.e. 'normal' and 'anomalous') are highly skewed and the *Class 8* population has size 14,000. So, we refrain from using any 'anomalous' class with samples less than 1,000. Therefore, in our derived dataset, we have only samples from *Class 8* forming the 'normal' class population and 7 different 'anomalous' classes. In our binary prediction module, we reiterate the experiments several times. At each session, *Class 8* is used as the 'normal' class and one of the remaining 7 classes is treated as the 'anomalous' class. Also to note that the signals in this collection are typically high-sampled and the ratio of the anomaly to non-anomaly classes is still very low. Therefore, to further balance the class population at every experimental session, 50 randomly selected sub-sampled signals (of length 500) from the entire signal comprising of nearly 3600 samples, are randomly selected to form the larger training collection. To maintain the balance we just randomly select an equal-sized subset of sub-sampled normal signals to represent the *Class 8* population.

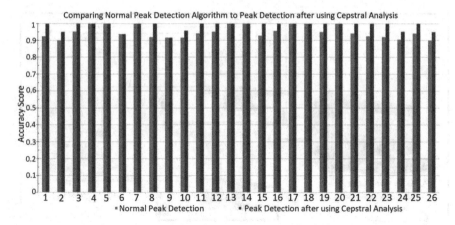

Fig. 4. Comparing the peak detection performance using the processed signal x against that achieved using Fused peak list by combining the peaks from x and the cepstrum signal c_x.

Note that in Mendeley Dataset [25], there are 7 anomaly classes and 1 normal class (namely, Class 1: Ventricular Bigeminy, Class 2: Ventricular Trigeminy, Class 3: Supraventricular Tachyarrhythmia, Class 4: Atrial Fibrillation, Class 5: Left Bundle Branch Block Beat, Class 6: Atrial Premature Beat, Class 7: Premature Ventricular Contraction, and Class 8: Normal Sinus Rhythm) and the ratio of the anomalies to the normal classes is exceptionally low. For the training and testing of the neural network, 50 randomly selected segments of 500 samples for every 3600 samples of the ECG signal were randomly selected. This procedure of subsampling was performed to ensure that the neural network produced by training on this data is not biased or overfitted due to the lack of anomaly-class data. Furthermore, this act of subsampling allows the neural network to produce a more fine-grained interval in which the anomalies are prevalent.

4.2   Prototype Implementation: *VitalChair*

The custom-built circuit used for the *Vitalchair* used in our experiments for real-life study, consists of several capacitors, resistors, and photodiodes[2]. It includes Arduino UNO; Breadboard; USB Cable; Power supplies; Jumper-wires (M/M, M/F); 1.0 M/4,7M Ohm Resistors; Piezoelectric; DS18B20 1-wire waterproof Temperature Sensors; Heart Rate pulse-sensors; different colored LEDs. To build the software module, I have used Arduino IDE and Python. Multiple biological signals including Electro-Cardiogram (ECG), Photoplethysmogram (PPG) from the wrist, Femoral Pulse (FP) are recorded using its corresponding sensor placed at different parts of the chair as illustrated in Fig. 1. The resulting signal from each sensor is passed onto an Arduino microcontroller attached to the bottom of

---

[2] https://cdn.shopify.com/s/files/1/0100/6632/files/PulseSensorAmpd_-_Schematic. pdf?1862089645030619491.

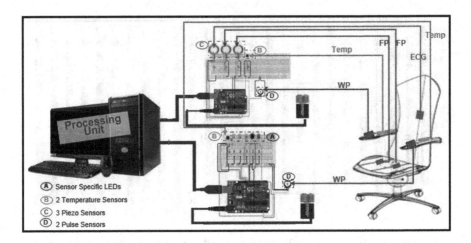

Fig. 5. A custom-built prototype of VitalChair, where vital signals are represented as: WP = Wrist Pulse, FP = Femoral Pulse, ECG = Electro-Cardiogram signal, and Temp = Body Temperature

the chair to collect readings from each sensor. Data was acquired onto a server connected to the Arduino over USB and analyzed using the Arduino software in real-time. The outputs of the sensors at different positions on the SmartChair are collected in a synchronized fashion for a comprehensive understanding of the seat occupant's overall wellbeing.

4.3   Performance Evaluation

Peak Detection Accuracy Metric. The results of the first type of experiments, evaluating the peak detection module of the proposed method, use *Accuracy* as the evaluation metric. Given g as the number of hand-picked peaks by an independent evaluator and p is the number of system-identified peaks, we compute the *Accuracy* $= 1 - \frac{|p-g|}{g}$ The quantitative results obtained in the OHSU ECG signal dataset and our in-house dataset are reported in Fig. 3(a) and (b) respectively. As observed in Fig. 3(a), the average accuracy achieved by the proposed prediction module over 28 participants is around 94.18%. Specifically for the participant id 26, the accuracy (approx 75%) is considerably lower compared to the rest, which is due to the missing data at several time instants that resulted in missing some significant peaks. The deteriorated peak detection performance propagated to influence the performance of the subsequent prediction module.

Peak Detection Performance. In Fig. 3(b), we notice that the accuracy of the 'calm' state is usually greater than the after exercise accuracy. This is the case because, after exercise, an individual's heart rate increases significantly, which causes many additional consecutive peak occurrences. However, the system perceives this extra flow of peaks as noises and thus, some of the peaks are not

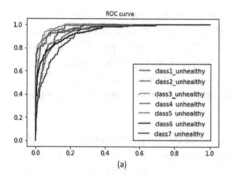
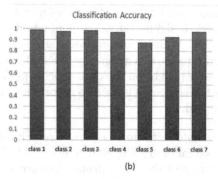

Fig. 6. The performance of the proposed prediction module on the Mendeley dataset, reported using class specific ROC Curves (in (a)) and the classification accuracy (in (b)), wherein Class 1: Ventricular Bigeminy, Class 2: Ventricular Trigeminy, Class 3: Supraventricular Tachyarrhythmia, Class 4: Atrial Fibrillation, Class 5: Left Bundle Branch Block Beat, Class 6: Atrial Premature Beat, and Class 7: Premature Ventricular Contraction with their AUC scores respectively as: 0.98, 0.98, 0.97, 0.95, 0.94, 0.95, and 0.92.

counted. This results in missing peaks that impact reducing the overall accuracy of the prediction module. However, this high-frequency heart-rate period only lasts for a couple of minutes and the individual (if indeed 'healthy') quickly regains their normal heart rate. To mitigate this noise impacted response, we pause the prediction task during the initial minute, so that any alert regarding the participant's health condition is generated only if it has been more than a minute since their seat occupancy.

As observed in Fig. 4, combining peaks from the processed signal x and the cepstrum signal c_x have been useful to improve the resulting peak detection performance of the proposed method by an average of 3%. In fact, in several instances (like participants 1, 8, 15, 22, and 23) the improvement reported was around 7–10%.

Anomaly Detection Performance Metrics. The *Classification Accuracy* and *Sensitivity* score are used as the compact evaluation metrics computed by relating FP (False Positives), FN (False Negatives), TP (True Positives) and TN (True Negatives) and defined as:

$$Classification\_Accuracy = \left(\sum_{i=1}^{N} \frac{TP+TN}{TP+TN+FP+FN} \right).100\%/N, \quad (4)$$

$$Sensitivity = \left(\sum_{i=1}^{N} \frac{TP}{TP+FN} \right).100\%/N, \quad (5)$$

where the scores are computed based on N-fold cross-validated test process, In our experiments, we have used $N = 5$. We also report the performance details using Area Under the Receiver Operating Curve, known as AUC score [68]. This metric is significant as the population distribution across different classes varies widely. While *Classification Accuracy* (or *Sensitivity*) may provide an overall performance at a given experimental parameter setting, the AUC metric provides greater insight on the class-specific performances of the proposed method. Also, *Sensitivity* score is used to report the comparative performance of the proposed method.

Anomaly Detection Performance. Figure. 6 reports the performance of the proposed method using *ROC* Curves, *AUC Scores* as the total area under the ROC curve, and the *Classification Accuracy* as the evaluation metrics [69]. As seen in the figure, note that, the average performance on all seven anomalous classes is around 95.29%. While the performance on Class 5 is approximately 87.22%, it is primarily attributed to the sparse signal (with also missing ECG values) obtained from participants.

4.4 Comparative Study

The performance of the proposed method is compared against that of several methods reported in [25], and the result is reported in Table 1. To attain an equivalent experimental setting, for this experiment, we combine all the 17 cardiac disorders into an anomaly class, while the healthy signals form the second class. As seen by comparing the results reported in the table, the proposed method shows an improved performance by reporting 3% increased *Sensitivity* score. An equivalent experiment is also performed using only 8 classes and as shown in the table, the proposed method attains an impressive performance gain of 2.5% compared to the best result reported on the data-set.

Table 1. A comparative study on the binary classification task performed using the Mendeley ECG 1000 Fragments Dataset [25].

Methods	Number of classes	*Sensitivity* score
Linear discriminant classification [22]	5	93%
Domain transfer SVM [21]	5	92%
Decision level fusion [23]	5	87%
Disease-specific feature selection [24]	5	86%
Morphological and dynamic features of ECG signals [70]	5	86%
Evolutionary neural system [25]	17	90%
Proposed method	8	95.5%
Proposed method	17	93%

Also in this scenario, it is also important to note that the performance varies from class to class (please refer to Fig. 6(b)). So, such course-level overall performance evaluation may not be sufficiently insightful in terms of getting sufficient insight on the effectiveness of the proposed model. For example, accurate identification of samples from Class 5 samples is harder than that of Class 6. Moreover, the above-mentioned paper obtains the accuracy in an obtrusive manner, which significantly reduces the amount of noise corrupting the signal. Therefore, the applicability of these methods is limited in various real-life environments, where signals can only be received in an unobtrusive manner. In contrast, the proposed method, which is generic and sufficiently robust to handle the noisy signal inputs, and allows for sequential learning by continual signal capturing process, is more effective and efficient. As described earlier, to further investigate the robustness of the method, we perform experiments in a real-life environment by deploying the software in the SmartChair, which collects signals by placing sensors at different parts of the chair. Also, the method is evaluated at different levels of stress and physical activity state of the participants to investigate the efficacy of the signal filtering and feature extraction methods.

5   Conclusion

In this paper, we have presented a framework that is able to accurately classify multiple input signals like ECG, PPG, and Femoral Pulse from a specific individual into two categories: healthy or unhealthy. Having been able to continuously monitor the patient's vital signals, this system has several life-changing effects, including the ability to identify pathology conditions before they can turn into a serious threat to the human's life or severe measures are required to cure them such as amputations. To demonstrate our proposed model's real-life feasibility, we have physically implemented this framework into a chair. However, the proposed method is sufficiently generic to be deployed into other frequently used furniture items like beds, sofas, etc. We plan to extend this work to include other means of extracting pathological information, like vocal signals, and synchronize them all to make a smart home system that will be able to accurately classify the disease-specific pathological condition the individual has using multi-modal information.

References

1. Mukhopadhyay, S.C.: Wearable sensors for human activity monitoring: a review. IEEE Sensor. J. **15**(3), 1321–1330 (2014)
2. Fletcher, R., Poh, M., Eydgahi, H.: Wearable sensors: opportunities and challenges for low-cost health care. In: 2010 Annual International Conference of the IEEE Engineering in Medicine and Biology Society (EMBC), vol. 1766 (1763)
3. Niswar, M., Nur, M., Ilham, A.A., Mappangara, I.: A low cost wearable medical device for vital signs monitoring in low-resource settings. Int. J. Electr. Comput. Eng. **9**, 2088–8708 (2019)
4. Huang, M.C., Liu, J.J., Xu, W., Gu, C., Li, C., Sarrafzadeh, M.: A self-calibrating radar sensor system for measuring vital signs. IEEE Trans. Biomed. Circuits Syst. **10**(2), 352–363 (2016)

5. Rathore, A.S., Li, Z., Zhu, W., Jin, Z., Xu, W.: A survey on heart biometrics. ACM Comput. Surv. (CSUR) **53**(6), 1–38 (2020)
6. Patil, O.R., Wang, W., Gao, Y., Xu, W., Jin, Z.: A low-cost, camera-based continuous PPG monitoring system using Laplacian pyramid. Smart Health **9**—-**10**, 2–11 (2018). CHASE 2018 Special Issue
7. Lim, Y.G., et al.: Monitoring physiological signals using nonintrusive sensors installed in daily life equipment. Biomed. Eng. Lett. **1**(1), 11–20 (2011). https://doi.org/10.1007/s13534-011-0012-0
8. Brüser, C., Antink, C.H., Wartzek, T., Walter, M., Leonhardt, S.: Ambient and unobtrusive cardiorespiratory monitoring techniques. IEEE Rev. Biomed. Eng. **8**, 30–43 (2015)
9. Kang, S., et al.: Sinabro: opportunistic and unobtrusive mobile electrocardiogram monitoring system. In: Proceedings of the 15th Workshop on Mobile Computing Systems and Applications, pp. 1–6 (2014)
10. Malik, A.R., Pilon, L., Boger, J.: Development of a smart seat cushion for heart rate monitoring using ballistocardiography. In: 2019 IEEE International Conference on Computational Science and Engineering (CSE) and IEEE International Conference on Embedded and Ubiquitous Computing (EUC), pp. 379–383 IEEE (2019)
11. Yu, X., et al.: A multi-modal sensor for a bed-integrated unobtrusive vital signs sensing array. IEEE Trans. Biomed. Circuits Syst. **13**(3), 529–539 (2019)
12. Wang, S., et al.: Noninvasive monitoring of vital signs based on highly sensitive fiber optic mattress. IEEE Sens. J. **20**(11), 6182–6190 (2020)
13. Pronk, N.: The problem with too much sitting: a workplace conundrum. ACSM's Health Fit. J. **15**(1), 41–43 (2011)
14. Arnrich, B., Setz, C., La Marca, R., Tröster, G., Ehlert, U.: What does your chair know about your stress level? IEEE Trans. Inf. Technol. Biomed. **14**(2), 207–214 (2009)
15. Zheng, Y., Morrell, J.B.: A vibrotactile feedback approach to posture guidance. In: 2010 IEEE haptics Symposium, pp. 351–358. IEEE (2010)
16. Baek, H.J., Chung, G.S., Kim, K.K., Park, K.S.: A smart health monitoring chair for nonintrusive measurement of biological signals. IEEE Trans. Inf. Technol. Biomed. **16**(1), 150–158 (2011)
17. Kumar, R., Bayliff, A., De, D., Evans, A., Das, S.K., Makos, M.: Care-chair: sedentary activities and behavior assessment with smart sensing on chair backrest. In: 2016 IEEE International Conference on Smart Computing (SMARTCOMP), pp. 1–18. IEEE (2016)
18. Griffiths, E., Saponas, T.S., Brush, A.B.: Health chair: implicitly sensing heart and respiratory rate. In: Proceedings of the 2014 ACM International Joint Conference on Pervasive and Ubiquitous Computing, pp. 661–671 (2014)
19. Ravichandran, R., Saba, E., Chen, K.Y., Goel, M., Gupta, S., Patel, S.N.: WiBreathe: estimating respiration rate using wireless signals in natural settings in the home. In: 2015 IEEE International Conference on Pervasive Computing and Communications (PerCom), pp. 131–139. IEEE (2015)
20. Zhang, Y., Chen, Z., Chen, W., Li, H.: Unobtrusive and continuous bcg-based human identification using a microbend fiber sensor. IEEE Access **7**, 72518–72527 (2019)
21. Bazi, Y., Alajlan, N., AlHichri, H., Malek, S.: Domain adaptation methods for ECG classification. In: 2013 International Conference on Computer Medical Applications (ICCMA), pp. 1–4 (2013)

22. Lin, C.C., Yang, C.M.: Heartbeat classification using normalized RR intervals and wavelet features. In: 2014 International Symposium on Computer. Consumer and Control, pp. 650–653 (2014)

23. Zhang, Z., Luo, X.: Heartbeat classification using decision level fusion. Biomed. Eng. Lett. 4(4), 388–395 (2014). https://doi.org/10.1007/s13534-014-0158-7

24. Zhang, Z., Dong, J., Luo, X., Choi, K.S., Wu, X.: Heartbeat classification using disease-specific feature selection. Comput. Biol. Med. 46, 79–89 (2014)

25. Pławiak, P.: Novel methodology of cardiac health recognition based on ECG signals and evolutionary-neural system. Expert Syst. Appl. 92, 334–349 (2018)

26. Hui, X., Kan, E.C.: Seat integration of RF vital-sign monitoring. In: 2019 IEEE MTT-S International Microwave Biomedical Conference (IMBioC), vol. 1, pp. 1–3. (2019)

27. Gui, Q., Ruiz-Blondet, M.V., Laszlo, S., Jin, Z.: A survey on brain biometrics. ACM Comput. Surv. (CSUR) 51(6), 1–38 (2019)

28. Anttonen, J., Surakka, V.: Emotions and heart rate while sitting on a chair. In: Proceedings of the SIGCHI Conference on Human Factors in Computing Systems, pp. 491–499 (2005)

29. Pinto, J.R., Cardoso, J.S., Lourenço, A., Carreiras, C.: Towards a continuous biometric system based on ECG signals acquired on the steering wheel. Sensors 17(10), 2228 (2017)

30. Sidek, K.A., Mai, V., Khalil, I.: Data mining in mobile ECG based biometric identification. J. Netw. Comput. Appl. 44, 83–91 (2014)

31. Kavsaoğlu, A.R., Polat, K., Bozkurt, M.R.: A novel feature ranking algorithm for biometric recognition with PPG signals. Comput. Biol. Med. 49, 1–14 (2014)

32. Li, M., Narayanan, S.: Robust ECG biometrics by fusing temporal and cepstral information. In: 2010 20th International Conference on Pattern Recognition, pp. 1326–1329. IEEE (2010)

33. Da Silva, H.P., Fred, A., Lourenço, A., Jain, A.K.: Finger ECG signal for user authentication: usability and performance. In: 2013 IEEE Sixth International Conference on Biometrics: Theory, Applications and Systems (BTAS), pp. 1–8. IEEE (2013)

34. Lin, S.L., Chen, C.K., Lin, C.L., Yang, W.C., Chiang, C.T.: Individual identification based on chaotic electrocardiogram signals during muscular exercise. IET Biometrics 3(4), 257–266 (2014)

35. Lin, F., Song, C., Zhuang, Y., Xu, W., Li, C., Ren, K.: Cardiac scan: a non-contact and continuous heart-based user authentication system. In: Proceedings of the 23rd Annual International Conference on Mobile Computing and Networking, pp. 315–328 (2017)

36. Gürkan, H., Guz, U., Yarman, B.S.: A novel biometric authentication approach using electrocardiogram signals. In: 2013 35th Annual International Conference of the IEEE Engineering in Medicine and Biology Society (EMBC), pp. 4259–4262. IEEE (2013)

37. Venkatesh, N., Jayaraman, S.: Human electrocardiogram for biometrics using DTW and FLDA. In: 2010 20th International Conference on Pattern Recognition, pp. 3838–3841. IEEE (2010)

38. Donida Labati, R., Muñoz, E., Piuri, V., Sassi, R., Scotti, F.: Deep-ECG: convolutional neural networks for ECG biometric recognition. Pattern Recogn. Lett. 126, 78–85 (2019)

39. Tavallali, P., Razavi, M., Pahlevan, N.: Artificial intelligence estimation of carotid-femoral pulse wave velocity using carotid waveform. Sci. Rep. 8, 1–12 (2018)

40. Ledezma, C.A., Zhou, X., Rodríguez, B., Tan, P.J., Díaz-Zuccarini, V.: A modeling and machine learning approach to ECG feature engineering for the detection of ischemia using pseudo-ECG. PLOS One **14**, 1–21 (2019)
41. da Silva Luz, E.J., Moreira, G.J., Oliveira, L.S., Schwartz, W.R., Menotti, D.: Learning deep off-the-person heart biometrics representations. IEEE Trans. Inf. Forensics Secur. **13**(5), 1258–1270 (2017)
42. Zhang, Q., Zhou, D., Zeng, X.: HeartID: a multiresolution convolutional neural network for ECG-based biometric human identification in smart health applications. Ieee Access **5**, 11805–11816 (2017)
43. Xiang, Y., Luo, J., Zhu, T., Wang, S., Xiang, X., Meng, J.: ECG-based heartbeat classification using two-level convolutional neural network and RR interval difference. IEICE Trans. Inf. Syst. **101**(4), 1189–1198 (2018)
44. Deshmane, M., Madhe, S.: ECG based biometric human identification using convolutional neural network in smart health applications. In: International Conference on Computing Communication Control and Automation (ICCUBEA), pp. 1–6 (2018)
45. Salloum, R., Kuo, C.C.J.: ECG-based biometrics using recurrent neural networks. In: 2017 IEEE International Conference on Acoustics, Speech and Signal Processing (ICASSP), pp. 2062–2066. IEEE (2017)
46. Everson, L., et al.: BiometricNet: deep learning based biometric identification using wrist-worn PPG. In: 2018 IEEE International Symposium on Circuits and Systems (ISCAS), pp. 1–5. IEEE (2018)
47. Salloum, R., Kuo, C.J.: ECG-based biometrics using recurrent neural networks. In: 2017 IEEE International Conference on Acoustics, Speech and Signal Processing (ICASSP), pp. 2062–2066 (2017)
48. Dezaki, F.T., et al.: Deep residual recurrent neural networks for characterisation of cardiac cycle phase from echocardiograms. In: Cardoso, M.J., et al. (eds.) DLMIA/ML-CDS-2017. LNCS, vol. 10553, pp. 100–108. Springer, Cham (2017). https://doi.org/10.1007/978-3-319-67558-9_12
49. Hui, X., Conroy, T.B., Kan, E.C.: Multi-point near-field RF sensing of blood pressures and heartbeat dynamics. IEEE Access **8**, 89935–89945 (2020)
50. Sidikova, M., et al.: Vital sign monitoring in car seats based on electrocardiography, ballistocardiography and seismocardiography: A review. Sensors **20**(19), 5699 (2020)
51. Singh, R.K., Sarkar, A., Anoop, C.S.: A health monitoring system using multiple non-contact ECG sensors for automotive drivers. In: 2016 IEEE International Instrumentation and Measurement Technology Conference Proceedings, pp. 1–6 (2016)
52. Kim, K.K., Lim, Y.K., Park, K.S.: The electrically noncontacting ECG measurement on the toilet seat using the capacitively-coupled insulated electrodes. In: The 26th Annual International Conference of the IEEE Engineering in Medicine and Biology Society, vol. 1, pp. 2375–2378. IEEE (2004)
53. Wu, K.F., Chan, C.H., Zhang, Y.t.: Contactless and cuffless monitoring of blood pressure on a chair using e-textile materials. In: 2006 3rd IEEE/EMBS International Summer School on Medical Devices and Biosensors, pp. 98–100. IEEE (2006)
54. Choi, M., Jeong, J., Kim, S., Kim, S.: Reduction of motion artifacts and improvement of R peak detecting accuracy using adjacent non-intrusive ECG sensors. Sensors **16**, 715 (2016)
55. Coutinho, D.P., Silva, H., Gamboa, H., Fred, A., Figueiredo, M.: Novel fiducial and non-fiducial approaches to electrocardiogram-based biometric systems. IET Biometrics **2**(2), 64–75 (2013)

56. Adib, F., Mao, H., Kabelac, Z., Katabi, D., Miller, R.C.: Smart homes that monitor breathing and heart rate. In: Proceedings of the 33rd Annual ACM Conference on Human Factors in Computing Systems, pp. 837–846. Association for Computing Machinery, New York (2015)

57. Welkowitz, W., Cui, Q., Qi, Y., Kostis, J.B.: Noninvasive estimation of cardiac output. IEEE Trans. Biomed. Eng. **38**(11), 1100–1105 (1991)

58. Smith, J., Camporota, L., Beale, R.: Monitoring arterial blood pressure and cardiac output using central or peripheral arterial pressure waveforms. In: Vincent, J.L. (ed.) Intensive Care Medicine, pp. 285–296. Springer, New York (2009). https://doi.org/10.1007/978-0-387-92278-2_27

59. Chen, J., et al.: High durable, biocompatible, and flexible piezoelectric pulse sensor using single-crystalline III-N thin film. Adv. Funct. Mater. **29**, 1903162 (2019)

60. Winder, S.: Analog and digital filter design. Elsevier, Amsterdam (2002)

61. Virtanen, P., et al.: SciPy 1.0: Fundamental algorithms for scientific computing in python. Nat. Methods **17**(3), 261–272 (2020)

62. O'Haver, T.: Pragmatic introduction to signal processing (2018)

63. Richig, J.W., Sleeper, M.M.: Electrocardiography of Laboratory Animals. Academic Press, San Diego (2018)

64. van Gent, P., Farah, H., Nes, N., Arem, B.: HeartPy: a novel heart rate algorithm for the analysis of noisy signals. Transp. Res. Part F Traffic Psychol. Behav. **66**, 368–378 (2019)

65. Pei, S.C., Lin, H.S.: Minimum-phase FIR filter design using real cepstrum. IEEE Trans. Circuits Syst. II Express Briefs **53**(10), 1113–1117 (2006)

66. Bretscher, O.: Linear Algebra with Applications. Prentice Hall, Eaglewood Cliffs (1997)

67. Rogovoy, N., et al.: The dialysis procedure triggers autonomic imbalance and cardiac arrhythmias: insights from continuous 14-day ECG monitoring, April 2019

68. Fan, J., Upadhye, S., Worster, A.: Understanding receiver operating characteristic (roc) curves. Can. J. Emerg. Med. **8**(1), 19–20 (2006)

69. Pedregosa, F., et al.: Scikit-learn: machine learning in Python. J. Mach. Learn. Res. **12**, 2825–2830 (2011)

70. Ye, C., Kumar, B.V., Coimbra, M.T.: Heartbeat classification using morphological and dynamic features of ECG signals. IEEE Trans. Biomed. Eng. **59**(10), 2930–2941 (2012)

Real-Time Visual Respiration Tracking with Radar Sensors

Shaozhang Dai$^{(\boxtimes)}$, Weiqiao Han, Malikeh P. Ebrahim, and Mehmet R. Yuce

Department of Electrical and Computer Systems Engineering, Monash University, Melbourne, Australia
{shaozhang.dai1,weiqiao.han,melika.pour.ebrahim,Mehmet.Yuce}@monash.edu

Abstract. Wireless detection of respiration rate (RR) plays a significant role in many healthcare applications. Most of the solutions provide simple waveforms and display the number of estimated RR. In this paper, a visualiser's approach for the wireless respiration tracking with commercial radar sensor, Walabot, is proposed. Walabot provides a real-time 2D heatmap from the reflected signals, and an abstract graph is extracted from the heatmap to represent the respiratory motion intuitively. Since monitored objects' movements may cause inaccurate measurements, two optimisation algorithms are developed to enhance accuracy. A respiration waveform is then obtained, and the average RR is calculated. The data is collected for different scenarios of breathing speed, including normal, hold, and deep. The computed RR accuracy is compared with the manually counted RR during the data collection as a reference. Overall, the calculated RR has high average accuracy, and the performance of the visualiser is precise and consistent. This solution also has the potential to monitor respirations for multiple subjects or in a through-wall situation.

Keywords: Data visualization · Wireless monitoring · Respiration rate

1 Introduction

Physiological signal monitoring has received significant attention in recent decades, especially for health care purposes. Breathing waveform, as one of the important vital signals, has an essential role in early diagnosis for respiratory diseases such as lung disease (too fast breathing), apnoea (sudden stop) [10], unusual respiration (e.g., Biot's Breathing, Cheyne-Stokes respiration) [2,17], and other related diseases [12,16]. Therefore, the early investigation and treatment are proven to be highly effective [1,15].

There are many processes to measure and monitor breathing with various sources of signals like mechanical movement on the torso [14], or airflow pressure by oral or nasal cannula [8]; however, most of the monitoring devices output only processed waveforms and the estimated respiratory rate [5,7,18]. People with little knowledge of physiology might have difficulty understanding how the breathing in each second contributes to the final respiratory waveform.

© ICST Institute for Computer Sciences, Social Informatics and Telecommunications Engineering 2022
Published by Springer Nature Switzerland AG 2022. All Rights Reserved
M. Ur Rehman and A. Zoha (Eds.): BODYNETS 2021, LNICST 420, pp. 158–167, 2022.
https://doi.org/10.1007/978-3-030-95593-9_13

This paper proposes a solution which provides an abstract visualiser for breathing monitoring to indicate different respiratory processes (inhalation and exhalation) with a commercial wireless radar. The algorithm is image-based so that the mechanical movement caused in the respiratory process can be extracted. In Sect. 2, the radar sensor and the analysis processes are presented. Section 3 shows the experimental results and the comparison with the manually counted RR as a reference. The conclusion and potential applications will be discussed in the last section.

2   Methods

2.1   Sensor System

Walabot is a low-cost commodity ultra-wideband (UWB) radar-based device which generates 2D and 3D image frames from the reflected signals. Walabot operates in the frequency range of 3.3–10.3 GHz, which can cover 10 m detection range based on the Frequency-Modulated Continuous Wave (FMCW) chip's gradient. It contains a 2D antenna array to produce and receive radio frequency (RF) waves, and the reflected signals are processed by the VYYR2401 A3 System- on-Chip integrated circuit. Doppler, azimuth and elevation positions [11] of the moving objects are extracted from the processed signal in the form of 2D and 3D heatmap image [3].

2.2   Sensor Overview

Object distance and angle are calculated from the received RF signals by the 2D array of antenna in polar coordinates (Theta-Phi-R), Fig. 1. With the intensity of

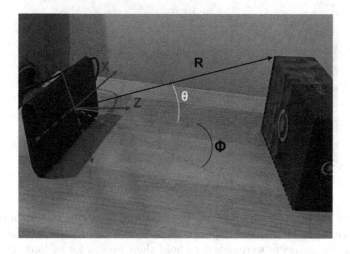

Fig. 1. Walabot parameters (Theta, Phi, and R)

the RF signals, a 3-dimensional heatmap image is constructed. The 2D heatmap is the projection of the 3D image along one axis. By placing the Walabot sensor in a correct orientation, the produced 2D heatmap can be used to extract the vital signals like respiration.

To eliminate the environmental impact on the heatmap, Walabot, in the calibration phase, produces RF signals and records reflected signals as a reference, so that reflections from static objects in the subsequent signals are removed. The obtained 2D heatmap is further simplified to a single point representing the moving object's centre. Since the centre point represents the overall movements of the detected moving objects, by tracking this centre point, vital information like respiration waveform is observed.

2.3   Experimental Protocol

The experimental setup for the data collection is shown in Fig. 2. The experimental data were collected on five healthy subjects, from 25 to 30 years old. The experiment was conducted indoor with controlled room temperature. Walabot was placed 60 cm above the bed with specifications adjusted to mainly the subjects' torso (Theta: 10 to −10°, Phi: 15 to −15°, and R: 50 cm to 70 cm). Generated 2D heatmap and the extracted respiratory waveform were recorded for future analysis. To compute the accuracy of the calculated result, each subject's respiratory rate was simultaneously counted as the reference signal.

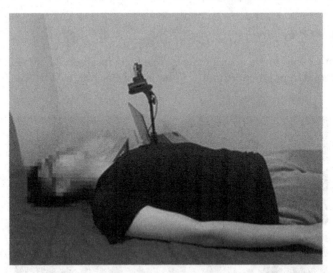

Fig. 2. Experiment setup for data collection

Subjects were required to lie on the bed and simulate the scenarios with different breathing speed. The experiment started with breathing normally for 3 min. Then, the subjects were asked to hold their breath for as long as possible. In the end, subjects need to have deep breathing for 3 min. The recorded signals were processed to extract respiratory waveform. The result was evaluated in Sect. 3 to analyse the breathing visualisation performance and the accuracy of the estimated respiration rate.

2.4   Signal Processing

The respiratory motion is measured by computing the relative displacement of the centre point in two contiguous heatmap frames. For example, the centre point locates at the top of the heatmap during inhalation and the point will move to the bottom of the heatmap during exhalation. Then the respiratory motion can be simulated by comparing the difference between these two locations. To emphasize the current respiratory process, a curve is generated by connecting the relative zero, representing the previous location of the target, and the current location. The amplitude of the displacement represents the respiratory motion magnitude, and the curve shape indicates either the target is in inhalation or exhalation. Figure 3 shows the generated visualisation graph where there are two threshold lines defining the valid displacement range, which means any movement detected outside this area will not be considered as breathing.

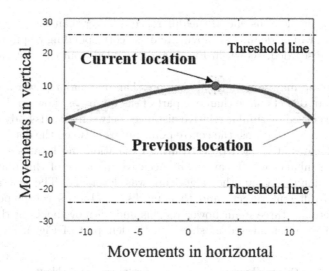

Fig. 3. Line graph of the abstract representation of breathing process

The respiration waveform fluctuates significantly and erratically during the target object's movement, as shown in Fig. 4. Therefore, to maintain the respiration monitoring accuracy, the respiration recording related to the target movements is eliminated. Only the respiration waveform of the target in static status is considered.

An algorithm was created to detect movements from the analysis of the heatmap. The algorithm compares the difference between the current detected

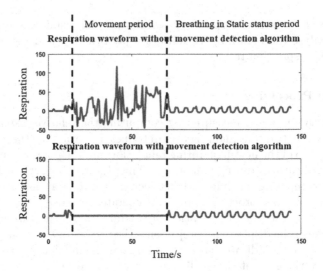

Fig. 4. Respiration waveform after movement signal is removed

heatmap and the previous one. If the difference is larger than the pre-set threshold, the target will be defined as moving and the corresponding respiration waveform will be discarded, shown in Fig. 4, and excluded from the respiration estimation.

The heatmap may sometimes show more than one major power area, which means Walabot detects more than one part of the target, as shown in Fig. 5. This issue may be caused by similar relative distances between various body parts and Walabot. In some situations, the centre point jumps between the detected power areas (e.g., locates at the left object during exhalation and locates at the right object during inhalation). To avoid the negative influence of this phenomenon in real-time monitoring, another algorithm was developed. The new algorithm distinguishes different targets and then marks all object's centre points. For example, there are three main power regions and all movements of these three objects need to be monitored as shown in the left part of Fig. 5. By applying

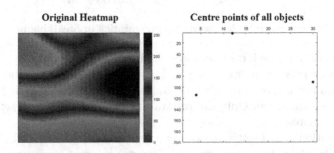

Fig. 5. An example of centre points extraction (Left: 2D heatmap; Right: extracted centre points)

the algorithm, the local maximum points, which is also the centre point of the power region, can be indicated as shown in the right part of Fig. 5. Then, the respiration waveform is generated by comparing the movements of all detected targets' centre points between consecutive frames. Figure 6 shows the flowchart of the signal processing procedures for the real-time respiration monitoring.

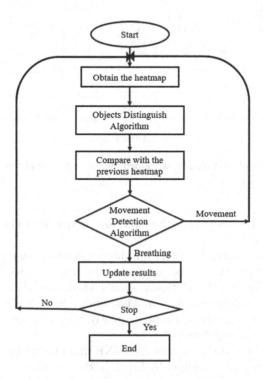

Fig. 6. The flowchart of the signal processing for respiration monitoring with radar sensor

3   Results and Discussion

An example of a monitored respiration waveform is shown in Fig. 7. The monitored subject was breathing normally for 3 min at first and then holding the breath for several seconds, followed by deep breathing for another 3 min. The respiration frequency in one minute is calculated as Eq. 1.

$$f = \frac{BreathingCounts}{T_{end} - T_{start}} * 60 \tag{1}$$

T_{start} is the start time in seconds of the calculated respiration period and T_{end} is the end time in seconds of the calculated respiration period. The result f is the respiration frequency of the calculated respiration period, and the unit is

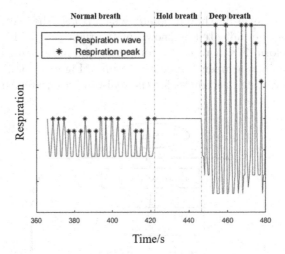

Fig. 7. An example of respiration waveform for normal, hold, and deep scenarios obtained from Walabot

times per minute. In this paper, all respiration frequency values are calculated by using this equation.

During the experiment, the line graph shows the breathing process intuitively. In Fig. 8, we only use two simple symbols (line and dot) to demonstrate the current breathing process. Inhalation is shown when the vertical displacement is positive, and vice versa for exhalation. The amplitude of displacement indicates whether the subject is breathing deeply or gently. Similarly, a straight line means that there is no breathing detected.

The normalised root-mean-square error (NRMSE) method is used to measure the device's accuracy, as described by Eq. 2. In the equation, n is the number of observations; RR_{ref} and RR_i are the respiration rates obtained from the manual counter and the estimated calculation, respectively. The NRMSE method can emphasise the magnitude of the variance if the reference is accurate and large errors will be accentuated in such case [4].

Table 1. NRMSE between the estimated RR and reference RR of 5 subjects for normal and deep breathing

Subject No.	Normal breathing (%)	Deep breathing (%)
1	1.26	2.32
2	3.48	3.82
3	2.26	4.36
4	3.53	5.74
5	2.77	4.17

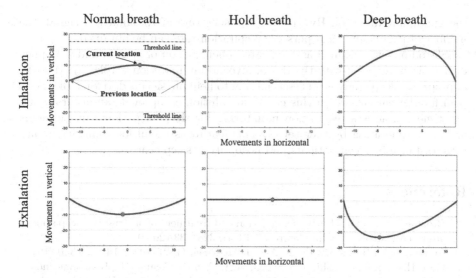

Fig. 8. Examples of the line graph for different breathing scenarios (column) and different breathing processes (row)

$$NRMSE = \frac{\sqrt{\frac{1}{n}\sum_{i=1}^{n}(RR_i - RR_{ref})^2}}{\frac{1}{n}\sum_{i=1}^{n}RR_{ref}} \tag{2}$$

Five subjects were observed for both normal breathing and deep breathing, and the result is shown in Table 1. The NRMSE shows an accurate estimation of RR obtained from the experiment. The maximum NRMSE is 5.74% in deep breathing for subject 4 and the minimum NRMSE is 1.26% in normal breathing for subject 1. In terms of RR per minute, the average difference between the estimation and manual count is less than 1 bit per minute.

4   Conclusion

This paper proposes an image-based visualisation solution for breathing monitoring with a real-time abstract representation of breathing processes and the estimated respiratory rate from the extracted respiratory waveform. The evaluated sensor is a UWB radar called Walabot which produces a real-time 2D heatmap from the reflected RF waves of all detected moving objects in range. The heatmap is simplified into a line graph emphasising the change of signals. This abstract graph highlights the physiological movement corresponding to the state of inhalation or exhalation.

The developed object distinguishing algorithm ensures the accurate and reliable result of respiration monitoring. Furthermore, the movements of each distinguished object can be collected and recorded. Then the movement frequency is obtained by convoluting the first signal with the rest of the signals and taking the maximum value [6]. By drawing the spectrum of the analysed signal, the number of people and each person's respiration rate can be obtained.

Sleep apnoea is defined as a repeated phenomenon of apnoea and hypopnea during sleep, together with the risk of myocardial infarction, stroke etc. [13]. An appropriate sleep study is an essential tool to help physicians develop a diagnosis plan for the patient [9]. In this case, our solution can provide an accurate and real-time contactless respiration monitoring for sleeping patients in the home and easily operating by themselves. This feature is useful for countries with a large distance between patients and hospitals or sleep centres.

References

1. Broadley, S.A., et al.: Early investigation and treatment of obstructive sleep apnoea after acute stroke. J. Clin. Neurosci. **14**(4), 328–333 (2007)
2. Conner, L.A.: Biot's breathing. Am. J. Med. Sci. (1827–1924) **141**(3), 350 (1911)
3. Guo, H., Zhang, N., Shi, W., Saeed, A.A., Wu, S., Wang, H.: Real-time indoor 3D human imaging based on MIMO radar sensing. In: 2019 IEEE International Conference on Multimedia and Expo (ICME), pp. 1408–1413. IEEE (2019)
4. Karlen, W., et al.: Improving the accuracy and efficiency of respiratory rate measurements in children using mobile devices. PloS One **9**(6), e99266 (2014)
5. Lee, Y.S., Pathirana, P.N., Steinfort, C.L., Caelli, T.: Monitoring and analysis of respiratory patterns using microwave doppler radar. IEEE J. Transl. Eng. Health Med. **2**, 1–12 (2014)
6. Levitas, B., Matuzas, J., Drozdov, M.: Detection and separation of several human beings behind the wall with UWB radar. In: 2008 International Radar Symposium, pp. 1–4. IEEE (2008)
7. Li, W., Tan, B., Piechocki, R.J.: Non-contact breathing detection using passive radar. In: 2016 IEEE International Conference on Communications (ICC), pp. 1–6. IEEE (2016)
8. Nakano, H., Tanigawa, T., Furukawa, T., Nishima, S.: Automatic detection of sleep-disordered breathing from a single-channel airflow record. Eur. Resp. J. **29**(4), 728–736 (2007)
9. Patil, S.P., Schneider, H., Schwartz, A.R., Smith, P.L.: Adult obstructive sleep apnea: pathophysiology and diagnosis. Chest **132**(1), 325–337 (2007)
10. Pereira, J., et al.: Breath analysis as a potential and non-invasive frontier in disease diagnosis: an overview. Metabolites **5**(1), 3–55 (2015)
11. Ram, S.S., Li, Y., Lin, A., Ling, H.: Doppler-based detection and tracking of humans in indoor environments. J. Franklin Inst. **345**(6), 679–699 (2008)
12. Rudrappa, M., Modi, P., Bollu, P.C.: Cheyne Stokes Respirations. StatPearls [Internet]. StatPearls Publishing, St. Petersburg (2020)
13. Strollo, P.J., Jr., Rogers, R.M.: Obstructive sleep apnea. New Engl. J. Med. **334**(2), 99–104 (1996)
14. Wang, C.W., Hunter, A., Gravill, N., Matusiewicz, S.: Unconstrained video monitoring of breathing behavior and application to diagnosis of sleep apnea. IEEE Trans. Biomed. Eng. **61**(2), 396–404 (2013)
15. Welte, T., Vogelmeier, C., Papi, A.: COPD: early diagnosis and treatment to slow disease progression. Int. J. Clin. Pract. **69**(3), 336–349 (2015)

16. Yamaoka-Tojo, M.: Is it possible to distinguish patients with terminal stage of heart failure by analyzing their breathing patterns? oscillatory breathing as a manifestation of poor prognosis in advanced heart failure. Int. Heart J. **59**(4), 674–676 (2018)
17. Yang, K.I., Kim, D.E., Koo, B.B.: Obstructive apnea with pseudo-cheyne-stokes breathing. Sleep Med. **7**(16), 891–893 (2015)
18. Yang, Z., Bocca, M., Jain, V., Mohapatra, P.: Contactless breathing rate monitoring in vehicle using UWB radar. In: Proceedings of the 7th International Workshop on Real-World Embedded Wireless Systems and Networks, pp. 13–18 (2018)

Body-Area Sensing in Maternity Care: Evaluation of Commercial Wristbands for Pre-birth Stress Management

Anna Nordin[1]([✉]) [iD], Karin Ängeby[3] [iD], and Lothar Fritsch[2] [iD]

[1] Karlstad University, Karlstad, Sweden
Anna.Nordin@kau.se
[2] Oslo Metropolitan University, Oslo, Norway
Lothar.Fritsch@OsloMET.no
[3] County Council of Värmland, Karlstad, Sweden
karin.angeby@regionvarmland.se

Abstract. Many women use digital tools during pregnancy and birth. There are many existing mobile applications to measure quantity and length of contractions during early labour, but there is a need to offer evidence-based, credible electronic and digital solutions to parents-to-be. This article presents ongoing research work in a research project regarding mobile telemetric supported maternity care. It summarizes an approach for stress management in late maternity and under birth preparation that is based on body area sensing, our investigation of the properties of commercially available wearable wristbands for body sensing, and the insights gained from testing the wristbands from the project's perspective. We found that sensing precision is very variable depending on the wristband model, while the flows of medical personal data exclusively are routed through vendor cloud platforms outside the EU. The impact of our findings for the use of commercial wristbands in European medical research and practice is discussed in the conclusion.

Keywords: Midwifery · Stress management · Body area networking · Mobile health · Wearables · Self-metering

1 Introduction

The process of childbearing and giving birth is complex, both physically and psychologically. The part of early labour called latent phase is often associated with painful contractions and perceived as a part of childbirth where women experience insecurity, stress and a feeling of being left out from professional care (Ängeby et al. 2018). Women admitted to obstetrical wards during early labour are often subjected to medical interventions (Mikolajczyk et al. 2016), neonatal resuscitation and extended maternal hospital stay (Miller et al. 2020). It is common that women in the latent phase visits obstetrical ward only to be sent home to await a more established labour. Women in labour often

© ICST Institute for Computer Sciences, Social Informatics and Telecommunications Engineering 2022
Published by Springer Nature Switzerland AG 2022. All Rights Reserved
M. Ur Rehman and A. Zoha (Eds.): BODYNETS 2021, LNICST 420, pp. 168–175, 2022.
https://doi.org/10.1007/978-3-030-95593-9_14

experience this as stressful and as a rejection from health care (Eri et al. 2015). Health care staff also experience stress when meeting women's needs in early labour (Eri et al. 2011). The wish for a positive birth experience is clearly prominent in literature (Downe et al. 2018) and in 2018, the World Health Organization issued a guideline raising positive birth experience as critical aspect during intra-partum care of high quality (WHO 2018).

2   Stress Reduction Project Vision

During the 20th century, women's birthplace moved from homes to hospital, and women's support from family during all phases of labor ceased. The emotional health and wellbeing of women during childbirth is equally of worth as the medical objectives according to the World Health Organization (WHO). Swedish maternity healthcare has focused on a positive birth experience as an important outcome (SALAR 2016). Women and their partners often feel stressed and omitted in early labor. They demand more support in the form of knowledge and strategies for pain management. The amount of information is extensive but the massive range of information makes it difficult to screen for the women. The amount of mobile applications to measure quantity and length of contractions during early labour is extensive, but with a main focus only in counting time in, and frequency of, contractions (Lupton and Pedersen 2016). The Give Birth Without Fear method was developed by physiotherapists and midwifes with the aim to offer women tools to give birth with confidence. Through a salutogenetic perspective, the method helps the woman to use her own body and mind to reduce stress and fear which inhibits the release of hormones important for labour. The four tools in the method; Breathing, Relaxation, the Voice and the Power of the Mind rests on knowledge of physiology and the importance of support during labour and enables the body's relaxation and release of the peace and calm hormone oxytocin. The Give Birth Without Fear method have been used by tens of thousands of women and it is also applied internationally in healthcare with the nursing model Confident Birth aiming to reduce stress and fear (Heli 2013). The Give Birth Without Fear method was further developed in a process where technicians, women, and their partners participated. From this work, the application called Contraction Coper was developed. The need of digital services for becoming parents got even more evident during the covid-19 pandemic since all parental education were canceled in Swedish primary health care and this further underlines the need of scientific evaluation of the Contraction Coper. A forthcoming project will examine the effect of Contraction Coper application on pregnant women's perceived concerns and stress during pregnancy and birth in a randomized controlled study. Subgroup analyses will be performed using wristband to measure heartrate, sleep, and activity as a proxy for discomfort since pain during contractions causes increase of pulse, sleep-arousal and change of bodily activities. Women and partners use digital tools to keep their bodily changes and the baby during pregnancy. The number of applications, wearable technology, and the uncertainty in scientific underpinning among many of them calls for mobile applications with scientific development and evaluation. As a feasibility study of the effects of wearable technology on stress during pregnancy, early labour and childbirth, the aim was to evaluate six wristbands regarding specifications, functionality, digital privacy, and integrity as well as technical implementation.

3   Technological View on Body Sensing with Wristbands

Our prototype will build a Body-Area-Network (BAN) with remote connectivity and with user interaction. illustrates the technological components. A BAN of one or more sensors connected through a smartphone serving as a data hub will provide the sensing and feedback unit for the pregnant woman (Fig. 1). The hub collects and stores sensor data and captures data steams for stress indicators and activities that will get analyzed. The data then is transferred to the research database. The user may receive feedback and suggestions for stress-reducing activities if healthcare providers offer interactive feedback. Statistics over stress indicators, collected from body sensing, can be presented to the user, together with suggestions for interactive stress reduction exercises.

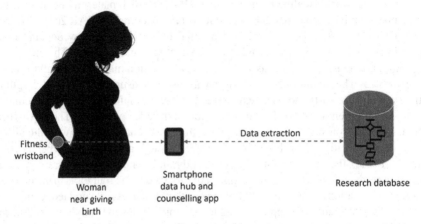

Fig. 1.   Body-area network (BAN) and IoT network for envisioned relaxation application.

3.1   Data Architecture

Since the goal of the project is research and development of effective stress-reduction measures, the data collection architecture is likely to get implemented in hybrid ways: Collection and feedback can partially get performed on the smartphone device that serves as the data hub. On the other hand, the health researcher will need access to a more in-depth picture of the patient's stress signals, as well as the captured control data over actual stress-reducing exercise efforts. Medical researchers involved in development may perform additional analysis of the generated data. Due to the data being medical personal data, its handling will need a solid privacy design, de-personalization routines and sufficient levels of secrecy deployed to data storages. Types of data captured from the users are:

- **Personal data processed** from **health system:** Patient identification; relevant medical data from patient journals, relevant background on pregnancy
- **Personal data collected from user and user sensors:** Location through GPS and location services; Movement through accelerometer sensors; Pulse rates (through

pulse sensing); Other sensor readings from wearables (potentially skin conductivity, temperature, humidity, EEG); Direct information collected from GUI with user interaction (surveys on well-being, stress, etc.)

- **Personal data derived from data using the above measurements or health APIs from sensor and wearable vendors:** Calories used during exercise; Quality of sleep metrics; Quantification metrics for activity, such as step counting and others; Psychometrics based on survey responses.

3.2 Other Requirements for Wearables

Wearables used by pregnant women need to fulfil requirements to be considered reliable and safe enough. Parameters of interest are: Reliability and precision of sensing and activity tracking functionality under different activities; Battery lifetime and charging cycle for each wearable; Comfort as well as feasibility of wearing; including adjustable straps or mounting; including waterproofness of wearables; Potential release of unhealthy substances from materials used to build devices; Usability of device, of its user interface, of charging procedure by human under stress.

3.3 Considerations in the Area of Software Engineering

For production, deployment and maintenance of the planned mobile wearable application, a number of requirements from the software engineering perspective will be necessary to consider: The wearables provide sufficient interfaces or APIs for data access and data extraction as well as developer support; Derived data as well as raw data is accessible, either directly from the device or through sufficiently rich cloud APIs; Information security and information privacy are sufficient for handling personal medical information. In summary, the BAN must fulfil requirements towards data quality, reliability, usability, safety, information security, information and data privacy, as well as technical and integration aspects in order to be considered in the project.

4 Evaluation of Commercial Wristbands

For a research prototype, a body-area network composed of commercial pulse measurement wristbands connected to a smartphone is targeted. For this purpose, seven commercially available wristbands were chosen for evaluation: Huawei band 4, Garmin Vivosport, Garmin Vivofit 4, Garmin Vivosmart 4, Samsung Galaxy Fit E, Xiaomi smartband 5, Fitbit companion. The Fitbit device did not arrive and was therefore excluded. Evaluation focused on: Accessible data from measurements, ease of technical integration, data flows, data protection, data sharing. Precision and battery features were assessed. The device evaluation was done in a student project in fall 2020 at Karlstad University (Zaman et al. 2021) that was supervised by the authors.

4.1 Technical Qualities, Sensors and Reliability

The technical features and precision of data delivered was evaluated. Activities were carried out with the wristbands to assess data quality. The bands were equipped with a variety of sensors, as shown in Table 1. Pulse sensor and accelerometer are present in all bands. Derived data is generated in the vendor's supporting cloud services. The portfolio of derived data is diverse. Data includes pace, elevation, calories used, stroke recognition, route tracking, weight tracking and fat-burning counter.

Table 1. Available sensors

	Huawei Band 4	Xiaomi Mi 5	Samsung Galaxy Fit E	Garmin Vi-vosmart 4	Garmin Vi-vosport	Garmin Vivofit 4
Pulse	Yes	Yes	Yes	Yes	Yes	No
GPS	No	No	No	No	Yes	No
Blood oxygen	Yes	No	No	No	Yes	No
Accelerometer	Yes	Yes	Yes	Yes	Yes	Yes
Barometer	No	Yes	No	Yes	Yes	No
Gyroscope	Yes	Yes	No	No	No	No

Pulse measurements were controlled with manual pulse counting with stop watches after a period of activity. The test group found error margins for pulse for Garmin Vivosmart 4 when the person was moving quick. Up to 25% error for the Huawei band were noticed. On average, a deviation of 10–20% between manual pulse rate and wristband pulse rates was observed. Most bands count too high, while Samsung's Fit E counted a few percent too low. Bands were worn on left and right arms respectively. They seemed to work on both arms equally with their respective error margins. For detailed tables with experimental data, see (Zaman et al. 2021).

Accelerometer-based step counting has its pitfalls, too. While all bands get the overall number of steps walked counted with a small error margin, their estimation of the distance walked is unreliable. Only Garmin Vivosport had built-in GPS, providing better total distance walked.

Battery lifetime varied considerably. Table 2 shows the battery life times. The longest time was 7 days. Charging periods were 1–2 h. Garmin's Vivofit 4 has a build-in non-chargeable battery with a projected lifetime of one year.

Sleep quality measurements were carried out by wearing several wristbands at the same time, while keeping notes of sleep interruptions and sleep/wakeup time in a log, which then was compared to the wristband's reports. A rating scale from 1 to 5 was used to judge precision, as well as how informative the sleep quality report was. The result is shown in Table 3. Capture of wake/sleep states was of varied precision. The sleep quality reports were perceived as partially useful.

Table 2. Battery lifetime of wristbands (charging time in hours in brackets)

Huawei Band 4	Garmin Vivosport	Garmin Vivosmart 4	Garmin Vivofit 4	Samsung Fit E	Xiaomi Mi5
7 (2)	4 (2)	6 (2)	365 (−)	4 (2)	5 (2)

Table 3. Result of assessment of sleep monitoring, scale 1–5. Best score: 5.

Type	Xiaomi Mi 5	GarminVivosoft 4	Samsung Galaxy Fit E	GarminVivosport	Huawei Band 4	GarminVivosmart
Accuracy	4.5	2.5	3	5	4	3.5
Informativity	4	1	3	4	5	4

Other Assessments. Waterproofness was one precondition for wearables. All wristbands were exposed to everyday situations exposing them to water (shower, dish washing). All function correct, however touch screens did not work correctly until completely dry. The impact of liquids on the quality of pulse measurements was not assessed. Comfort of wearing versus reliability of measurements was only inspected superficially, since for most bands a certain way of wearing must be considered for their functioning.

4.2 Ease of Integration

Wristband vendors provide proprietary APIs for integration. All except Xiaomi provided development partner programs that govern and regulate access to APIs. Huawei did not answer to access requests in both Sweden and Norway. Samsung provides access through its health API. Garmin provided educational access. Garmin's architecture enables callback access through a server callback URL. Huawei facilitates access through the Health Kit API. Samsung lists a health SDK that provides registered partners access to Samsung's Health Data Store at the Samsung Health Cloud. Conditions for API access are different for each vendor. Their expectation is a signed developer contract with non-disclosure agreement to access the cloud APIs. Data extraction is done through cloud APIs, not directly from the bands. Garmin and Huawei's architectures expect callback URLs in order to deliver data through HTTP requests to a custom application server. The APIs are based on established web technologies. Their technical integration, at least for the two aforementioned vendors, should not pose problems. The detailed functioning of the Samsung API could not get evaluated.

4.3 Data Protection and Data Sharing

Mapping the data flows of sensitive medical personal data was one of the goals of our evaluation. The privacy policies were inspected. The findings were that Samsung, Huawei and Garmin all address European regulation and GDPR compliance in their policies, however to varying degrees. Xiaomi defines the location of legal disputes as China, even though they reference GDPR as compliance framework for personal data. Privacy policies are written for various mobile products, not specifically for the wristbands. They hardly define storage location or storage period of the collected data. Various channels for data subject intervention are mentioned, often as e-mail addresses. Personal data is indexed by wristband device ID, by smartphone identity data (which can deliver many identity attributes, see (Momen and Fritsch 2020)), and through accounts on vendor cloud platforms. Platforms provide interfaces to fitness monitoring social media platforms, which can cross-reference tracking data. Overall, from a medical privacy perspective, it will be a demanding task to secure wristband tracking data on its way through the platform ecosystem of the respective vendor that is distributed onto servers outside the domain of Europe's GDPR, as sensitive medical data is seldom permitted stored outside the EU by local regulators. Alternative strategies, such as the registration of pseudonymous user profiles and accounts must be considered, as well as the sanitization person-relatable data, such as GPS location. Regarding information security, the products only provide very basic security. Transmission security with SSL/TLS, API software tokens and password authentication are the technologies used. No multi-factor authentication, no end-user cryptography, no data authentication or integrity protection beyond transport security was visible in the documentation. The wristband products do not seem to have been developed with a medical privacy context in mind. Our findings are consistent with a detailed report by Canadian privacy researchers (Hilts et al. 2016).

5   Conclusion

Our evaluation of commercial wristbands arrives at several important conclusions. First, the precision of sensor measurements has a considerable error margin, which must get evaluated for its implications for the stress management supervision context. While wristbands were powered over several days, and generally robust and waterproof, their quality of derived data such as sleep quality had a wide spectrum of precision.

Data access is provided through the vendors' respective cloud platforms. Data cannot directly get accessed from the wearables. Therefore, vendor apps must get installed on smartphones, which then push the apps to the vendor tracking cloud platform. There, derived data is generated, and APIs provide access to apps and fitness tracking platforms. We did not notice any specific functionality for the management of medical privacy. Software development support was available for most vendors. Garmin's equipment was most accessible for software development. Generally, vendors were looking for large-scale partners rather than development projects or experimental access to their software platforms. The platforms appear being planned for a larger ecosystem of consumer devices getting developed around them. Functionality envisions data sharing with fitness tracking social media platforms. A more thorough analysis of the privacy consequences of such architectural features must be done before experimenting with medical data. A negative finding was the cloud-based data access options for all evaluated wristbands. This causes major data protection issues, as personal data, and potentially sensitive medical data, is exported to 3rd-country cloud storage. Therefore, the body-area network architecture would either need audited data processor agreements, or cloud servers hosted in Europe. None of the commercial wristbands offered this option in their documentation. We need therefore resume our search for wearables that are both matured consumer-safe products and offer direct access to the data.

Acknowledgement. The work leading to this publication was funded through the Digital Well Research project by Region Värmland, Sweden.

References

Ängeby, K., Sandin-Bojö, A.-K., Persenius, M., Wilde-Larsson, B.: Early labour experience questionnaire: psychometric testing and women's experiences in a Swedish setting. Midwifery **64**, 77–84 (2018)

Mikolajczyk, R.T., Zhang, J., Grewal, J., Chan, L.C., Petersen, A., Gross, M.M.: Early versus late admission to labor affects labor progression and risk of cesarean section in nulliparous women. Front. Med. **3**, 26 (2016). https://doi.org/10.3389/fmed.2016.00026

Miller, Y., Armanasco, A., McCosker, L., Thompson, R.: Variations in outcomes for women admitted to hospital in early versus active labour: an observational study. BMC Preg n. Childbirth **20**, 469 (2020). https://doi.org/10.1186/s12884-020-03149-7

Eri, T.S., Bondas, T., Gross, M.M., Janssen, P.A., Green, J.M.: A balancing act in an unknown territory: a metasynthesis of first-time mothers' experiences in early labour. Midwifery **31**(3), e58–e67 (2015). https://doi.org/10.1016/j.midw.2014.11.007

Eri, T.S., Blystad, A., Gjengedal, E., Blaaka, G.: 'Stay home for as long as possible': Midwives' priorities and strategies in communicating with first-time mothers in early labour. Midwifery **27**(6), e286–e292 (2011)

Downe, S., Finlayson, K., Oladapo, O., Bonet, M., Gülmezoglu, A.M.: What matters to women during childbirth: a systematic qualitative review. PLoS ONE **13**(4), 1–17 (2018)

WHO recommendations: intrapartum care for a positive childbirth experience. Geneva: World Health Organization: Licence: CC BY-NC-SA 3.0 IGO (2018)

Sveriges Kommuner och Regioner (SALAR): Förlossningsvård och kvinnors hälsa i fokus. E. Estling. Sveriges Kommuner och Landsting, Stockholm (2016)

Lupton, D., Pedersen, S.: An Australian survey of women's use of pregnancy and parenting apps. Women Birth **29**(4), 368–375 (2016)

Heli, S.: Confident Birth: Pinter & Martin Publishers, London (2013)

Zaman, S., Tunc, E., Bahmiary, D.: Wristband evaluation. techical report, 55 pages, Karlstad University, Faculty of Health, Science and Technology, Sweden (2021). http://urn.kb.se/res olve?urn=urn:nbn:se:kau:diva-83399

Momen, N., Fritsch, L.: App-generated digital identities extracted through an droid permission-based data access a survey of app privacy. In: Reinhardt, D., Langweg, H., Witt, B.C., Fischer, M. (Hrsg.) SICHERHEIT 2020, pp. 15–28. Gesellschaft für Informatik e.V., Bonn (2020). https://doi.org/10.18420/sicherheit2020_01

Hilts, A., Parsons, C., Knockel, J.: Every Step You Fake: A Comparative Anal ysis of Fitness Tracker Privacy and Security. Open Effect Report (2016). https://openeffect.ca/reports/Every_Step_You_Fake.pdf

Home-Based Pulmonary Rehabilitation of COPD Individuals Using the Wearable Respeck Monitor

D. K. Arvind$^{(\boxtimes)}$, T. Georgescu, C. A. Bates, D. Fischer, and Q. Zhou

Centre for Speckled Computing, School of Informatics, University of Edinburgh, Edinburgh, Scotland, UK
dka@ed.ac.uk

Abstract. Patients with Chronic Obstructive Pulmonary Disease (COPD) are advised to perform pulmonary rehabilitation exercises regularly to help manage their long-term condition. This paper describes a home-based pulmonary rehabilitation system comprising of the Respeck respiratory and physical activity monitor and a mobile App. The Respeck is a wireless sensor device worn as a plaster on the chest that monitors continuously the respiratory rate (breaths/minute) and respiratory effort/flow, and the intensity of physical activity during the rehabilitation exercises. A pulmonary rehabilitation application on the mobile device orchestrates the daily pulmonary rehabilitation exercises and harvests the respiratory and physical activity data during the exercises for onward transmission to the server for storage and analysis. This paper describes the design of an end-to-end system for guided self-management. A method is described for relating the Respeck respiratory data to the self-administered COPD Assessment Test (CAT) score reflecting the individual's self-assessment of their condition.

Keywords: Wearable sensors · Wireless respiratory monitoring · Home-based pulmonary rehabilitation · Machine learning

1 Introduction

Chronic Obstructive Pulmonary Disease (COPD) is an umbrella term for respiratory conditions such as emphysema, chronic bronchitis and upper airways obstruction. In 2015, 3·2 Million (M) people (95% uncertainty interval [UI] 3·1M to 3·3M) died from COPD worldwide, an increase of 11·6% (95% UI 5·3 to 19·8) compared with 1990. From 1990 to 2015, the prevalence of COPD increased by 44·2% (41·7% to 46·6%) [1]. The national prevalence of COPD in European countries ranges between 0.2% to 28%. This wide range could be due to a number of reasons: real differences in prevalence between countries and the use of different methods of diagnosis. The top-5 countries in Western Europe with patients diagnosed as living with COPD are: France – 3.5M; UK – 3M; Germany – 2.7M; Italy – 2.6M; Spain – 1.5M; Belgium – 0.4M [2].

© ICST Institute for Computer Sciences, Social Informatics and Telecommunications Engineering 2022
Published by Springer Nature Switzerland AG 2022. All Rights Reserved
M. Ur Rehman and A. Zoha (Eds.): BODYNETS 2021, LNICST 420, pp. 176–191, 2022.
https://doi.org/10.1007/978-3-030-95593-9_15

In the UK projections until 2030 indicate that the number of COPD patients will increase by 39% in England and by 17% in Scotland, *i.e.*, 0.95M (95% uncertainty interval 0.94M–0.96M) in 2011 to 1.3M (1.1–1.4M) in 2030; for Scotland, the estimate is 0.10M (0.10–0.11M) people with diagnosed COPD in 2011, increasing to 0.12M (0.11–0.13M) in 2030 [3].

The direct healthcare costs for COPD can be divided into maintenance costs for the care of COPD patients and the additional costs for moderate to severe exacerbations. Between 2011–2030, the costs of COPD in England will rise by £800 Million from £1.5 Billion in 2011 to £2.3 Billion in 2030; similarly, the rise in costs in Scotland is projected to increase by £48 Million from £159 Million in 2011 to £207 Million in 2030. We have established that COPD is a financial burden for the healthcare system in European countries which is projected to rise at least until 2030 [3].

COPD is generally caused by smoking, long-term severe asthma, and environmental conditions, such as extended exposure to airborne particulate matter, and fumes from biomass burning for cooking and heating [4]. COPD sufferers experience wheezing, breathlessness, and complications due to pneumonia which affects their quality of life and productivity at work [5].

COPD is a chronic condition and number of steps can be taken by subjects to manage their condition. These include methods to improve breathing and alleviate breathlessness using abdominal breathing exercises, and a physical exercise programme called pulmonary rehabilitation (PR) to improve muscle strength and lung fitness. The 2016 update of quality standard from the UK National Institute for Health and Care Excellence (NICE) recommended that post-exacerbation patients should be offered a PR programme within four weeks of their hospital discharge to aid in restoring functional performance of the respiratory system, resuming every-day physical activities, improving quality of life, and reducing the risk of re-hospitalisation due to relapse [6].

PR involves a six-week course of weekly supervised group exercise classes and nutrition advice. It is important that the COPD patients also exercise at home in between the classes, and continue them regularly beyond the six-week course [7]. The resulting increase in aerobic performance through endurance training and daily physical activity is known to lead to improvements in their quality of life [7].

This paper describes a PR system comprising of a wearable sensor device and an Android App: the 3-axis accelerometer-based Respeck device [8] validated in clinical trials [9, 10] worn as a patch on the chest monitors the respiratory rate and respiratory effort, and the intensity of physical exercises during PR [11]; the Android application (the Rehab App) on the phone orchestrates the exercises and collects and transmits the anonymized subject data to the server using WiFi or mobile internet. The Care Team of community respiratory nurses, pulmonary physiotherapists and general practitioners have access to the key to the subject's personal information and can view up-to-date status on the subject via the dashboard in a password-protected secure website. The PR system is one component of a larger COPD care package which employs machine learning algorithms running on the GoogleCloud server to analyse the continuous, minute-level Respeck data for patterns in breathing and activity levels which could forecast deterioration in the patient's condition leading to exacerbation and possible hospitalisation. The aim is for the Care Team to intervene in a timely fashion to arrest deterioration and avoid hospitalization, and manage the patients in the comfort of their home.

The PR system has the following objectives: (i) to enable patients to perform their PR exercises daily at home and at a time of their convenience; (ii) to inform the Care Team on a dashboard that their charges are complying with the exercise regime; (iii) to establish the relationship between the COPD Assessment Test (CAT) [12] reflecting the individual's perceived condition and the breathing data from the Respeck device.

The novel contributions of this paper are: the implementation of a home-based pulmonary rehabilitation system using a combination of a wearable Respeck device and an Android App, and relating the COPD subject's respiratory data with their CAT score.

2 Related Work

The adherence to the PR programme is an issue of concern to researchers and healthcare professionals [13, 14]. Keating *et al.* used qualitative methods to study the experiences of PR uptake or lack of it#, by interviewing 19 COPD patients who had declined to participate in a PR program, and the 18 COPD patients who had dropped out of their programme [15]. The lack of perceived benefits and transport considerations were major issues for the patients. Other factors were lack of self-confidence due to fear of being breathless and exacerbation of existing medical conditions, and the role of the referring physician and the healthcare team of physiotherapists and respiratory nurses in encouraging the patient to adhere with the PR regime.

The PR system presented in this paper addresses these issues squarely. A home-based PR system removes the need for COPD subjects to travel to the clinics as they can exercise in the comfort of their home at a time of their choosing. Up-to-date information is shared, lack of exercise sessions is flagged and the Care Team can make inquires on the patient's condition and reasons for non-compliance. The patients can also gain comfort that the Respeck data collected during the exercises, such as the elevation of respiratory rate after an exercise and the resting time between exercises could provide early warning in deterioration in their condition.

Vela *et al.* [16] emphasise the need to understand the patients' heterogeneities and co-morbidities such as cardiovascular diseases, Type 2 diabetes, metabolic syndrome, anxiety, and depression. The design of the PR system allows customisation of the exercise sessions to suit their conditions on the day and taking account of their co-morbidities.

3 Pulmonary Rehabilitation System

The primary function of the home-based PR system is to guide the patients to perform the exercises regularly. There are four main components: the Respeck respiratory and physical activity monitor (Fig. 1); the Android phone and App; the cloud-based server; and, the Dashboard, as illustrated in Fig. 2. The application running on a smartphone or a tablet (for patients with tremor in their fingers who will require a larger surface for the user interface) orchestrates the exercises with animations and voice instructions to illustrate the exercises which the patients mimic. Secondly, up-to-date information on the COPD patient's condition is required to be shared with the Care Team. This is achieved by the wireless Respeck respiratory and physical activity monitor (Fig. 1) worn as an adhesive patch on the chest during the PR exercises.

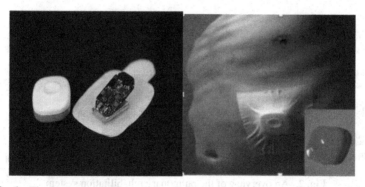

Fig. 1. The Respeck wireless monitor (left) worn as a plaster on the chest (right).

The Respeck device contains a three-axis accelerometer operating at 12.5 Hz, a 32-bit ARM processor for on-board processing of the sensor data, and a Bluetooth 4.0 radio for communicating with the mobile phone. It has been designed for continuous wear with minimal intervention from the patient. It is turned on continuously; the data is transmitted automatically to the mobile device using store-and-forward methods; low energy design ensures that the battery can run for a period of 4–6 months of continuous operation before recharging the device overnight using a wireless charger.

Data from the Respeck device is uploaded wirelessly to the server in real-time and analysed to provide the Care Team with up-to-date information on the conformance to the exercise regime in terms of frequency of exercise sessions, and the respiratory health condition (trends in respiratory rate) of their cohort. This enables the Care Team to prioritise their resources in a timely fashion for those who need them. Thirdly, the PR system addresses the important issue of extending the reach of the Care Team to provide remote observation of COPD patients without invading their privacy.

3.1 The Apps

Figure 3 illustrates the four main component Android applications: the Pairing App, the AirRespeck App, the Pulmonary Rehabilitation App, and, the Diary Application; and, the Respeck sensor device worn as a plaster on the chest of the COPD individual.

The Pairing App. The Pairing App associates the Respeck device of the subject and their unique personal identifier with the phone running the Pulmonary rehab application. This ensures that the data sent from the phone is tagged with the subject identifier during the course of the transfer to the Server, storage and future analysis. All the data is annotated with this unique identifier. This ensures that no personal information is stored on the server to ensure patient anonymity and adherence to the General Data Protection Regulation (GDPR). Only the Care Team has the key to relate the unique identifier to the subject's name and medical records on a need-to-know basis.

The AirRespeck Application. The AirRespeck App handles the secure and reliable transfer wirelessly of respiratory rate/flow extracted from the accelerometer sensor data in the Respeck device and its display in the App and onward transmission to the server.

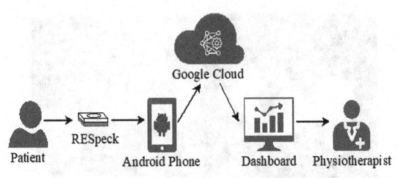

Fig. 2. An overview of the pulmonary rehabilitation system

The live data received from the Respeck is also forwarded to the Rehab application via a Broadcast.

The Pulmonary Rehabilitation (Rehab) Application. The Rehab Application on the mobile device orchestrates the rehabilitation exercises, both visually using animations and aurally via a voice interface for COPD individuals who tend to be elderly with deteriorating visual and aural faculties. The exercises are interspersed with resting periods for the patients to recover their breath. The rates of recovery of the breathing rate after each exercise recorded over several rehab sessions are used to characterise changes in the patient's condition over time and provide insights to the Care Team. In summary, the data from the App confirms whether the patient is conforming to the exercise regime, and provides assessment of the patient's well-being. The Rehab App enables patients to customise the exercise regime by choosing from the list of 10 exercises and selecting their durations. After the exercise selection, an animation of the current exercise is displayed, illustrating the correct way of performing the exercise. After finishing each exercise the patient is invited to rest until their breathing recovers and during this period their "quiet breathing at rest" is collected. The breathing rates and the rest times between each exercise are collected for each session. At the end of an exercise session, the patient can view their average breathing rate during the resting periods in comparison with previous sessions. All the exercise session statistics are returned to the AirRespeck App and uploaded to the server for analysis and the results displayed on the dashboard for the Care Team.

The Diary Application. COPD Assessment Test (CAT) [12] captures the patient's perception of their condition as recorded in the Diary App. It contains 8 questions with 6 possible answers with scores attached for each question - 0 being the best score and 5 being the worst. The scores are then aggregated to report a final CAT score: higher the score, the worse was the patient's self-assessment of their condition. The score is transmitted back to the AirRespeck App, which uploads it to the server to be displayed alongside the exercise data to the Care Team. Figure 4 illustrates the CAT scores for a COPD individual over a period of 6 months.

The Server. The server receives respiratory rate data from Airespeck App on the phone every minute, which is stored in the Google Datastore. It also contains the raw accelerometer data uploaded manually from the subject's phone by the healthcare team. The raw data can be analysed for classifying a larger range of physical activity recognition using more computationally intensive machine learning models than can be afforded on the phones.

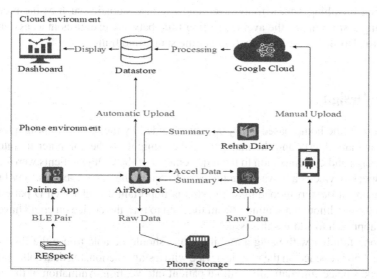

Fig. 3. Components of the pulmonary rehabilitation system.

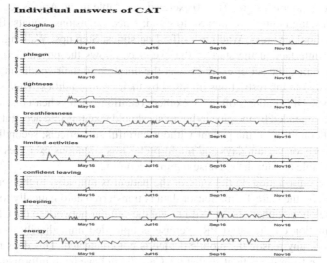

Fig. 4. The individual scores for the CAT questions for a single COPD subject for a period of 6 months.

The Dashboard. The continuous minute-averaged breathing data and PR data processed on the phone and automatically uploaded to the server, and the manually-uploaded raw data are displayed on a password-protected dashboard which can be viewed only by the Care Team personnel. The dashboard shows time-series data of the continuous monitoring breathing rate, activity level, and exercise statistics such as the breathing rate during resting times, the average resting time between exercises in a session. The dashboard also shows the CAT scores over the same time frame.

4   The Design

The design of the home-based PR system was guided by the following principles. The target users are elderly and the majority of them might not be computer literate. The ease of usage and customisation to the requirements of the COPD patients were central. The Respeck device is always on and does not require the patient to press any buttons to start using it or start uploading data. This is important as older COPD patients are likely to forget although a reminder from the App to turn the device on could have been another approach to address this issue.

Anyone familiar with using a mobile phone should be able to use the PR system. Once the App is opened on the mobile device with a single action, the data collection and upload takes place automatically without patient intervention. Animation of the current exercise reminds the user with a countdown to time the exercise. All visual information is also conveyed by a voice interface which calls out the exercises and counts down for patients with poor eyesight. The 10 exercises available in the App as recommended by the British Lung Foundation are: Sit to stand; Knee extensions; Squats; Heel raises; Bicep curls; Shoulder press; Wall push offs; Leg slides; Step ups; Walking. As shown in Fig. 5, the interface at the start of the exercises allows the physiotherapist or the patient to customise the set of exercises, set the duration to their condition on the day and personalise it to the restrictions imposed by their co-morbidities. This is important on two counts: COPD patients often have other conditions such as heart disease and any exercises recommended by the physiotherapists should take this into account and attend to the overall condition of the patient without harmful side-effects; secondly, patients might feel poorly on certain days and might prefer less strenuous exercises on the day and should be able to alter the exercise regime accordingly.

Up-to-date information on the state of the patient is uploaded to the server which can be viewed by the Care Team. Sensor data is transferred automatically to the server via the mobile phone either via the WiFi or via the cellular network to the Cloud-based server. Information on the latest PR exercise is uploaded immediately or stored and forwarded if for any reason the mobile device is not connected. This does not rely on any intervention from the patient so that the Care Team have fresh information on their cohort of patients.

The design of the home-based pulmonary rehabilitation system was guided by the requirements of the end-users and the healthcare team comprising of physiotherapists, respiratory nurses, primary care physicians and the hospital pulmonologists. A participatory approach to design was followed in which a focus group of the healthcare team

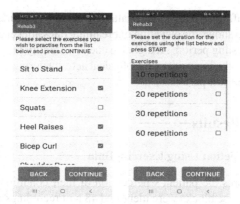

Fig. 5. Pulmonary rehabilitation app: selection of exercises and number of repetitions.

met to tease out the specification and early COPD patient users provided feedback on the design which was refined iteratively resulting in the final deployment design.

Some early adopters wanted two changes: on certain days the patients wanted to take a long walk in lieu of the exercises and wanted this facility to be included in the App design. Another set of patients wanted a dashboard at the start where they could choose which set of exercises they wanted to follow on that day and modify the period of each exercise accordingly.

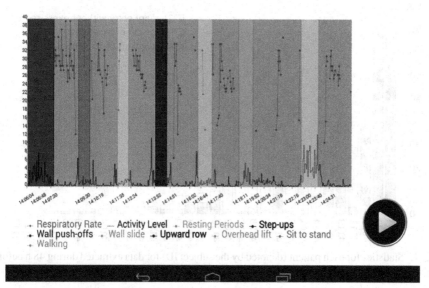

Fig. 6. A display of the recovery of the Respeck respiratory rate during the resting periods and intensity of exercise activity during pulmonary rehabilitation.

The display of information for the healthcare team was guided by their clinical requirements. Figure 6 shows the elevation of breathing rates after each exercise and their recovery during the resting period. At a glance one can identify the relative durations of the different exercises, the intensity of the physical activity during the exercises, and the duration of intervening rest periods.

5 Analysis and Results

5.1 CAT Score Prediction Using Exercise Data

The CAT score captures the patient's perception of their condition as recorded in the Diary App. Valid exercise blocks were identified 48 h of recordings around a CAT diary submission, as each CAT submission had to be associated with exactly one exercise block. In total, 20 out of the 31 investigated patients submitted diary entries with a preceding valid exercise block. Figure 7 shows the distribution of valid and invalid exercise blocks for each patient ID. The distribution of CAT scores is bimodal, with a high prevalence of high and low scores and a moderately represented middle ground, as illustrated in Fig. 8. This is due to the diary entries being consistently filled in by only a few patients which are either at the healthier end of the scale (4002, 4113) or at the unhealthy end of the scale (4019, 4103). The lack of CAT scores below 5 is explained by the fact that the study included only patients already diagnosed with COPD, and would therefore have a CAT score greater than 5.

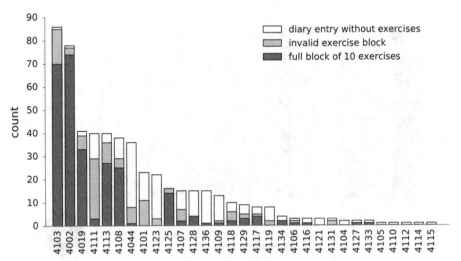

Fig. 7. Statistics for each patient (denoted by the subject ID) for data extracted during 48 h before a diary entry.

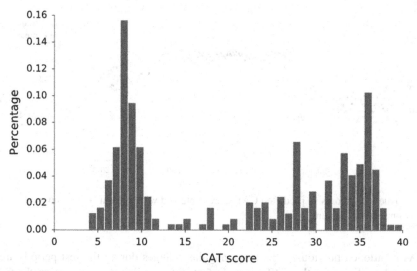

Fig. 8. The distribution of CAT scores for all diary entries succeeding a valid exercise block in a time window of 48 h.

5.1.1 Labels and Feature Extraction

The following hypothesis was formulated: the CAT score can be predicted by the features extracted from the Respeck data during the PR exercises. The features considered for this task were:

1. The diary entries to derive the CAT score
2. The respiratory rate
3. Respiratory rate recovery slopes after an exercise session
4. The length of the rest periods between exercises
5. The intensity of activity during an exercise
6. Exercise execution features, such as speed and angle changes (denoting quick and large movements).

The feature correlation was calculated using the Pearson correlation coefficient and the features were ranked by their absolute coefficient value.

The highest coefficient value (-0.84) is achieved by the mean angles during the rest periods, suggesting that healthier patients might move around more during the rest periods. Other highly correlated features are the resting time length (0.78) and the breathing rate after each exercise (0.47–0.63). The prediction baseline was set as predicting the mean CAT score of all CAT score available in the dataset. The error measures used are the mean absolute error (MAE) and the root mean-square error (RMSE). The MAE measure weighs all deviations the same, whereas RMSE penalizes larger errors quadratically more than lower ones.

The baseline results obtained from predicting the mean CAT score are 11.34 for MAE and 12.03 for RMSE.

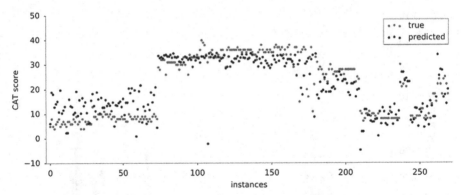

Fig. 9. True CAT scores vs predicted CAT scores obtained with a linear regression model fitted to only one activity feature.

As mentioned previously, the mean angular changes during the rest periods are a very good predictor for the CAT score. In fact, fitting a linear regression on the CAT scores using just this feature as an input can predict the labels with a MAE of 5.44 and a RMSE of 6.6, which is significantly better than the baseline, as shown in Fig. 9. The activity features during the exercise periods have a lower r-value than the activity features during rest periods, but the correlation of −0.38 for both the activity measure and angle changes during exercises suggests that healthier subjects typically perform more ample and faster movements than subjects with a worse health condition.

The length of the rest periods after each exercise had a high correlation coefficient of 0.78, suggesting that healthier patients (lower CAT scores) take a shorter time to rest between exercises. The length feature also obtained a MAE of 6.78 and a RMSE of 7.69 when used to predict the CAT score with a linear model.

The mean respiratory rate during resting periods has a correlation coefficient of 0.72 and suggests that a higher breathing rate during resting periods is an indicator of the worsening condition of a patient. Individual exercises have different average resting breathing rate measurements and our experiments show that the 'Sit to stand' exercise has the highest correlation coefficient, whereas the 'Shoulder press' exercise has the lowest correlation coefficient.

The variance of the respiratory rate is also a good predictor, with a score of 0.66, implying that patients with a more varying breathing rate report higher CAT scores.

In addition to the intuitive features discussed so far, spectra features consider the frequency components of the Respeck signal. Each spectrum covers a frequency range of about 0.05 Hz, and each exercise is decomposed in this range of frequencies. A high positive correlation value for a particular spectrum suggests that patients in a bad condition tend to move in that particular frequency range.

Figure 10 shows the distribution of frequencies for each exercise (x-axis) and their correlation coefficient (y-axis). For the walking exercise, the main frequency component is the walking speed, and the graph suggests that a speed of 0.5–1 Hz (1 step every 1 or 2 s) is highly correlated with less healthy patients. In contrast, healthy patients walk with a speed of 2 Hz (2 steps per second) up to a speed of 6 Hz (5–6 steps every second). The "sit to stand" exercise has very few positive coefficients, and the graph suggests that less healthy patients perform the movement in the 0.1–0.2 Hz category, implying one sit-to-stand motion in 5–10 s.

5.1.2 Linear Regression

As stated previously, a baseline model using solely the mean angles during the resting time feature as a predictor obtained a result of 5.64 (MAE) and 6.88 (RMSE).

The models trained on this task were an Ordinary Least Squares (OLS) regression, then included regularization factors to avoid overfitting in the Lasso Regression and Ridge Regression models. Finally, an Elastic Net was fitted to the data which contains both L1 and L2 regularisation factors.

The hyperparameter optimisation was achieved by splitting the dataset randomly into training (80%) and test (20%) sets. The training set was further split by 10-fold cross-validation. The RMSE measure used to determine the best hyperparameter for each model. Table 1 presents the results for all trained models, with reported MAE and RMSE scores on the test set. The extremely high MAE and RMSE values for OLS regression illustrate the negative effect of overfitting the data when training the model without regularisation terms.

5.1.3 Regression with Artificial Neural Networks

Regression using Artificial Neural Networks (ANN) was attempted using an ANN with one hidden layer and one unit cell for the output. The activation function for the hidden layer was chosen to be TanH for its empirically tested performance. The learning rate was set to 0.001 fixed across epochs and no regularisation terms were applied. The effect of adding more units to the hidden layer was investigated, and discovered that even the lowest values of RMSE, achieved at 3–7 units in the hidden layers, achieved worse results than the ridge regression.

Adding another hidden unit to the network proved to be beneficial, as it obtained a lower RMSE than the linear models, as shown in Fig. 11. The best performance was achieved for 40 units in the first hidden layer, and 85 units in the second hidden layer, with an RMSE of 4.144. Adding even more hidden layers only reduced the performance of the model. The RMSE and MAE performances of the 2 hidden-layer-network configuration on the test set, averaged over five runs, were 4.98 and 3.119, respectively.

To further optimise the performance, a neural network ensemble was implemented which ran the same neural network several times, with different weight initialisations, and took the mean of the individual predictions as the final prediction. Figure 12 shows the RMSE score for number of networks in the ensemble, the minimum being reached at an ensemble of 6 networks.

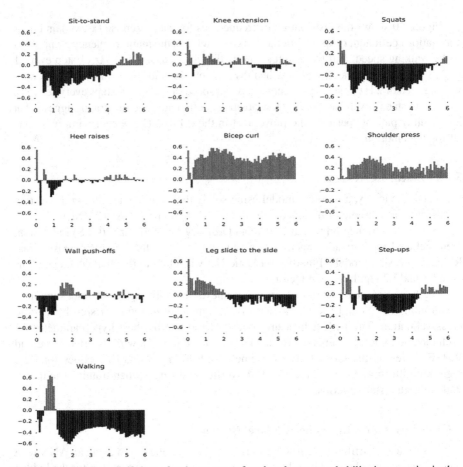

Fig. 10. Correlation coefficients for the spectra of each pulmonary rehabilitation exercise in the frequency range of 0 to 6 Hz.

Table 1. Best MAE and RMSE for the four linear regression models, reported on the test set.

Model	MAE	RMSE	Parameters
OLS	2955527104.13	3958822894.18	-
Lasso	3.83	5.19	$\alpha = 0.36$
Ridge	3.53	4.61	$\alpha = 106.5$
Elastic net	3.53	4.61	$\alpha = 0.55$, L1 ratio = 0.0

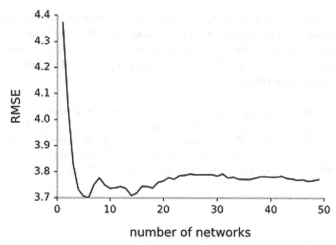

Fig. 11. RMSE for different number of networks in the ensemble when using the mean predictions of the networks

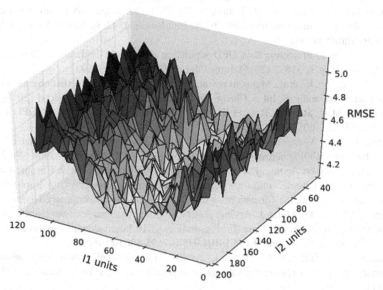

Fig. 12. RMSE for different number of units in the two hidden layers (l1 and l2).

6   Conclusion

This paper has presented a novel approach to home-based pulmonary rehabilitation. The fiscal burden of COPD on the healthcare system was established and the reasons for poor adherence has been explained. The combination of a wearable device with a mobile App provides an IoT solution which addresses the barriers to poor compliance. The design issues together with data analysis using machine learning and the display of information to the healthcare team has been described. In conclusion, the home-based pulmonary rehabilitation system helps COPD patients to perform their daily exercises at home and for the healthcare team to monitor compliance and changes in the health status of the patients using the respiratory rate from the Respeck device as the key parameter. Future work will involve the use of the Respeck and the pulmonary rehabilitation system in large scale clinical deployment.

Acknowledgements. The authors wish to thank the anonymous volunteers in the London boroughs of Sutton and Merton. The work was supported by the Centre for Speckled Computing, and co-authors TG, CAB and DF were partially supported by the following grants: EPSRC-funded INHALE project (grant EP/T003189/1), the MRC/AHRC-funded PHILAP project (grant MC_PC_MR/R024405/1), and the NERC/MRC-funded DAPHNE project (grant NE/P016340).

References

1. Global, regional, and national deaths, prevalence, disability-adjusted life years, and years lived with disability for chronic obstructive pulmonary disease and asthma, 1990–2015: a systematic analysis for the global burden of disease study 2015. Lancet **5**(9), 691–706 (2017)
2. Gibson, G.J., Loddenkemper, R., Lundbäck, B., Sibille, Y.: Respiratory health and disease in Europe: the new European lung white book. Eur. Respir. J. **42**(3), 559–563 (2013). https://www.erswhitebook.org/
3. McLean, S., et al.: Projecting the COPD population and costs in England and Scotland: 2011 to 2030. Sci. Rep. **6**, 31893 (2016). https://doi.org/10.1038/srep31893
4. Li, J., Sun, S., Tan, R., et al.: Major air pollutants and risk of COPD exacerbations: a systematic review and meta-analysis. Int. J. Chron. Obstruct Pulmon. Dis. **11**, 3079–3091 (2016)
5. Calverley, P.M.A., Stockley, R.A., et al.: Reported pneumonia in patients with COPD. CHEST **139**(3), 505–512 (2011)
6. Halpin, D.M.G., Miravitlles, M., Metzdorf, N., et al.: Impact and prevention of severe exacerbations of COPD: a review of the evidence. Int. J. COPD **12**, 2891–2908 (2017)
7. Centre for Policy on Ageing, Pulmonary Rehabilitation for patients with Chronic Obstructive Pulmonary Disease. http://www.cpa.org.uk/information/reviews/CPA-Rapid-Review-Pulmonary-Rehabilitation-for-patients-with-Chronic-Obstructive-Pumonary-Disease.pdf
8. Bates, C.A., Ling, M., Mann, J., Arvind, D.K.: Respiratory rate and flow waveform estimation from tri-axial accelerometer data. In: Proceedings 2010 International Conference on Body Sensor Networks, Singapore. IEEE. ISBN 978-0-7695-4065-8/10 (2010)
9. Drummond, G., Bates, C.A., Mann, J., Arvind, D.K.: Validation of a new non-invasive automatic monitor of respiratory rate for postoperative subjects. Br. J. Anaesth. **107**, 4629 (2011)
10. Drummond, G.B., Fischer, D., Lees, M., Bates, A., Mann, J., Arvind, D.K.: Classifying signals from a wearable accelerometer device to measure respiratory rate. ERJ Open Res. **7**(2), 00681-2020 (2021). https://doi.org/10.1183/23120541.00681-2020
11. Mann, J., Rabinovich, R., Bates, A., Giavedoni, S., MacNee, W., Arvind, D.K.: Simultaneous activity and respiratory monitoring using an accelerometer. In: Proceedings 2011 International Conference on Body Sensor Networks. BSN 2011, Dallas. IEEE (2011)
12. Dodd, J., Hogg, L., Nolan, J., et al.: The COPD assessment test (CAT): response to pulmonary rehabilitation. A multicentre, prospective study. THORAX **66**(5), 425–429 (2011)
13. Jones, S.E., Green, S.A., Clark, A.L., et al.: Pulmonary rehabilitation following hospitalisation for acute exacerbation of COPD: referrals, uptake and adherence. THORAX **69**(2), 181–182 (2014)

14. Hayton, C., Clark, A., Olive, S., et al.: Barriers to pulmonary rehabilitation: characteristics that predict patient attendance and adherence. Respir. Med. **107**(3), 401–407 (2013)
15. Keating, A., Lee, A.L.: Holland AE Lack of perceived benefit and inadequate transport influence uptake and completion of pulmonary rehabilitation in people with chronic obstructive pulmonary disease: a qualitative study. J. Physiother. **57**(3), 183–190 (2011)
16. Vela, E., Tényi, Á., Cano, I., et al.: Population-based analysis of patients with COPD in Catalonia: a cohort study with implications for clinical management. BMJ Open (2018). https://doi.org/10.1136/bmjopen-2017-017283

Data Analytics for Healthcare Systems

SVM Time Series Classification of Selected Gait Abnormalities

Jakob Rostovski$^{(\boxtimes)}$ [iD], Andrei Krivošei [iD], Alar Kuusik [iD], Ulvi Ahmadov [iD], and Muhammad Mahtab Alam [iD]

TJS Department of Electronics, Tallinn University of Technology,
Ehitajate tee 5, 19086 Tallinn, Estonia
jakob.rostovski@taltech.ee

Abstract. Gait analysis is widely used for human disability level assessment, physiotherapeutic and medical treatment efficiency analysis. Wearable motion sensors are most widely used gait observation devices today. Automated detection of gait abnormalities, namely incorrect step patterns, would simplify the long term gait assessment and enable usage of corrective measures as passive and active physiotherapeutic assistive devices. Automatic detection of gait abnormalities with wearable devices is a complex task. Support Vector Machines (SVM) driven machine learning methods are quite widely used for motion signals classification. However, it is unknown how well actual implementations work for specific gait deviations of partially disabled people. In this work we evaluate how well SVM method works for detecting specific incorrect step patterns characteristics for the most frequent neuromuscular impairments. F1 score from 66% to 100% were achieved, depending on the gait type. Gait pattern deviations were simulated by the healthy volunteers. Angular speed motion data as an input to SVM was collected with a single Shimmer S3 wearable sensor.

Keywords: Gait analysis · Machine learning · SVM · Wearable sensors · Medical applications

1 Introduction

According to World Health Organisation (WHO) report about one billion persons are affected by neurological disorders worldwide [2]. Neurological diseases ranging from migraine to stroke and Alzheimer are the leading cause of Disability Adjusted Life Years (DALY) loss [8]. For example, there is a high risk of falling down for patients with gait impairments from neurological disease [20,24]. Therefore it is important to assess neurological disease patient gait deviations and, if possible, correct step patterns using certain assistive devices. It is shown that even simple mechanical devices like ankle-foot orthoses certainly can reduce the risk of falling [27]. However, it is shown that Functional Electrical Stimulation (FES) devices that activate in proper moments corresponding muscles, are

© ICST Institute for Computer Sciences, Social Informatics and Telecommunications Engineering 2022
Published by Springer Nature Switzerland AG 2022. All Rights Reserved
M. Ur Rehman and A. Zoha (Eds.): BODYNETS 2021, LNICST 420, pp. 195–209, 2022.
https://doi.org/10.1007/978-3-030-95593-9_16

more effective for fall prevention [14] and generic gate improvements [16]. Essentially, long term gate deviation analysis and efficient run-time control of FES devices requires automated recognition of "incorrect" steps or other gate deviations. According to our previous research [22] we have concluded that Support Vector Machines (SVM) based methods are most widely used ones for automated gait analysis, followed by Convolutional Neural Networks (CNN). The benefits of SVM include capability to operate with relatively small data sets and high computational efficiency [10,11]. For human activity recognition has been reported by Almaslukh et al. [1] quite impressive accuracy, close to 97%. There are several other results indicating 90% accuracy, listed in [22]. However, there is a very limited research conducted of analysing how well machine learning methods, particularly SVM, performs in detecting realistic gait deviations, caused by actual neural diseases. Current work focuses on describing test results collected by us in this domain, that are still relying on simulated gait deviations.

Gait of each person is virtually unique. It can be described by a set of parameters such as: step length, length of individual step phases, muscle force and etc. [18]. Especially high variability and deviations from the "normal" gait pattern can be seen in persons gait, who are suffering from neuromuscular diseases [15]. Therefore it is extremely difficult to analyze patients' gate patterns. Certain diseases cause jumpy gait changes - like freezing episodes of Parkinson Disease (PD) [4], other diseases, like Multiple Sclerosis (MS) may contain long duration relapse episodes with individual impact and have slow progression [23]. From the perspectives of physiotherapists, each person has own "normal" (or target) gate that has to be used as a reference in gate assessment procedure.

Various stationary (3D camera systems), portable (pressure mats) and wearable (motion sensors) instrumental solutions are used for gait analysis. However, wearable motion sensors, containing multidimensional Inertial Motion Units (IMUs), are the most widely used gait assessment devices in the recent years [25]. IMUs are also used for gait assessment of neurological disease patients [12,19,21].

Main goal of this research work is to detect abnormality in the gait, caused by some kind of disease, as fast as possible, to prevent person from falling. Current paper proposes analysis of gait using SVM, to classify the normal and abnormal steps. Even if such a full step classification does not solve the main goal, abnormality estimation in the real-time, it will be used as pre-processing stage to produce reference set of good steps for the real-time abnormality detection algorithm. Therefore the current paper proposes time series based "good" and "bad" steps SVM classifier implementation, which is built on the *tslearn* Python library [26] and applied to the time-series gyroscope gait data, which is different from feature based SVM classification, used in other works. Thus, it is possible to compare achieved results to the feature based approach, found in other works.

This paper consist of 5 sections: after the introductory state-of-art overview in Sect. 2 the motion data collection methodology is described; in Sect. 3 proposed application of the SVM based algorithm implementation, applied to the time-series gait data, is presented; the results are presented in the Subsect. 4 and discussion and conclusion are in the Sect. 5.

2   Gait Data Collection

The fundamental part of each instrumented gait analysis is collection of human walking patterns, which provide relevant information about the gait changes of the subjects. The human gate contains of seven phases [3] (Fig. 1). The ultimate long term goal is to detect deviations of each phase separately for fastest gate corrections. However, current study focuses on classification of whole steps only.

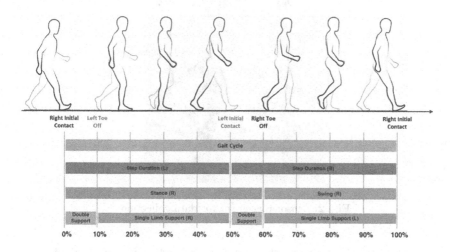

Fig. 1. The seven phases of human gait cycle [3]

During the current study, Shimmer S3 (Dublin, Ireland) wearable sensors were used for lower limb motion data capture. Sensors were configured to work 256 Hz sampling rate, measurement data was recorded on device's memory, later modulus was calculated from three-dimensional 16-bit gyroscope signal to reduce the amount of data feed to machine learning algorithm. Two different sensor placements were initially tested (Fig. 2): right below of the knee that is the location of foot drop FES devices directly stimulating the most important lower limb muscles, namely tibialis anterior and fibularis longus, and on forefoot, which is the most widely used placement of inertial sensors for gate cycle monitoring [9]. According to initial visual analysis of recorded signals, forefoot data was selected for the further analysis.

During the data collection, correct ("good") and incorrect ("bad") steps were mixed according to following procedure:

1. *Normal gait + one abnormal step*
2. *Normal gait + one abnormal step + normal gait*
3. *Normal gait + N · abnormal step + normal gait + N · abnormal step*, where $N = 0, 1, 2, 3, 4 \ldots$

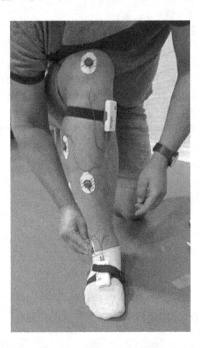

Fig. 2. Sensor placement for data collection

To add more variability to the test data, recording was performed on two types of surfaces: hard and soft (sand) surface. Each recording contains deviations of one specific disability type that is described below. Recordings were annotated using a semiautomatic tool: all correct and incorrect steps were labeled in the data file.

2.1 Data Collection of Simulated Gait Abnormalities

The ultimate goal of present study is to evaluate how well an actual SVM implementation can detect gait deviation caused by neurological impairments. Abnormalities were simulated by 2 healthy persons of different gender, both 23 years old. Simulations were replicating actual patients' videos and instructions of a professional physiotherapist. The chosen, most frequent, gait abnormalities were following:

Steppage gait - seen in patients gait with foot drop (weakness of foot dorsiflexion). This is caused due to an attempt to lift the leg high enough during walking, so that the foot does not drag on the floor [3]. This disability is most widely targeted with foot drop assistive devices.

Hemiplegic gait - includes impaired natural swing at the hip and knee with leg circumduction. The pelvis is often tilted upward on the involved side to permit adequate circumduction.

Diplegic gait - a specific subcategory of the wide spectrum of motion disorders
gathered under the name of cerebral palsy.

Ataxic gait - commonly defined as a lack of coordination in body movements or
a loss of balance, which is not due to muscle weakness.

Parkinsonian gait - is a feature of Parkinson's disease in later stages. It's often
considered to negatively impact the quality of life more than other Parkinson's
symptoms. Parkinsonian gait is usually small, shuffling steps.

Hyperkinetic gait - is seen with certain basal ganglia disorders, including Syden-
ham's chorea, Huntington's Disease, and other forms of chorea, athetosis, or
dystonia. The patient will display irregular, jerky, involuntary movements in
all extremities. Walking may accentuate their baseline movement disorder [3].

Comparative analysis of applying SVM algorithm to data is in the next
section.

3   SVM Performance Assessment

Considering that the SVM is well known in classification applications and, particularly, in gait analysis [1,5,13,17,28], this method, however, can not be used
directly with time series (output of IMU motion sensor), where the input vectors can be of different lengths (feature dimensions). Therefore, time series oriented implementation (*tslearn* [26]) of the SVM classifier (call it as tsSVM)
was selected for the current research work and applied to the human gait steps
ensemble extracted from the time series data to classify correct and anomaly
(incorrect) steps.

TsSVM implementation uses Global Alignment Kernel (GAK) [6], which
allows to apply the SVM classifier to time-series data with different duration of
samples.

The GAK is related to the soft-Dynamic Time Warping (soft-DTW) [7]
through Eq. (1), which is used to align time series samples in time. In ker-
nel equation, $\mathbf{x} = (\mathbf{x_0}, \ldots, \mathbf{x_{n-1}})$ and $\mathbf{y} = (\mathbf{y_0}, \ldots, \mathbf{y_{m-1}})$ are two time series of
respective lengths **n** and **m**. Hyper-parameter γ is related to the bandwidth
parameter σ of GAK through $\gamma = 2\sigma^2$.

$$k(x, y) = exp(\frac{softDTW_\gamma(x, y)}{\gamma}) \tag{1}$$

In Eq. (2) soft-DTW could be observed with hyper-parameter γ, that controls
smoothing of the resulting metric (squared DTW corresponds to the limit case
$\gamma \to 0$), where $(\mathbf{a_1}, \ldots, \mathbf{a_n})$ is time series.

$$soft - min_\gamma(a_1, \ldots, a_n) = -\gamma log \sum_i e^{-a_i/\gamma} \tag{2}$$

The GAK's smoothing hyper-parameter γ was experimentally chosen depending on the data set to get the best actual performance. Usually it was between 20 and 150. Tslearn toolbox was used to convert one-dimensional magnitude, calculated from gyroscope data from data set into time series with same length. Then data set was divided into training and test sets with proportion of 70% to 30% respectively. After that, training was performed and the following results were achieved.

First some preprocessing was required to be able to use the algorithm. Data was divided into individual steps, using timestamps in labels. After that they were combined into required form and normalized in duration by adding Nan's to the shorter steps. Then proper hyperparameter γ was chosen by iteration over potential numbers.

4   Results

In proposed approach 3D gyroscope angular velocity data was used as the initial input, which then was transformed into the magnitude time series format. Assuming that gyroscope axes are called gX, gY and gZ, the magnitude is calculated as in Eq. 3, where t_i is given moment of time, and normalized by Min-max feature scaling 4 for every time series instance:

$$gM(t_i) = \sqrt{gX(t_i)^2 + gY(t_i)^2 + gZ(t_i)^2} \qquad (3)$$

$$gM(t)_{norm} = \frac{gM(t) - gM(t)_{min}}{gM(t)_{max} - gM(t)_{min}} \qquad (4)$$

Calculated gyroscope magnitude time series (Eq. 3) is used as an input for the tsSVM algorithm.

To understand the results lets observe support vectors on Fig. 3 for two classes, they represent common step forms, corresponding to a particular class. For each class support vectors looks similar, only for class 2 excess vectors could be observed, what affects results. Ataxic gait test data set had 14 samples: 6 abnormal steps (positive) and 8 normal steps (negative). After training the SVM on 32 samples, two false positives were detected using test data set (Table 1).

This could have happened due to residual "abnormality" in normal steps following abnormal steps. On the Fig. 8c noisier step could be seen than the step on the Fig. 8a. Similar situation could be observed for steppage gait test 1, where there is to much deviation for normal steps (Fig. 5a and Fig. 5c), what could be considered as data collection error. This leads to misclassification of abnormal steps which result in 0% f1 score (Fig. 4). On the other hand, if normal steps are consistent, as for steppage gait test 2 (Fig. 7), classification of abnormal steps is preformed correctly and f1 score of 100% is achieved (Fig. 6).

Lets have closer look at step shapes. For example on Fig. 8a first peak represents a moment, when toe is starting to move in the end of stance phase (40%–60% of phase on Fig. 1), then it is start of a swing phase, till the second

Table 1. Classification quality for data. Where, TP is True Positive, TN is True Negative, FP is False Positive and FN is False Negative

Gait type, test number	TP	TN	FP	FN	F1 score
Ataxic, test 2	4	8	2	0	80%
Diplegic, test 1	3	7	0	0	100%
Diplegic, test 3	2	9	0	0	100%
Hemiplegic, test 2	1	9	0	1	67%
Hyperkinetic, test 2	4	8	0	2	80%
Parkinsonian, test 1	7	8	0	1	93%
Parkinsonian, test 2	6	7	1	0	92%
Steppage, test 1	0	10	0	2	*0%
Steppage, test 2	2	10	0	0	100%

*This test has bad data samples, reasons are described in results section.

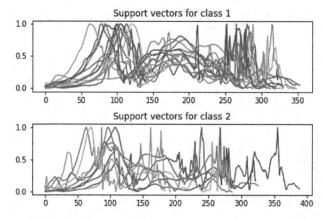

Fig. 3. Support vectors for ataxic gait, test 2. X-axis is the time [ms], Y-axis is normalized gyroscope magnitude values (see Eq. 4).

peak (60%–100%), which represents toe movement, to prepare for initial contact and third peak is, when toe lands on the ground flat (0%–20%), after that it is a stance phase between the toe movement (20%–40%). For abnormal step (Fig. 8b) clear separation between peaks is lost. According to description of ataxic gait type, clear swing phase is lost, what could be observed.

As it was mentioned above, on Fig. 8 and Fig. 10 peaks for normal and abnormal gait steps are located differently and have different amplitudes. F1 score for ataxic gait was 80% (Fig. 3) and for diplegic gait it was 100%, (Fig. 9) that shows SVM capability of classifying steps. Good results could be observed also for parkinsonian and hyperkinetic gaits, 93% and 80% respectively, because normal and abnormal steps have very different magnitude and shape. For diplegic gait abnormal step (Fig. 10b) it could be seen, that third peak is unclear, that

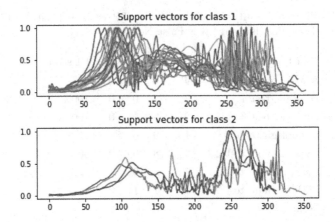

Fig. 4. Support vectors for steppage gait, test 1. X-axis is the time [ms], Y-axis is normalized gyroscope magnitude values (see Eq. 4).

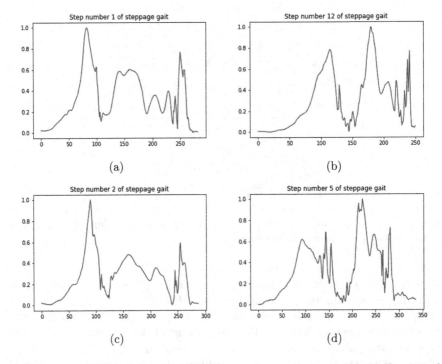

Fig. 5. Normal (left) and abnormal (right) steps for steppage gait, test 1. X-axis is the time [ms], Y-axis is normalized gyroscope magnitude values (see Eq. 4).

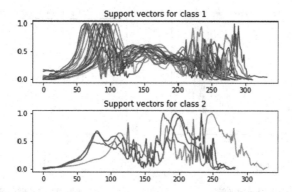

Fig. 6. Support vectors for steppage gait, test 2. X-axis is the time [ms], Y-axis is normalized gyroscope magnitude values (see Eq. 4).

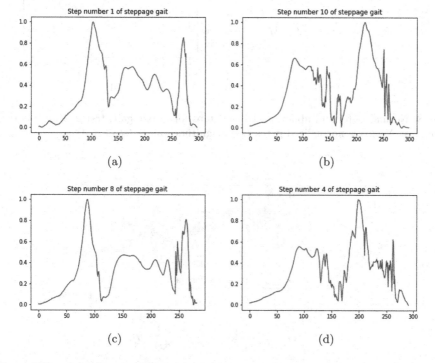

Fig. 7. Normal (left) and abnormal (right) steps for steppage gait, test 2. X-axis is the time [ms], Y-axis is normalized gyroscope magnitude values (see Eq. 4).

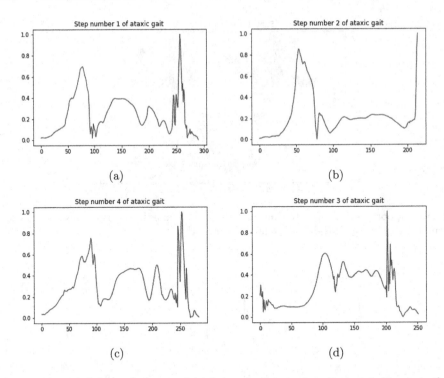

Fig. 8. Normal (left) and abnormal (right) steps for ataxic gait, test 2. X-axis is the time [ms], Y-axis is normalized gyroscope magnitude values (see Eq. 4).

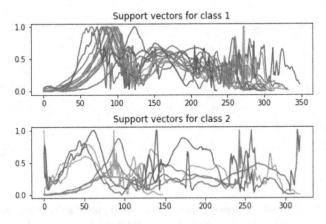

Fig. 9. Support vectors for diplegic gait, test 1. X-axis is the time [ms], Y-axis is normalized gyroscope magnitude values (see Eq. 4).

shows that there is no full contact of toe with ground on that gait type (Figs. 4, 6 and 9).

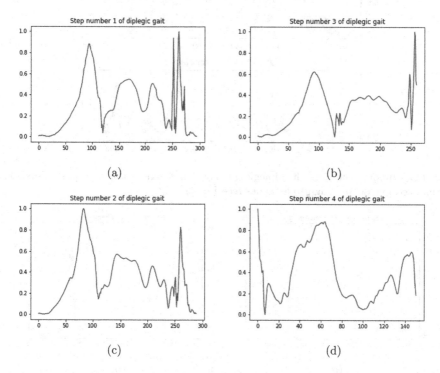

Fig. 10. Normal (left) and abnormal (right) steps for diplegic gait, test 1. X-axis is the time [ms], Y-axis is normalized gyroscope magnitude values (see Eq. 4).

Also for diplegic gait type it could be observed, that normal steps have more common features and abnormal steps have different number of peaks and magnitude. That helps tsSVM to differentiate them better and gives higher score. Because of the nature of this anomalous gait, several abnormal steps were performed in the row, that means that number of abnormal steps was more than in some other data sets.

Normal and abnormal steps for hemiplegic gait can be observed in the Fig. 12. They have similarly placed local maximums but with different amplitudes. This is due to abnormal movement, mainly affecting upper body, thus sensor have little impact by that movement. Normal steps have some variation, especially after abnormal step. This leads to misclassification and f1 score of 67% (Fig. 11).

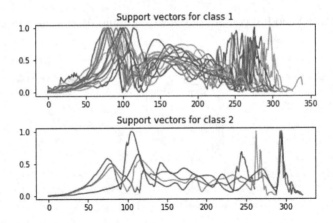

Fig. 11. Support vectors for hemiplegic gait, test 2. X-axis is the time [ms], Y-axis is normalized gyroscope magnitude values (see Eq. 4).

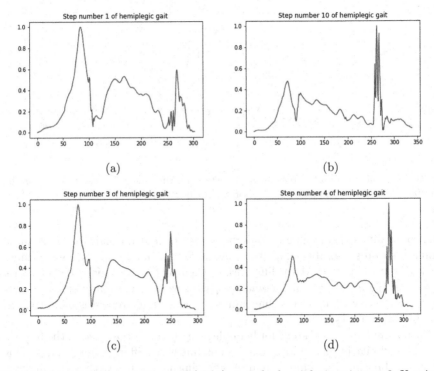

Fig. 12. Normal (left) and abnormal (right) steps for hemiplegic gait, test 2. X-axis is the time [ms], Y-axis is normalized gyroscope magnitude values (see Eq. 4).

5   Discussion and Conclusion

Ready made tsSVM could be well used for step classification, even using rather small amount of training data (tens of steps), as can be seen in results. The issues still occur, when the dataset is too small, and/or major variability in normal steps is present. As mentioned before, this situation is quite likely to appear with actual patient data. Some issues may arise, if gait deviation is happening in the upper part of the body. That would only lead to small deviations in forefoot placed sensor data, and could easily lead to misclassification of steps. A straightforward solution would be to add more body sensors, but that would increase systems cost and significantly reduce comfort of usage of this system. Obtained results could be useful in determining how different gait types abnormalities affect quality of classification of machine learning algorithms. It is clear, that good reference data presence (correct steps) is crucial for SVM, and, most likely for the other ML based classification methods as well.

Type of gait deviation has significant affect on quality of chosen algorithm results. Achieved average step classification accuracy was near to 80%, what is below the numbers published in literature. We assume, that classification performance of real patient data would be even worse. However, besides of performance improvements, with better training data selection and usage, we would develop an algorithm, that can detect anomalies during the gait phases instead of the whole steps. That is crucial to be able to correct gait on basis of needs. In the future we estimate, that applying certain ML techniques, possibly SVM, during the real-time operation of the next generation of FES devices, would make them less intervening and increase patients' comfort.

In real life human gait steps can not be modelled by using two class classifiers, thus multi-class classifier is crucial to distinguish the abnormal steps, related to some kind of disease, from normal steps. Normal steps could be divided into several classes as well, e.g. normal walking steps, turning steps and etc.

Thus, the further work will be focused on the construction of the multi-class classification algorithm for reference step obtaining. That would be used to develop real-time abnormality detection algorithm, that is able to detect abnormal gait in different contexts.

Acknowledgements. This work has been supported by Estonian Research Council, via research grant No PRG424 and from TAR16013 EXCITE "Estonian Centre of Excellence in ICT Research".

References

1. Almaslukh, B.: An effective deep autoencoder approach for online smartphone-based human activity recognition. Int. J. Comput. Sci. Netw. Secur. **17**, 160–165 (2017)
2. Bertolote, J.: Neurological disorders affect millions globally: WHO report. World Neurol. **22**(1) (2007)

3. di Biase, L., et al.: Gait analysis in Parkinson's disease: an overview of the most accurate markers for diagnosis and symptoms monitoring. Sensors **20**(12) (2020). https://doi.org/10.3390/s20123529. https://www.mdpi.com/1424-8220/20/12/3529

4. Buongiorno, D., Bortone, I., Cascarano, G.D., Trotta, G.F., Brunetti, A., Bevilacqua, V.: A low-cost vision system based on the analysis of motor features for recognition and severity rating of Parkinson's disease. BMC Med. Inform. Decis. Mak. **19**, 1–13 (2019)

5. Camps, J., et al.: Deep learning for freezing of gait detection in Parkinson's disease patients in their homes using a waist-worn inertial measurement unit. Knowl.-Based Syst. **139**, 119–131 (2018). https://doi.org/10.1016/j.knosys.2017.10.017

6. Cuturi, M.: Fast global alignment kernels. In: Proceedings of the 28th International Conference on Machine Learning (ICML 2011), pp. 929–936 (2011)

7. Cuturi, M., Blondel, M.: Soft-DTW: a differentiable loss function for time-series (2018)

8. Feigin, V.L., et al.: Global, regional, and national burden of neurological disorders during 1990–2015: a systematic analysis for the global burden of disease study 2015. Lancet Neurol. **16**(11), 877–897 (2017)

9. Gil-Castillo, J., Alnajjar, F., Koutsou, A., Torricelli, D., Moreno, J.C.: Advances in neuroprosthetic management of foot drop: a review. J. Neuroeng. Rehabil. **17**(1), 1–19 (2020)

10. Gurchiek, R.D., et al.: Remote gait analysis using wearable sensors detects asymmetric gait patterns in patients recovering from ACL reconstruction. In: 2019 IEEE 16th International Conference on Wearable and Implantable Body Sensor Networks (BSN), pp. 1–4 (2019)

11. Hsieh, C., Shi, W., Huang, H., Liu, K., Hsu, S.J., Chan, C.: Machine learning-based fall characteristics monitoring system for strategic plan of falls prevention. In: 2018 IEEE International Conference on Applied System Invention (ICASI), pp. 818–821 (2018)

12. Hsu, W.C., et al.: Multiple-wearable-sensor-based gait classification and analysis in patients with neurological disorders. Sensors **18**(10), 3397 (2018)

13. Huang, J., Stamp, M., Troia, F.D.: A comparison of machine learning classifiers for acoustic gait analysis. In: International Conference on Security and Management, SAM 2018 (2018)

14. Kluding, P.M., et al.: Foot drop stimulation versus ankle foot orthosis after stroke: 30-week outcomes. Stroke **44**(6), 1660–1669 (2013)

15. Kuusik, A., Gross-Paju, K., Maamägi, H., Reilent, E.: Comparative study of four instrumented mobility analysis tests on neurological disease patients. In: 2014 11th International Conference on Wearable and Implantable Body Sensor Networks Workshops, pp. 33–37. IEEE (2014)

16. Miller, L., et al.: Functional electrical stimulation for foot drop in multiple sclerosis: a systematic review and meta-analysis of the effect on gait speed. Arch. Phys. Med. Rehabil. **98**(7), 1435–1452 (2017)

17. Murad, A., Pyun, J.Y.: Deep recurrent neural networks for human activity recognition. Sensors **17**(11), 2556 (2017)

18. Murray, M.: Gait as a total pattern of movement. Am. J. Phys. Med. **46**(1), 290–333 (1967). http://europepmc.org/abstract/MED/5336886

19. Pau, M., et al.: Clinical assessment of gait in individuals with multiple sclerosis using wearable inertial sensors: comparison with patient-based measure. Mult. Scler. Relat. Disord. **10**, 187–191 (2016)

20. Pirker, W., Katzenschlager, R.: Gait disorders in adults and the elderly. Wiener klinische Wochenschrift, **129**(3), 81–95 (2016). https://doi.org/10.1007/s00508-016-1096-4

21. Ramdhani, R.A., Khojandi, A., Shylo, O., Kopell, B.H.: Optimizing clinical assessments in Parkinson's disease through the use of wearable sensors and data driven modeling. Front. Comput. Neurosci. **12**, 72 (2018)

22. Saboor, A., et al.: Latest research trends in gait analysis using wearable sensors and machine learning: a systematic review. IEEE Access **8**, 167830–167864 (2020)

23. Sandroff, B.M., Sosnoff, J.J., Motl, R.W.: Physical fitness, walking performance, and gait in multiple sclerosis. J. Neurol. Sci. **328**(1–2), 70–76 (2013)

24. Stolze, H., Klebe, S., Zechlin, C., Baecker, C., Friege, L., Deuschl, G.: Falls in frequent neurological diseases. J. Neurol. **251**(1), 79–84 (2004)

25. TarniȚă, D.: Wearable sensors used for human gait analysis. Rom. J. Morphol. Embryol. **57**(2), 373–382 (2016)

26. Tavenard, R., et al.: Tslearn, a machine learning toolkit for time series data. J. Mach. Learn. Res. **21**(118), 1–6 (2020). http://jmlr.org/papers/v21/20-091.html

27. Wang, C., Goel, R., Zhang, Q., Lepow, B., Najafi, B.: Daily use of bilateral custom-made ankle-foot orthoses for fall prevention in older adults: a randomized controlled trial. J. Am. Geriatr. Soc. **67**(8), 1656–1661 (2019)

28. Zhen, T., Mao, L., Wang, J., Gao, Q.: Wearable preimpact fall detector using SVM. In: 2016 10th International Conference on Sensing Technology (ICST), pp. 1–6 (2016)

Comparing the Performance of Different Classifiers for Posture Detection

Sagar Suresh Kumar[1], Kia Dashtipour[1,2(✉)], Mandar Gogate[2],
Jawad Ahmad[2], Khaled Assaleh[3], Kamran Arshad[3], Muhammad Ali Imran[1,4],
Qammer Abbasi[1], and Wasim Ahmad[1]

[1] James Watt School of Engineering, University of Glasgow, Glasgow, UK
[2] School of Computing, Edinburgh Napier University, Edinburgh, UK
k.dashtipour@napier.ac.uk
[3] Faculty of Engineering and IT, Ajman University, Ajman 346, UAE
[4] Artificial Intelligence Research Center (AIRC), Ajman University, Ajman, UAE

Abstract. Human Posture Classification (HPC) is used in many fields such as human computer interfacing, security surveillance, rehabilitation, remote monitoring, and so on. This paper compares the performance of different classifiers in the detection of 3 postures, sitting, standing, and lying down, which was recorded using Microsoft Kinect cameras. The Machine Learning classifiers used included the Support Vector Classifier, Naive Bayes, Logistic Regression, K-Nearest Neighbours, and Random Forests. The Deep Learning ones included the standard Multi-Layer Perceptron, Convolutional Neural Networks (CNN), and Long Short Term Memory Networks (LSTM). It was observed that Deep Learning methods outperformed the former and that the one-dimensional CNN performed the best with an accuracy of 93.45%.

Keywords: Machine learning · Deep learning · Detecting Alzheimer

1 Introduction

Human Posture Classification (HPC) has applications in a wide range of fields such as human computer interfacing, security surveillance, rehabilitation, remote monitoring, and so on [20]. There are broadly two kinds of sensor schemes that can be used for HPC: wearable and contactless. Wearable methods use sensors such as accelerometers, gyroscopes, magnetometers or even sensors that use physiological data such as Electromyogram (EMG), on different locations of the body while contactless ones rely on image or video processing, and also sensors in the proximity of the patient. Generally, wearable methods are obtrusive and cause discomfort. This is especially true for the elderly and the physically compromised. Hence, the research area of contactless HPC has gained popularity in the past few years [4,7,11,19,26,40,41,45].

HPC has been used to identify and correct several medical ailments in the past. Matar et al. used contactless bed-sheet pressure sensors to detect bed-posture and prevent pressure ulcers [38]. Lee et al. used inertial sensors to

© ICST Institute for Computer Sciences, Social Informatics and Telecommunications Engineering 2022
Published by Springer Nature Switzerland AG 2022. All Rights Reserved
M. Ur Rehman and A. Zoha (Eds.): BODYNETS 2021, LNICST 420, pp. 210–218, 2022.
https://doi.org/10.1007/978-3-030-95593-9_17

monitor squat exercises to prevent knee and leg injuries [33]. In camera based methods, Microsoft Kinect devices, which provides depth images using a combination of RGB and IR cameras and outputs the 3D coordinates of 32 joints, are quite popular. These solutions have benefited from the developments Machine and Deep Learning [3]. However, most of the past papers just use one or two classifiers without addressing in detail the classification schemes that produce optimal results. Hence, this work extensively compares the performance of different machine and deep learning classifiers and attempts to ascertain the optimum classifier(s) for posture data.

The rest of the paper is structured as follows. Section 2 provides the background information related to posture detection. Section 3 presents the proposed methodology. Section 4 provides the experimental results of the proposed posture detection and discussion, and finally Sect. 5 concludes the paper.

2 Related Work

Sidrah et al. [34] developed a novel approach based on hybrid approach used machine learning and deep learning approaches to detect human posture detection. However, the proposed approach can detect falling and standing and it cannot detect multiple posture detection. Panini et al. [42] presented an approach based on posture human detection in domotic application. The machine learning is used to generate the probability maps. The statistic classifier used to compare the probability maps and histogram profiles extracted from moving of people. The experimental results show that the results are robust and computational time are lowers as compared to state-of-the-art approaches such as [2, 8–10, 12–18, 27, 29, 30].

Ma et al. [37] proposed a cushion-based posture detection system used to process sensor for human detection in the wheelchair. The method is consists of three different steps such as classification for posture, backward selection of sensor configuration, and comparison with state-of-the-art approaches [1, 5, 6, 21–25, 28, 31, 32, 35, 36, 46, 47].

Nasirahmadi et al. [39] proposed an approach to identify whether a two-dimensional imaging system along with deep learning approaches to detecting standing and lying postures with CNN and ResNet features extraction of RGB images were used. Sacchetti et al. [44] developed an approach to classify human posture detection in classroom ambience. The posture can be divided into confident and non confident aiming for teacher evaluation, interested/non interested. The approach presents some concepts about postures and how effectively detect openpose library and finally neural network is used measure the effectiveness of the approach.

3 Methodology

In this section, we discussed the proposed methodology for human posture detection. The Fig. 1 displays the overview framework of the approach.

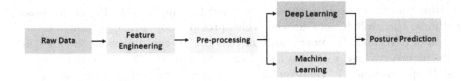

Fig. 1. Overview proposed approach

3.1   Classifiers

A wide range of machine and deep learning classifiers were used and are illustrated in Table 1 and Table 2. The Waikato Environment for Knowledge Analysis (WEKA) platform was used in this study to implement these algorithms. Among machine learning algorithms, the Naive Bayes Classifier's prior probabilities were set to 0, the Logistic Regression model used L2 loss, the K-nearest neighbours algorithm used 30 neighbours, and the the Random Forests classifier used 100 decision trees.

Convolutional Neural Network: For comparison, the novel CNN framework is developed. The implemented CNN consists of input, hidden and output layers. Our proposed CNN framework contains convolutional, max pooling and fully connected layers. The 10-layered CNN framework achieved the most promising results. The Fig. 2 shows the architecture for CNN.

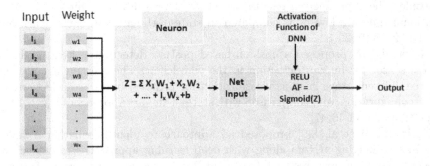

Fig. 2. Overview architecture of CNN

Long Short Term Memory (LSTM): The long short term memory (LSTM) proposed architecture contains input layer, two different stacked LSTM and one output as fully connected layer. Particularly, the LSTM architecture consists of two different stacked bidirectional layers (contains 128 cells and 64 cells) with dropout 0.2 and a dense layer with two neurons and softmax activation.

Among deep learning algorithms, both 1D and 2D Convolutional Neural Networks were used and their structures consisting of max pooling, convolution, and fully connected layers (total 10) are illustrated. Both unidirectional and bidirectional Long Short Term Memory (LSTM) Networks were used consisting of 2 stacked layers of 128 and 64 cells and a dense layer of softmax activation function. The Multilayer Perceptron (MLP) consisted of 2 hidden layers and used the ReLu activation function. K fold cross validation was used and K values of 10, 5, and 2 were tested.

4   Results and Discussion

The Deep Learning based classifiers have outperformed the Machine Learning Classifiers in general, as shown in Table 1 and 2. As expected, as the number of K-folds decreased, the accuracies decreased as well. Among Machine Learning methods, the Support Vector Machine with Radial Basis Function (RBF) Kernel performed the best with an overall accuracy of 83.42% while the Naive Bayes performed the worst with an accuracy of 74.56%. In Deep Learning methods, CNNs and LSTMs were superior to the traditional MLP networks. Although the latter 2 had similar accuracies, the 1D-CNN performed the best with an accuracy of 93.45%. Thus, future work should focus on optimizing the structure and performance of this network in posture detection.

Dataset: The data from [43] was used in this study, in which Microsoft Kinect V2 cameras were used to extract posture information of six users and three activities: sitting, standing, and lying down. Although the cameras obtain 75 points, which represent the x,y, and z coordinates of 25 body joints, 7 location independent features are extracted from them to reduce the computational load. These include the height,left hip angle, right hip angle, left knee angle, right knee angle, chest angle, and chest-knee angle. They were calculated from the body joints depth coordinates using cosine formula.

Table 1 shows the summary of results of machine learning and their performance using 10-fold cross validation. As shown in Table 1 the SVM outperforms other machine learning classifiers.

Table 1. Machine Learning classifiers and their performance with 10 fold cross validation

Classifier	Accuracy	Recall	Precision	F1 score
SVM (RBF)	83.42%	0.83	0.82	0.81
Naive Bayes	74.56%	0.74	0.73	0.74
Logistic Regression	80.91%	0.80	0.79	0.80
KNN	76.98%	0.76	0.75	076
Random Forests	77.08%	0.77	0.76	0.77

Table 2 shows the summary of results of deep learning and their performance using 10-fold cross validation. As shown in Table 2 the 1D-CNN outperforms other deep learning classifiers such as 2D-CNN, LSTM, BiLSTM.

Table 2. Deep Learning classifiers and their performance with 10-fold cross validation

Classifier	Accuracy	Recall	Precision	F1 score
MLP	82.56%	0.82	0.82	0.82
1D-CNN	93.45%	0.93	0.92	0.93
2D-CNN	91.59%	0.91	0.90	0.91
LSTM	88.19%	0.88	0.87	0.88
BiLSTM	90.87%	0.90	0.90	0.90

Table 3 shows the summary of results of machine learning and their performance using 5-fold cross validation. As shown in Table 3 the MLP outperforms other machine learning classifiers.

Table 3. Machine Learning classifiers and their performance with 5-fold cross validation

Classifier	Accuracy	Precision	Recall	F-measure
MLP	81.56	0.81	0.8	0.81
SVM	81.02	0.81	0.8	0.81
Naive Bayes	71.36	0.71	0.7	0.71
Logistic Regression	71.26	0.71	0.7	0.71
KNN	74.87	0.75	0.74	75
Random Forest	76.34	0.76	0.76	0.76

Table 4 shows the summary of results of deep learning and their performance using 5-fold cross validation. As shown in Table 4 the 1D-CNN outperforms other deep learning classifiers.

Table 4. Deep Learning classifiers and their performance with 5-fold cross validation

Classifier	Accuracy	Precision	Recall	F-measure
1D-CNN	91.51	0.91	0.91	0.91
2D-CNN	90.96	0.91	0.9	0.91
LSTM	89.56	0.89	0.88	0.89
BiLSTM	88.98	0.89	0.88	0.89

Table 5 shows the summary of results of machine learning and their performance using 2-fold cross validation. As shown in Table 5 the SVM outperforms other machine learning classifiers.

Table 5. Machine Learning classifiers and their performance with 2-fold cross validation

Classifier	Accuracy	Precision	Recall	F-measure
MLP	80.42	0.8	0.79	0.8
SVM	81.01	0.81	0.81	0.81
Nave Bayes	70.94	0.7	0.7	0.7
Logistic Regression	70.59	0.7	0.7	0.7
KNN	74.29	0.74	0.74	74
Random Forest	75.63	0.75	0.74	0.75

Table 6 shows the summary of results of deep learning and their performance using 2-fold cross validation. As shown in Table 6 the 1D-CNN outperforms other deep learning classifiers.

Table 6. Deep Learning classifiers and their performance with 2-fold cross validation

Classifier	Accuracy	Precision	Recall	F-measure
1D-CNN	90.23	0.9	0.89	0.9
2D-CNN	89.67	0.89	0.88	0.89
LSTM	88.19	0.88	0.87	0.88
BiLSTM	87.76	0.87	0.86	0.87

5   Conclusion

The human posture detection is important in remote monitoring of patient. However, most of the current approaches cannot perfectly detect different human postures such as sitting, standing and lying down. Therefore, in this study, we proposed an approach based on the machine learning and deep learning approaches to detect different posture detection.

Acknowledgement. This work is supported in part by the Ajman University Internal Research Grant.

References

1. Adeel, A., Gogate, M., Hussain, A.: Contextual deep learning-based audio-visual switching for speech enhancement in real-world environments. Inf. Fusion **59**, 163–170 (2020)
2. Ahmed, R., et al.: Deep neural network-based contextual recognition of Arabic handwritten scripts. Entropy **23**(3), 340 (2021)

3. Alaoui, H., Moutacalli, M.T., Adda, M.: AI-enabled high-level layer for posture recognition using the azure Kinect in Unity3D. In 2020 IEEE 4th International Conference on Image Processing, Applications and Systems (IPAS), pp. 155–161 (2020)

4. Alqarafi, A.S., Adeel, A., Gogate, M., Dashitpour, K., Hussain, A., Durrani, T.: Toward's Arabic multi-modal sentiment analysis. In: Liang, Q., Mu, J., Jia, M., Wang, W., Feng, X., Zhang, B. (eds.) CSPS 2017. LNEE, vol. 463, pp. 2378–2386. Springer, Singapore (2019). https://doi.org/10.1007/978-981-10-6571-2_290

5. Asad, S.M., et al.: Mobility management-based autonomous energy-aware framework using machine learning approach in dense mobile networks. Signals 1(2), 170–187 (2020)

6. Asad, S.M., Dashtipour, K., Hussain, S., Abbasi, Q.H., Imran, M.A.: Travelers-tracing and mobility profiling using machine learning in railway systems. In: 2020 International Conference on UK-China Emerging Technologies (UCET), pp. 1–4. IEEE (2020)

7. Churcher, A., et al.: An experimental analysis of attack classification using machine learning in IoT networks. Sensors 21(2), 446 (2021)

8. Dashtipour, K., Gogate, M., Adeel, A., Algarafi, A., Howard, N., Hussain, A.: Persian named entity recognition. In: 2017 IEEE 16th International Conference on Cognitive Informatics and Cognitive Computing (ICCI* CC), pp. 79–83. IEEE (2017)

9. Dashtipour, K., Gogate, M., Adeel, A., Hussain, A., Alqarafi, A., Durrani, T.: A comparative study of Persian sentiment analysis based on different feature combinations. In: Liang, Q., Mu, J., Jia, M., Wang, W., Feng, X., Zhang, B. (eds.) CSPS 2017. LNEE, vol. 463, pp. 2288–2294. Springer, Singapore (2019). https://doi.org/10.1007/978-981-10-6571-2_279

10. Dashtipour, K., Gogate, M., Adeel, A., Ieracitano, C., Larijani, H., Hussain, A.: Exploiting deep learning for Persian sentiment analysis. In: Ren, J., et al. (eds.) BICS 2018. LNCS (LNAI), vol. 10989, pp. 597–604. Springer, Cham (2018). https://doi.org/10.1007/978-3-030-00563-4_58

11. Dashtipour, K., Gogate, M., Adeel, A., Larijani, H., Hussain, A.: Sentiment analysis of Persian movie reviews using deep learning. Entropy 23(5), 596 (2021)

12. Dashtipour, K., Gogate, M., Cambria, E., Hussain, A.: A novel context-aware multimodal framework for persian sentiment analysis. arXiv preprint arXiv:2103.02636 (2021)

13. Dashtipour, K., Gogate, M., Li, J., Jiang, F., Kong, B., Hussain, A.: A hybrid Persian sentiment analysis framework: integrating dependency grammar based rules and deep neural networks. Neurocomputing 380, 1–10 (2020)

14. Dashtipour, K., Hussain, A., Gelbukh, A.: Adaptation of sentiment analysis techniques to Persian language. In: Gelbukh, A. (ed.) CICLing 2017, Part II. LNCS, vol. 10762, pp. 129–140. Springer, Cham (2018). https://doi.org/10.1007/978-3-319-77116-8_10

15. Dashtipour, K., Hussain, A., Zhou, Q., Gelbukh, A., Hawalah, A.Y.A., Cambria, E.: PerSent: a freely available Persian sentiment Lexicon. In: Liu, C.-L., Hussain, A., Luo, B., Tan, K.C., Zeng, Y., Zhang, Z. (eds.) BICS 2016. LNCS (LNAI), vol. 10023, pp. 310–320. Springer, Cham (2016). https://doi.org/10.1007/978-3-319-49685-6_28

16. Dashtipour, K., et al.: Multilingual sentiment analysis: state of the art and independent comparison of techniques. Cogn. Comput. 8(4), 757–771 (2016)

17. Dashtipour, K., Raza, A., Gelbukh, A., Zhang, R., Cambria, E., Hussain, A.: PerSent 2.0: Persian sentiment lexicon enriched with domain-specific words. In: Ren, J., et al. (eds.) BICS 2019. LNCS (LNAI), vol. 11691, pp. 497–509. Springer, Cham (2020). https://doi.org/10.1007/978-3-030-39431-8_48

18. Dashtipour, K., et al.: Public perception towards fifth generation of cellular networks (5G) on social media. Front. Big Data (2021)

19. Gepperth, A.R.T., Hecht, T., Gogate, M.: A generative learning approach to sensor fusion and change detection. Cogn. Comput. **8**(5), 806–817 (2016). https://doi.org/10.1007/s12559-016-9390-z

20. Ghazal, S., Khan, U.S.: Human posture classification using skeleton information. In: 2018 International Conference on Computing, Mathematics and Engineering Technologies (iCoMET), pp. 1–4 (2018)

21. Gogate, M., Adeel, A., Hussain, A.: Deep learning driven multimodal fusion for automated deception detection. In: 2017 IEEE Symposium Series on Computational Intelligence (SSCI), pp. 1–6. IEEE (2017)

22. Gogate, M., Adeel, A., Hussain, A.: A novel brain-inspired compression-based optimised multimodal fusion for emotion recognition. In: 2017 IEEE Symposium Series on Computational Intelligence (SSCI), pp. 1–7. IEEE (2017)

23. Gogate, M., Adeel, A., Marxer, R., Barker, J., Hussain, A.: DNN driven speaker independent audio-visual mask estimation for speech separation. arXiv preprint arXiv:1808.00060 (2018)

24. Gogate, M., Dashtipour, K., Adeel, A., Hussain, A.: CochleaNet: a robust language-independent audio-visual model for real-time speech enhancement. Inf. Fusion **63**, 273–285 (2020)

25. Gogate, M., Dashtipour, K., Hussain, A.: Visual speech in real noisy environments (vision): A novel benchmark dataset and deep learning-based baseline system. In: 2020 Proceedings of the Interspeech, pp. 4521–4525 (2020)

26. Gogate, M., Hussain, A., Huang, K.: Random features and random neurons for brain-inspired big data analytics. In: 2019 International Conference on Data Mining Workshops (ICDMW), pp. 522–529. IEEE (2019)

27. Guellil, I., et al.: A semi-supervised approach for sentiment analysis of Arab(ic+izi) messages: Application to the Algerian dialect. SN Comput. Sci. **2**(2), 1–18 (2021). https://doi.org/10.1007/s42979-021-00510-1

28. Huma, Z.E., et al.: A hybrid deep random neural network for cyberattack detection in the industrial internet of things. IEEE Access **9**, 55595–55605 (2021)

29. Hussain, A., et al.: Artificial intelligence-enabled analysis of UK and us public attitudes on Facebook and twitter towards COVID-19 vaccinations. medRxiv (2020)

30. Hussien, I.O., Dashtipour, K., Hussain, A.: Comparison of sentiment analysis approaches using modern Arabic and Sudanese dialect. In: Ren, J., et al. (eds.) BICS 2018. LNCS (LNAI), vol. 10989, pp. 615–624. Springer, Cham (2018). https://doi.org/10.1007/978-3-030-00563-4_60

31. Ieracitano, C., et al.: Statistical analysis driven optimized deep learning system for intrusion detection. In: Ren, J., et al. (eds.) BICS 2018. LNCS (LNAI), vol. 10989, pp. 759–769. Springer, Cham (2018). https://doi.org/10.1007/978-3-030-00563-4_74

32. Jiang, F., Kong, B., Li, J., Dashtipour, K., Gogate, M.: Robust visual saliency optimization based on bidirectional markov chains. Cogn. Comput. 1–12 (2020)

33. Lee, J., Joo, H., Lee, J., Chee, Y.: Automatic classification of squat posture using inertial sensors: deep learning approach. Sensors **20**(2), 361 (2020)

34. Liaqat, S., Dashtipour, K., Arshad, K., Assaleh, K., Ramzan, N.: A hybrid posture detection framework: integrating machine learning and deep neural networks. IEEE Sens.J. **21**(7), 9515–9522 (2021)
35. Liaqat, S., Dashtipour, K., Arshad, K., Ramzan, N.: Non invasive skin hydration level detection using machine learning. Electronics **9**(7), 1086 (2020)
36. Liaqat, S., Dashtipour, K., Zahid, A., Assaleh, K., Arshad, K., Ramzan, N.: Detection of atrial fibrillation using a machine learning approach. Information **11**(12), 549 (2020)
37. Ma, C., Li, W., Gravina, R., Fortino, G.: Posture detection based on smart cushion for wheelchair users. Sensors **17**(4), 719 (2017)
38. Matar, G., Lina, J.M., Kaddoum, G.: Artificial neural network for in-bed posture classification using bed-sheet pressure sensors. IEEE J. Biomed. Health Inf. **24**(1), 101–110 (2020)
39. Nasirahmadi, A., et al.: Deep learning and machine vision approaches for posture detection of individual pigs. Sensors **19**(17), 3738 (2019)
40. Nisar, S., Tariq, M., Adeel, A., Gogate, M., Hussain, A.: Cognitively inspired feature extraction and speech recognition for automated hearing loss testing. Cogn. Comput. **11**(4), 489–502 (2019). https://doi.org/10.1007/s12559-018-9607-4
41. Ozturk, M., Gogate, M., Onireti, O., Adeel, A., Hussain, A., Imran, M.A.: A novel deep learning driven, low-cost mobility prediction approach for 5G cellular networks: the case of the control/data separation architecture (CDSA). Neurocomputing **358**, 479–489 (2019)
42. Panini, L., Cucchiara, R.: A machine learning approach for human posture detection in domotics applications. In: 12th International Conference on Image Analysis and Processing, 2003. Proceedings, pp. 103–108. IEEE (2003)
43. Qassoud., Bolic., Rajan.: Posture-and-fall-detection-system-using-3d-motion-sensors (2018)
44. Sacchetti, R., Teixeira, T., Barbosa, B., Neves, A.J., Soares, S.C., Dimas, I.D.: Human body posture detection in context: the case of teaching and learning environments. SIGNAL 2018 Editors **87**, 79–84 (2018)
45. Shiva, A.S., Gogate, M., Howard, N., Graham, B., Hussain, A.: Complex-valued computational model of hippocampal CA3 recurrent collaterals. In: 2017 IEEE 16th International Conference on Cognitive Informatics and Cognitive Computing (ICCI* CC), pp. 161–166. IEEE (2017)
46. Taylor, W., Shah, S.A., Dashtipour, K., Zahid, A., Abbasi, Q.H., Imran, M.A.: An intelligent non-invasive real-time human activity recognition system for next-generation healthcare. Sensors **20**(9), 2653 (2020)
47. Yu, Z., et al.: Energy and performance trade-off optimization in heterogeneous computing via reinforcement learning. Electronics **9**(11), 1812 (2020)

Distance Estimation for Molecular Communication in Blood Vessel

Yu Li[1], Zhongke Ma[2], Hao Yan[2(✉)], Jie Luo[1], and Lin Lin[1]

[1] College of Electronics and Information Engineering,
Tongji University, Shanghai, China
{1930703,2132942,fxlinlin}@tongji.edu.cn
[2] School of Electronic, Information and Electrical Engineering,
Shanghai Jiao Tong University, Shanghai, China
yan_hao@sjtu.edu.cn

Abstract. Molecular communication (MC) is proposed as a promising communication paradigm for nanonetworks. The knowledge of the distance between transmitter and receiver is of great importance in MC to achieve good system performance. The distance estimation work has been carried out based on the free diffusion channel of MC. The blood vessel, which is different from the free diffusion channel, is also very important for many MC applications such as drug delivery. However, the distance estimation schemes for the channel of blood vessel have not been investigated. In this work, we propose a distance estimation scheme for the blood vessel channel of MC. A more realistic model of the flow velocity in the blood vessel is presented. The corresponding channel impulse response (CIR) of the blood vessel channel is derived. Moreover, the effectiveness of the proposed distance estimation scheme is validated by simulations.

Keywords: Molecular communication · Blood vessel · Blood velocity · Distance estimation

1 Introduction

Molecular communication (MC) is a promising paradigm to interconnect nanomachines in a nanonetwork due to its advantages of bio-compatibility and energy efficiency [4,16]. One of the most important applications of the MC is the drug delivery system where drug particles (micro- or nano- meter in size) propagate from the injected site to the targeted site via blood vessels [10]. However, the study of MC in the channel of blood vessel is quite limited. Therefore, it is very necessary and important to investigate MC system in the blood vessel channel.

H. Yan—This work was supported in part by National Natural Science Foundation, China (61971314, 62071297), in part by Science and Technology Commission of Shanghai Municipality (19ZR1426500, 19510744900) and in part by Sino-German Center of Intelligent Systems, Tongji University.

M. Ur Rehman and A. Zoha (Eds.): BODYNETS 2021, LNICST 420, pp. 219–229, 2022.
https://doi.org/10.1007/978-3-030-95593-9_18

In MC, the distance between the transmitter and the receiver is quite an important parameter [11]. Different distance between nanomachines results in different channel impulse response (CIR) which has great impacts on the performance of the MC system [7]. For example, the distance has to be known in order to achieve clock synchronization among nanomachines [12]. The distance is also a key parameter to determine the transmission rate and the number of molecules to be released for the optimal channel capacity [17]. In the MC applications such as the drug delivery system, the distance between the drug carrier nanomachine and the destination is quite important. Therefore, the distance between the transmitter and the receiver is of great importance and appropriate distance estimation schemes are quite necessary.

The studies on the distance estimation schemes in MC mainly focus on the distance estimation in free diffusion channel. For the free diffusion channel, the scheme based on the peak concentration of the received signal is the most frequently used method [6,13]. The receiver measures the concentration of the molecules and records the time when the concentration reaches its maximum. The distance is then calculated with the peak time and the concentration value. Another scheme is to use the energy to estimate the distance [18]. It performs better in accuracy compared with the peak concentration scheme, though it is more complex. In [15], round trip time and signal attenuation protocols are proposed. These two schemes estimate distance by measuring the round trip time or the signal attenuation of the received feedback signal. These schemes are designed for the free diffusion channel. However, the blood vessel is neither a simple free diffusion channel nor a flow-assisted channel with a constant flow speed. The velocity of the blood flow in blood vessels changes periodically [3]. Therefore, the state-of-the-art distance estimation schemes designed for free diffusion channel are not suitable for blood vessel channels. To the best of our knowledge, there is no specific distance estimation scheme for the blood vessel channel. The investigation of distance estimation schemes in blood vessel channels is quite necessary.

In this paper, we propose a distance estimation scheme for the channel of the blood vessels in the MC system. We establish a more realistic model of the blood velocity in vessels for MC. Based on the proposed blood velocity model, the CIR of the blood vessel is derived. We find that both the periodical property of the blood velocity and the molecule releasing time relative to the period of the blood velocity affect the CIR. By acquiring the period of the blood velocity and the molecule releasing time relative to the period, the distance is accurately estimated. The effectiveness of the proposed scheme is validated by the simulation.

The remainder of the paper is organized as follows. In Sect. 2, we put forward the blood velocity pattern and introduce the system model. Section 3 proposes the scheme for the estimation of the distance between the transmitter and the receiver. Simulation results are shown in Sect. 4. Finally, the conclusion is drawn in Sect. 5.

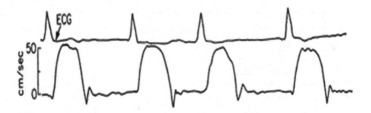

Fig. 1. The blood velocity in human beings' pulmonary artery. ECG means electrocardiogram.

2   System Model

2.1   Model of Blood Velocity

Considering the fact that the heart beats periodically, the pressure difference at the two ends of the vessel also changes periodically. Accordingly, the blood velocity changes periodically. Figure 1 shows an example of the blood velocity pattern in a human being's pulmonary artery [5]. The upper curve is the ECG curve, and the lower curve is the velocity pattern. The blood velocity changes periodically and its waveform is close to a rectangle wave. According to [5], no matter how long the period is, the duty cycle of the blood velocity is always about 37.5% of the period.

In the state-of-the-art MC studies, the blood velocity is always modeled as a constant velocity, and the channel of the blood vessel is correspondingly considered as a flow-assisted diffusion channel with a constant flow velocity. Such approximation is quite different from reality and not accurate at all. Herein, we propose a more accurate model of the blood velocity. As the blood velocity curve in Fig. 1 is close to a rectangle wave, we adopt the rectangle wave as the approximation shown in Fig. 2 to better model the blood velocity in vessels. Its period is defined as T and the amplitude is V_0. Assume the signal molecules are released at $t = 0$. τ is the time duration between the initial time $t = 0$ and the first rising edge of the periodical rectangle wave. This parameter is useful in the distance estimation scheme in Sect. 3. The function of the modeled blood velocity can be written as

$$V(t) = \begin{cases} V_0 & kT + \tau < t < kT + 0.375T + \tau, \\ 0 & kT + 0.375T + \tau < t < kT + T + \tau, \end{cases} \tag{1}$$

where $k = 0, 1, 2, 3, \ldots$ and the duty cycle is 37.5%.

For a particular vessel, V_0 is a fixed value. For example, in human beings' capillary vessels, the approximate amplitude is $V_0 = 0.4\,\text{mm/s}$ [9]. But the period of the blood velocity T is variable. This is because that the heart rate differs among people. And even for the same person, the heart rates are different in different body states, such as when people are resting or doing exercise.

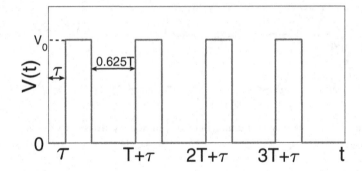

Fig. 2. The proposed model of the blood velocity in blood vessel.

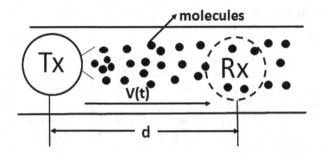

Fig. 3. Illustration of an end-to-end MC system in a 3D fluid environment.

2.2 System Model

An end-to-end MC system in a 3D fluid environment is considered in this paper. It is illustrated in Fig. 3. A passive receiver is located at a Euclidean distance of d from the transmitter. The synchronization between the transmitter and the receiver is assumed to be achieved [14]. The transmitter releases N molecules into the channel. The molecules propagate in the channel affected by both the diffusion and blood velocity $V(t)$. Finally, the molecules arrive at the receiver at different times. The passive receiver detects the concentration of the molecules that enter its sensing range, but does not affect the movement of the molecules. Based on the detected signal, the distance d is estimated by the scheme proposed in Sect. 3. In the system, the time instant that the transmitter releases the molecules is set as $t = 0$. Usually the time interval τ between the releasing time and the time of the first rising edge of the blood velocity is stochastic, because the transmitter can release molecules at any time which is irrelevant to the blood flow.

In a free diffusion channel, the channel impulse response (CIR) at the receiver is given in [8] as

$$h(t) = \frac{1}{(4\pi Dt)^{\frac{3}{2}}} exp(-\frac{d^2}{4Dt}), \tag{2}$$

where D is the diffusion coefficient. In the channel of blood vessel where exist both free diffusion and blood flow assisted diffusion with velocity $V(t)$ in (1), the CIR can be derived as

$$h(t) = \frac{1}{(4\pi Dt)^{\frac{3}{2}}} exp\{-\frac{[d - \int_0^t V(t)\, dt]^2}{4Dt}\}. \tag{3}$$

If the transmitter releases N signal molecules, the concentration of the signal molecules detected by the receiver then comes to

$$C(t) = \frac{N}{(4\pi Dt)^{\frac{3}{2}}} exp\{-\frac{[d - \int_0^t V(t)\, dt]^2}{4Dt}\}. \tag{4}$$

An example of signal concentration detected by the receiver is shown in Fig. 4, associated with $V(t)$ to illustrate their relationship. When $V(t) = 0$, due to the free diffusion, the molecules perform Brownian motion. When $V(t) \neq 0$, the drift with velocity V_0 dominates the movement of molecules. The diffusion still takes effect, but its impact is quite limited. Affected by such $V(t)$, it is noticed that the plot of signal concentration in Fig. 4 is quite different from the signal concentration in free diffusion channel or that in the constant flow-assisted channel. The concentration curve in Fig. 4 looks like cutting the concentration curve of constant flow-assisted channel into several pieces and connecting these pieces with line segments which are parts of the concentration curve of free diffusion channel where concentration changes slowly. These two different types of pieces appear alternately and correspond to the time that $V(t) = V_0$ and $V(t) = 0$ respectively. The amplitude changes at $V(t) = V_0$ are faster than the amplitude changes at $V(t) = 0$. We define these points at the junction of the two types of pieces as feature points of the concentration curve. Hence, at the feature points, the change of its first derivative is relatively larger than that of other parts.

The concentration curve in the bottom panel of Fig. 4 is an example of the channel response in blood vessels with fixed values of parameter T and τ. Different from the response in the free diffusion channel and constant flow-assisted channel with fixed d, the CIR for the channel with periodic blood velocity also varies with different values of T and τ.

3   Distance Estimation Scheme

As discussed in Sect. 2, the CIR of the blood vessel channel is different from the CIRs of free-diffusion channel and constant flow-assisted channel. Therefore, the distance estimation schemes for free-diffusion channel and constant flow-assisted channel are not applicable to the blood vessel channel. Herein, we propose a distance estimation scheme for the blood vessel channel.

Our proposed scheme utilizes the CIR of blood vessel channel in (3) to estimate the distance in blood vessels. The transmitter releases N molecules which propagate in the blood vessel. The receiver measures the concentration $C(t)$

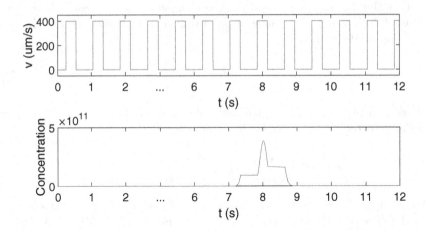

Fig. 4. The concentration curve of the blood vessel and the corresponding $V(t)$.

of signal molecules and records the corresponding time when the concentration reaches its maximum. The problem is that $V(t)$ is unknown in (3). In order to calculate the distance d, $V(t)$ should be estimated first. With the peak time, peak concentration, and $V(t)$, the distance is calculated through the CIR in (3).

The whole scheme includes two parts: 1. Calculate variables T and τ to obtain $V(t)$ in (1); 2. Estimate the distance d with (3). In this paper, the situation that $d < V_0 \times 0.375T$ is not considered. That is to say, we do not consider the situation that the transmitter and receiver locate too close such that the peak concentration of molecules arrives within a single period of blood velocity.

The receiver measures the concentration of signal molecules and records the time when the concentration reaches its maximum.

3.1   Calculate T and τ

To calculate T in (1), our strategy is to find the feature points of the concentration curve. The time interval between two feature points at two neighboring rising edges or two neighboring falling edges is the period of the blood velocity T.

Firstly, we discuss how to find the feature points. The receiver takes samples of the concentration of signal molecules around it. We denote the sampling values as $C(\Delta)$, $C(2\Delta)$, $C(3\Delta)$, ..., $C(n\Delta)$, where Δ is the sampling interval. Since there are noises in the MC system which affect the accuracy of the received signal. Therefore, smoothing is performed in the first step. After smoothing, the first and second derivatives of the concentration are calculated as

$$S(i) = \frac{C[(i+1)\Delta] - C(i\Delta)}{\Delta}, \tag{5}$$

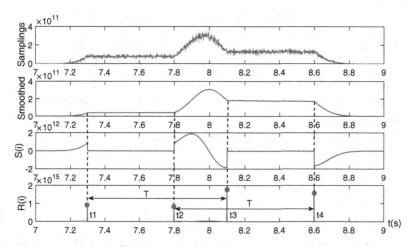

Fig. 5. Illustration of the calculation process of T. The plot of the concentration $C(i)$, the first derivative $S(i)$, and the absolute value of the second derivative $R(i)$ are shown in the top two panels, the middle and bottom panels respectively in the figure. The real distance is $1270\,\mu\mathrm{m}$ and other parameters are the same as defined in Table 1.

and

$$R(i) = \frac{S[(i+1)\Delta] - S(i\Delta)}{\Delta}, \tag{6}$$

where $i = 1, 2, 3, \ldots$

Figure 5 is used to illustrate the above processes. The top panel shows the sampled concentration with noise at the receiver. The second panel is the smoothed signal of the concentration curve. The third and bottom panels are the first derivative and the absolute of the second derivative of the smoothed signal. It is seen that the absolute values of the second derivative at the feature points are much higher than those at non-feature points. We also find that among all feature points before or after the peak concentration, those feature points closer to the peak concentration have larger second derivative values than the feature points further away from the peak. This is because the amplitude of the concentration curve far away from the peak is lower and changes more slowly. The first derivative of the feature point far away from the peak is smoother and the second derivative is smaller. The greater the amplitude of the concentration curve near the peak, the more drastic the change in the first derivative, and therefore the greater the second derivative.

Thus, it can be seen that the feature points of the four largest second derivatives are consecutive feature points around the peak of concentration curve as shown in Fig. 5. If we arrange their time values in chronological order as t_1, t_2, t_3, and t_4 such that $t_1 < t_2 < t_3 < t_4$, we have that $T = t_4 - t_2 = t_3 - t_1$. For accuracy, t_1, t_2, t_3, and t_4 are all used in the calculation of the period of blood velocity T as

Table 1. Simulation parameters

Parameter	Symbol	Value
Diffusion coefficient of information molecules	D	$10^{-10}\,\mathrm{m^2/s}$ [1]
Number of molecules	N	1.1×10^{10}
Volume of spherical reception space of receiver	V_R	$0.0056\,\mathrm{\mu m^3}$
Real distance	d	300–$2100\,\mathrm{\mu m}$
Interval between releasing time and rising edge	τ	0.1–$0.7\,\mathrm{s}$ [2]
Symbol interval	T_b	$2.7\,\mathrm{ms}$

$$T = \frac{(t_4 - t_2) + (t_3 - t_1)}{2}. \tag{7}$$

The relationships between t_1, t_2, t_3, and t_4 are also used in the calculation of τ. We have prior knowledge that the duty cycle is 37.5%. Therefore, the feature points are not equally spaced. According to such property of the duty cycle, in the case that $t_4 - t_3 > t_3 - t_2$, t_2 and t_4 are the time of rising edges. In the case that $t_4 - t_3 < t_3 - t_2$, t_1 and t_3 are the time of rising edges. According to the definition of τ, it is the time interval between the releasing time of molecules and the time of the first rising edge of the blood velocity. Therefore, the remainder of any rising edge time divided by the period T is the required τ, which can be expressed as

$$\tau = \begin{cases} t_2 - \lfloor t_2/T \rfloor \times T & \text{if } t_4 - t_3 > t_3 - t_2, \\ t_1 - \lfloor t_1/T \rfloor \times T & \text{if } t_4 - t_3 \leq t_3 - t_2, \end{cases} \tag{8}$$

where $\lfloor \cdot \rfloor$ denotes the floor function.

With T calculated in (7) and τ in (8), $V(t)$ in (1) and (3) is obtained.

3.2 Distance Estimation

The receiver takes samples of the concentration. After smoothing is performed to remove the noise, the time t_{max} and the amplitude C_{max} when the concentration reaches its maximum are recorded. And $V(t)$ is calculated as discussed in Sect. 3.1. With $V(t)$, C_{max}, and t_{max}, the distance d is calculated by (3) as

$$d = \sqrt{-4Dt_{max}ln[\frac{C_{max}}{N}(4\pi Dt_{max})^{\frac{3}{2}}] + \int_0^{t_{max}} V(t)\,dt}. \tag{9}$$

4   Simulation Results

In this section, the proposed distance estimation scheme for blood vessel channel is examined through Monte Carlo simulation. The system parameters in Table 1 are adopted as default parameters without stated otherwise.

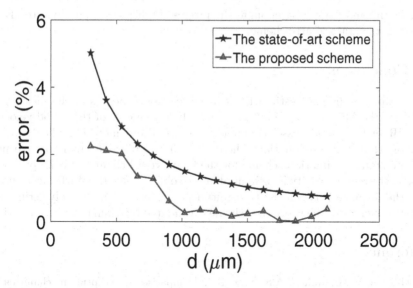

Fig. 6. Comparison of our proposed scheme with the existing constant flow-assisted scheme [6].

To quantitatively evaluate the performance of the proposed scheme, the relative estimation error (error for short in the following part) is used as the performance metric which is defined as

$$error = \frac{|d_{est} - d|}{d}, \tag{10}$$

where d_{est} is the estimated distance by the proposed scheme. A smaller error indicates a better performance.

The effectiveness of the proposed distance estimation scheme is investigated by comparing it with the state-of-art distance estimation scheme in [6]. In the comparison scheme, the blood velocity $V(t)$ is set as a known constant as in the state-of-the-art MC studies. The constant velocity value is set as the average of the blood velocity which is $V(t) = V_0 \times 0.375$. In such a case, the channel is a constant flow-assisted channel. The receiver measures the concentration of the molecules and records the time when the concentration reaches its maximum. The distance is calculated with the peak time and concentration value through the CIR in (3) with a known velocity $V(t) = V_0 \times 0.375$.

The result is shown in Fig. 6. The proposed distance estimation scheme with a more realistic model of the blood vessel channel performs better than the comparison scheme. The effectiveness of the proposed scheme is demonstrated. The result also shows that, when the distance becomes larger, the error decreases and the difference between the state-of-art scheme and the proposed one becomes smaller. This is because as the distance becomes larger, the arriving time of molecules becomes longer and more periods are covered before arrival. The overall inaccuracy of approximating the blood velocity with its average is reduced.

But, for distances not long enough, the proposed scheme has an obvious advantage over the state-of-art scheme.

5   Conclusion

In this work, a distance estimation scheme for the blood vessel channel is proposed for the MC system. Due to the periodical property of the blood velocity, the CIR of the blood vessel channel is not fixed and more complicated. The state-of-art distance estimation schemes are not applicable anymore. We propose a distance estimation scheme for the blood vessel channel. In the proposed scheme, the blood velocity is estimated first to obtain the CIR. With the accurate CIR, the distance between the transmitter and receiver is accurately estimated. The effectiveness of the proposed scheme is validated by simulation investigation.

References

1. Al-Zu'bi, M.M., Mohan, A.S., Ling, S.S.: Comparison of reception mechanisms for molecular communication via diffusion. In: 2018 9th International Conference on Information and Communication Systems (ICICS), pp. 203–207. IEEE (2018)
2. Banerjee, S., Paul, S., Sharma, R., Brahma, A.: Heartbeat monitoring using IoT. In: 2018 IEEE 9th Annual Information Technology, Electronics and Mobile Communication Conference, (IEMCON), pp. 894–900. IEEE (2018)
3. Du, T., Hu, D., Cai, D.: Outflow boundary conditions for blood flow in arterial trees. PloS One 10(5), e0128597 (2015)
4. Farsad, N., Yilmaz, H.B., Eckford, A., Chae, C.B., Guo, W.: A comprehensive survey of recent advancements in molecular communication. IEEE Commun. Surv. Tutor.. 18(3), 1887–1919 (2016). Third Quarter
5. Gabe, I.T., Gault, J.H., Ross, J., et al.: Measurement of instantaneous blood flow velocity and pressure in conscious man with a catheter-tip velocity probe. Circulation 40(5), 603–614 (1969)
6. Huang, J.T., Lai, H.Y., Lee, Y.C., Lee, C.H., Yeh, P.C.: Distance estimation in concentration-based molecular communications. In: 2013 IEEE Global Communications Conference (GLOBECOM), pp. 2587–2591 (2013)
7. Huang, S., Lin, L., Guo, W., Yan, H., Xu, J., Liu, F.: Initial distance estimation and signal detection for diffusive mobile molecular communication. IEEE Trans. Nanobiosci. 19(3), 422–433 (2020)
8. Kilinc, D., Akan, O.B.: Receiver design for molecular communication. IEEE J. Sel. Areas Commun. 31(12), 705–714 (2013)
9. Koutsiaris, A.G., et al.: Blood velocity pulse quantification in the human conjunctival pre-capillary arterioles. Microvasc. Res. 80(2), 202–208 (2010)
10. Lin, L., Huang, F., Yan, H., Liu, F., Guo, W.: Ant-behavior inspired intelligent nanonet for targeted drug delivery in cancer therapy. IEEE Trans. NanoBiosci. 19(3), 323–332 (2020)
11. Lin, L., Luo, Z., Huang, L., Luo, C., Wu, Q., Yan, H.: High-accuracy distance estimation for molecular communication systems via diffusion. Nano Commun. Netw. 19, 47–53 (2019)
12. Lin, L., Zhang, J., Ma, M., Yan, H.: Time synchronization for molecular communication with drift. IEEE Commun. Lett. 21(3), 476–479 (2017)

13. Luo, Z., Lin, L., Fu, Q., Yan, H.: An effective distance measurement method for molecular communication systems. In: Proceedings of the 2018 International Conference on on Sensing, Communication and Networking (SECON Workshops), pp. 1–4. IEEE (2018)
14. Luo, Z., Lin, L., Ma, M.: Offset estimation for clock synchronization in mobile molecular communication system. In: Proceedings of the IEEE WCNC, pp. 1–6. IEEE (2016)
15. Moore, M.J., Nakano, T., Enomoto, A., Suda, T.: Measuring distance from single spike feedback signals in molecular communication. IEEE Trans. Signal Process. **60**(7), 3576–3587 (2012)
16. Nakano, T.: Molecular communication: a 10 year retrospective. IEEE Trans. Mol. Biol. Multi-scale Commun. **3**(2), 71–78 (2017)
17. Pierobon, M., Akyildiz, I.F.: Capacity of a diffusion-based molecular communication system with channel memory and molecular noise. IEEE Trans. Inf. Theory **59**(2), 942–954 (2013)
18. Wang, X., Higgins, M.D., Leeson, M.S.: Distance estimation schemes for diffusion based molecular communication systems. IEEE Commun. Lett. **19**(3), 399–402 (2015)

Innovating the Future Healthcare Systems

Opti-Speech-VMT: Implementation and Evaluation

Hiranya G. Kumar[1](✉)(iD), Anthony R. Lawn[1,2], B. Prabhakaran[1](iD),
and William F. Katz[1](iD)

[1] University of Texas at Dallas, Richardson, TX 75080, USA
{hiranya,bprabhakaran,wkatz}@utdallas.edu
[2] Topaz Labs, 14285 Midway Road, Suite 125, Addison, TX 75001, USA

Abstract. We describe Opti-Speech-VMT, a prototype tongue tracking system that uses electromagnetic articulography to permit visual feedback during oral movements.Opti-Speech-VMT is specialized for visuo-motor tracking (VMT) experiments in which participants follow an oscillating virtual target in the oral cavity using a tongue sensor. The algorithms for linear, curved, and custom trajectories are outlined, and new functionality is briefly presented. Because latency can potentially affect accuracy in VMT tasks, we examined system latency at both the API and total framework levels. Using a video camera, we compared the movement of a sensor (placed on an experimenter's finger) against an oscillating target displayed on a computer monitor. The average total latency was 87.3 ms, with 69.8 ms attributable to the API, and 17.4 ms to Opti-Speech-VMT. These results indicate minimal reduction in performance due to Opti-Speech-VMT, and suggest the importance of the EMA hardware and signal processing optimizations used.

Keywords: Speech · Tongue · Visual feedback · Electromagnetic articulography · Avatar · 3D model · Latency

1 Introduction

In previous work, we described Opti-Speech, a technique for animating a 3D model of the human tongue in real time [1]. The system was designed for research and training in second language learning and for clinical applications in speech language pathology. We used motion capture data from an electromagnetic articulography (EMA) system and an off-the-shelf 3D animation software (Maya) to create the visual representation. The goal of the Opti-Speech project was to create a real-time tongue representation with the necessary resolution for designating tongue shapes and positions common to a variety of speech sounds. In our application, "joint" positions and rotations were used to drive a hierarchical rig of virtual joints that in turn deformed a geometric mesh of a virtual tongue. Based on practical considerations (number of EMA sensors that can be comfortably placed on the lingual surface) and prior research on the number of

M. Ur Rehman and A. Zoha (Eds.): BODYNETS 2021, LNICST 420, pp. 233–246, 2022.
https://doi.org/10.1007/978-3-030-95593-9_19

EMA sensors that can effectively describe speech sounds [2,3], we determined that five markers could provide the necessary resolution for identifying tongue shapes and positions common to a variety of speech sounds. We created a flexible rig of joints in Autodesk Maya to allow the markers to drive a polygonal tongue that was then brought into Autodesk MotionBuilder software. Through a custom plugin for MotionBuilder, the motion data from our EMA system is streamed in real-time and constrained to the marker setup of the rig. The resulting movement of the tongue mesh allows the subject to watch a 3D model of their own tongue movements in real time (Fig. 1).

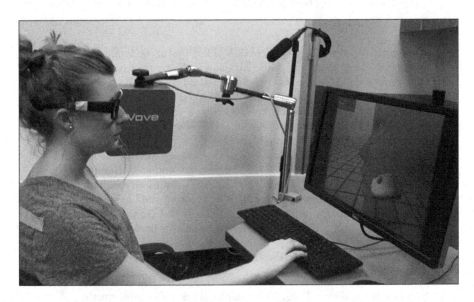

Fig. 1. A participant using the Opti-Speech system with NDI WAVE hardware.

Several studies were conducted using the first prototype system, including training [4–6], and visuomotor tracking [7,8] paradigms. These studies revealed the limitations of our first prototype Opti-Speech system, including an inability to introduce moving targets and to present different trajectories for these moving targets. These additional features are useful for studies of speech motor control, including comparisons of speech and non-speech movements. In addition, these features will help in clinical studies that present more sophisticated moving target patterns for patients to emulate.

In this paper, we introduce Opti-Speech-VMT (Opti-Speech for Visual Motor Tracking experiments) providing: (i) a variety of static and moving targets, (ii) different trajectories for the moving target, including curved and custom trajectories. Since the latency of the system could have effects on users in speech and tracking experiments, we investigated the Opti-Speech-VMT and total system latency periods. The results indicated that Opti-Speech-VMT contributed minimal latency (17.464 ms) and that total system delay was substantially larger (87.319 ms). Most importantly, these latency periods fall below the range reported to have potential adverse effects on speech performance.

2   Related Work

Although the effects of visual feedback on speech have been extensively reviewed in several studies [9–18], few studies have focused on the framework used to obtain the feedback. Most of the studies on effects of visual feedback on speech learning have relied on ultrasound imaging [9–12]. Ultrasound (US) imaging allows a participant to directly visualize the interior of the oral cavity as a two-dimensional image. It comes with a few advantages: the output from an US system doesn't need processing to be used as visual feedback for the participant, the detection system itself is non-intrusive, and the equipment is portable. In addition, there have been recent developments in tongue tracking and segmentation in US images. Laporte et al. (2018) [13] developed an US tongue tracking system that uses simple tongue shape and motion models with a flexible contour representation to estimate the shape of the tongue. Karimi et al. (2019) [14] discuss an algorithm requiring no training or manual intervention which uses image enhancement, skeletonization and clustering to come up with a set of candidate points that can then be used to fit an active contour to the image, subsequently initializing a tracking algorithm. Mozaffari et al. (2020) [15] make use of Deep Learning techniques (Encoder-decoder CNN models) for automatic tracking of tongue contours in real-time in US images.

A disadvantage of US feedback systems is that the imaging provided is typically low-resolution, monochrome, and noisy, and therefore not very intuitive. In addition, the visual feedback cannot be customized by the user to add functionality such as interactive feedback, adding targets, manipulating input data, etc., which limits usability for different types of speech experiments.

EMA-based systems have also been used for visual feedback studies [16–18], although to lesser extent than US-based systems, due to their lack of portability and high costs. Shtern et al. (2012) [16] and Tilsen et al. (2015) [17] describe EMA real-time feedback systems for articulatory training. Real-time kinematic data from the EMA system is used to create an interactive 3D game for speech learning/rehabilitation, based on the Unity Game Engine.

Suemitsu et al. (2015) [18] make use of EMA hardware for real-time visual feedback to support learning the pronunciation of a second language. Specifically, they studied the production of an unfamiliar English vowel, (/æ/), by five native Japanese speakers. An array of EMA sensors was used to obtain each participant's tongue and lip fleshpoint positions, and an image of the tongue surface was estimated using cubit spline interpolation. Participants compared their head-corrected, near real-time data with an/æ/target obtained from a multiple linear regression model based on previous X-ray microbeam data and additional EMA data.

The project that most directly relates to ours is a visual feedback framework (Kristy et al. [19]) based on Blender, a free and open-source software for 3D development. This framework is able to visualise and record data from a EMA system or from a file. It uses NDI WAVE hardware and performs data-processing steps (including head correction, smoothing, and transformation to local coordinate system) before generating the visual feedback. A Python program is used to fetch and process data using the NDI Wave API.

Although the EMA-based game systems mentioned above do provide the user with visual feedback of their tongue movements, they have a near-static environment with a minimal feature set. As such, these systems lack several important features, including an ability to add interactive targets, easily control the visual elements on the screen, vary the sensor placement, and conduct visuomotor tracking experiments.

3   Opti-Speech-VMT

Visuomotor tracking (VMT) tasks involve a participant following a rhythmic external signal with a limb or speech articulator (typically the lip/jaw). It is common to designate targets of different speeds and levels of predictability to assess the role of feedforward/feedback processing in motor control. In addition, the direction of movement may be of interest [5,6].

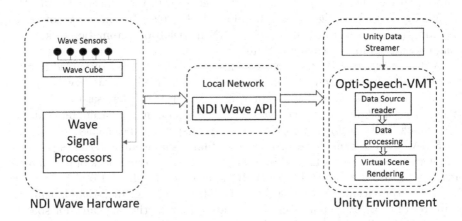

Fig. 2. A flowchart describing the workflow of the Opti-Speech-VMT system used with NDI Wave hardware.

3.1   General Features

Opti-Speech-VMT is built using the open source software Unity (version 2020.1.12f1) in Windows 10, and is compatible with the latest version of Unity and Windows (as of this date). Due to the application being built in Unity, which is a cross-platform tool, it can be migrated to other Unity supported platforms (such as Linux, MacOS, etc.) with minimal effort. Figure 3 shows the GUI of

Opti-Speech-VMT. All the menus are collapsible, to allow a clean user interface. Some menus have been expanded in the figure to show the available options for the user.

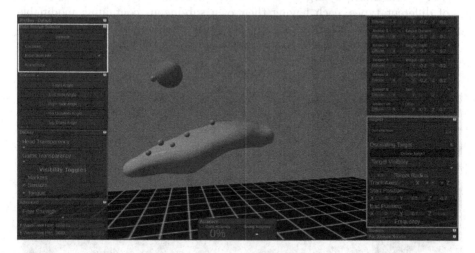

Fig. 3. A screenshot of the Opti-Speech-VMT GUI showing the tongue avatar with fully transparent skull and jaw models.

Various features offered by Opti-Speech-VMT are:

1. **Data source selector**: Opti-Speech-VMT supports multiple data sources simultaneously. The Data source selector menu (highlighted in a yellow box in Fig. 3) allows the user to select from multiple data sources that could be connected to the system. Currently supported sources are:
   (a) File reader: Allows the user to play back a recorded sweep from a file
   (b) WaveFront: Allows user to stream data from NDI WAVE hardware.
   (c) Carstens (under development): Allows user to stream data from Carstens AG500 series articulography systems.
   Additional data sources can be added to the application by following the developer manual available with the project.
2. **Display menu**: The display menu (highlighted in a blue box in Fig. 3) allows the user to hide, show, and control the transparency of various elements on the screen, such as the tongue model, skull, jaws, markers, and sensors. Figure 4 shows an example with transparency for the skull and jaws set to around 50%. Users can set the values according to the participant's preferences or the experiment's requirements.
3. **Sensor List**: The Sensors List menu (highlighted in a red box in Fig. 3) allows the user to map the software sensor markers to physical sensors connected to the system. This mapping can be changed in real-time, which saves the user time and effort by not needing to ensure that the physical sensors are placed in a particular order. The menu also allows the user to set sensor-specific

offsets in case adjustments are needed to the positions of the virtual sensors (without requiring the user to adjust the physical sensors).

4. **Targets**: The targets menu (highlighted in a green box in Fig. 3) allows the user to add multiple targets to the scene simultaneously. The targets can be of different types, each having their own sub-menus containing modifiable parameters specific to the target type. Additional targets with custom trajectories can also be added to the application using the guide provided in the Developers manual.

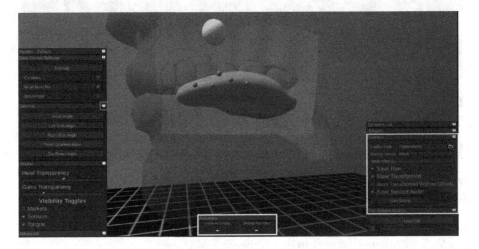

Fig. 4. A screenshot of the Opti-Speech-VMT GUI showing the tongue avatar with translucent skull and jaw models.

5. **Sweeps**: This menu (highlighted in a lime green box in Fig. 4) allows the user to record sweeps of an experiment. The sweeps record the data of all the objects present in the scene per timestamp. This includes status and positions of all the sensors, and the position and parameters of the targets and markers and other data needed by the application to replay the sweep (using the File Reader Data Source in Data Selector menu). Since the timestamp has a resolution of 1 millisecond, the data recorded are high resolution and allow for a precise replay of the sweep. The data are saved in a .tsv (tab-separated values) format, which is easy to read with any text editor or Microsoft Excel. Audio data synchronized with the timestamps can also be saved using options available in the menu.

6. **Tongue model**: The tongue model used in Opti-Speech-VMT is not rigid. This allows the shape and size of the tongue model to automatically change based on the positions of the physical sensors on the participant's tongue. While the model is not intended to be biomechanically/anatomically realistic for medical (e.g., surgical reconstruction planning) purposes, it closely represents tongue surface dimensions and movements sufficient for real-time applications.

7. **Accuracy Window**: The accuracy window (highlighted in a yellow box in Fig. 4) shows the cycle and sweep accuracies of the tongue movement with respect to a given target. This can be used as a visible metric for the participant to understand their performance on a per-cycle and per-sweep level.

8. **Other menus**: Apart from the above-mentioned menus, other menus are mainly designed for convenience. This includes the **Profiles menu** (above the Data Source Selector menu), which allows the users to save experiment settings in a profile and quickly load them to effortlessly repeat an experiment, the **Camera menu**, which has preset camera angles that help the user change the camera view to any of the available ones with just one click, and the **Advanced menu**, which allows a user to specify network settings used to communicate with connected EMA hardware and also specify Filter Strength to smooth out the raw sensor data incoming from the API. This can help smooth out the 'jittering' of virtual sensors that can result from the hardware being highly sensitive.

9. **Documentation**: Detailed documentation of the application is also available for user reference and further development of the application. The documentation is split into the "Researcher manual", meant for users of the application, and the "Developer manual", meant for developers who wish to modify or extend the functionalities of the application. The white speech bubbles (highlighted in a red box in Fig. 4) at the top right corner of each of the menus directly takes the user to the section of the documentation describing the usage of that specific menu. An example of the documentation for the Data Source selector menu is shown in Fig. 5.

3.2   Target Features

Static/Moving Targets: As in the original Opti-Speech prototype, Opti-Speech-VMT provides a static target for tongue tracking by allowing the operator to designate a virtual sphere in the oral cavity that a participant "hits" using a selected sensor on their tongue avatar. When the target is hit, it changes color, providing the participant with visual feedback of accuracy. Opti-Speech-VMT includes a "moving target" option that programs a single target to oscillate between two positions in the oral cavity. The direction, distance traversed, speed, and predictability of the oscillating target motion are all set by the operator during a session. The speed is controlled by a "frequency" option available in the menu. An option to add "randomness" to the target speed, which makes the speed variable and unpredictable between oscillations, is also available in the menu.

Trajectories: Target trajectories can be linear, curved, or "custom". This allows the experimenter to set tongue targets in linear oscillating patterns that are traditionally reported in VMT studies, as well as curved patterns that are more speech-like, as previous studies have reported curved (arc-like) patterns taken by the tongue in reaching spatial endpoints [20]. The custom trajectory

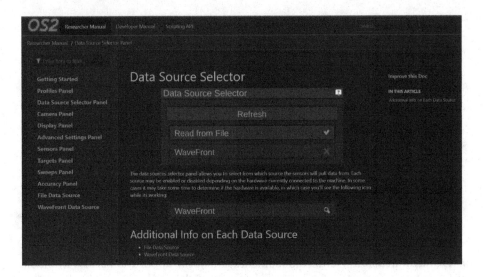

Fig. 5. An example of the documentation provided with Opti-Speech-VMT.

option can be used to create a variety of movement patterns, such as may be required in different studies of motor control.

Linear trajectories are based on a sinusoidal function, as described in Eq. 1 and Eq. 2. We use Eq. 1 with a Linear Interpolation (Lerp) function (Eq. 2) and user-provided start and end positions to get the position of the target at any given time (currTime). Employing a sinusoidal function instead of a standard linear function for linear oscillating motion allows us to generate a trajectory that slows down the target near the start and end positions, instead of abruptly reversing the direction of motion. This makes the trajectory closer to natural tongue motion.

$$f(freq, time) = \frac{Cos(2 * \pi * freq * time/1000) + 1}{2} \tag{1}$$

$$current\ position = Lerp(startPosition, endPosition, f(freq, time)) \tag{2}$$

Where,

- freq = frequency of oscillation (oscillations/second).
- nRebounds = number of times the target has changed directions till now.
- startPosition = User defined start position of the target.
- currPosition = current position of the target at the given time.
- pauseTime = User defined time to pause after reaching start/end position (in ms).
- time = Current timestamp from the application

Curved trajectories are implemented using an ellipse equation, as shown in (Eq. 3). The trajectory is currently restricted to the YZ plane only. Apart from the frequency of oscillation, this equation also needs the major and minor axis of the ellipse as user inputs. To emulate a more natural tongue movement, we add a small user-defined pause towards the end and start positions of the trajectory. The adding of a pause time makes the algorithm significantly more complicated.

$$currPosition = (c.x, c.y + r.y * Sin(angle), c.z + r.z * Cos(angle)) \quad (3)$$

$$if\ tempAngle >= 90,\ angle = tempAngle,\ else\ angle = 180 - tempAngle \quad (4)$$

$$tempAngle = (freq * 180 * localTime/1000)\ mod\ 180 \quad (5)$$

$$localTime = time - nRebounds * pauseTime \quad (6)$$

$$c = startPosition - r \quad (7)$$

Where,

- c = 3D coordinates of the center of the ellipse.
- r = User defined 3D vector with the radius of the ellipse along each axis.
- freq = frequency of oscillation (oscillations/second).
- nRebounds = number of time the target has changed directions till now.
- startPosition = User defined start position of the target.
- currPosition = current position of the target at the given time.
- pauseTime = User defined time to pause after reaching start/end position (in ms).
- time = Current timestamp from the application

The curved trajectories are currently limited to the YZ plane (Y axis being vertical and Z axis being horizontal with respect to the oral cavity) for simplicity and since most common 2D tongue motions are restricted to the YZ (mid-sagittal) plane.

Custom motion trajectories replicate a prerecorded tongue movement. Tongue movement can be recorded using the 'Record Sweep' functionality offered by the application. The menu allows the Target to replicate the movements of any of the sensors recorded in the sweep. This can be used to have the patient emulate pronunciation of a particular syllable/word. All the trajectories that cannot be described by a simple mathematical equation can be recorded by the user in a sweep and replicated by this function for experiments and/or training.

4   Measurement of Latency

For a visual feedback system, latency is an important metric. A significant lag between the tongue's motion and the visual feedback on the screen can have significant effects on the subject's experience and response as well as on the experimental results [21–23].

For instance, studies of the effects of visual and/or auditory feedback on pointing and steering tasks (Friston et al. [22]), sequence reproduction on a keyboard (Kulpa et al. [21]), and sentence repetition (Chesters et al. [23]) report a broad range at which latencies affect motor behavior, ranging from 16–400 ms. Friston et al. [22] also note that measurement of latencies below 50 ms, in tasks that involve indirect physical interaction, has only recently become possible due to advancements in technology. Regarding tongue visual feedback, Suemitsu et al. [18] describe "no perceptually apparent latency between sensor motion and its visualization" for their system based on a Carstens AG500 EMA system. While perceptual benchmarks are important, it would also be useful to have measurements of the latency of visual feedback frameworks to help further studies in this domain. We therefore designed an experiment to measure the latency of the Opti-Speech framework at different levels.

4.1   Visual Feedback Task

The experiment makes use of a camera to monitor the real sensor and the computer screen (60 Hz refresh rate) showing the API and Opti-Speech-VMT sensors. The camera records a video of the sensor moving in an oscillating trajectory in the plane of observation of the camera. The perspectives of the camera in the rendering software (API and Opti-Speech-VMT) are adjusted to match that of the camera recording the experiment, such that they have the same plane of observation. A tripod-mounted phone camera (Samsung Galaxy S20FE) was used in 1920×1080 60 FPS video recording mode, with all other video settings set to auto. Video was recorded in a well-lit environment to facilitate color-based tracking.

We directly measured two types of latency periods: the latency at the API level (API Latency), which is the time taken by the EMA hardware to process raw signals from the sensors into sensor positions, and latency at the framework level (total latency), which is the total time taken for a change in real sensor position to reflect in Opti-Speech-VMT's visual tongue avatar. We use these latency values to compute Opti-Speech-VMT latency (Eq. 8), which is the time taken by Opti-Speech-VMT to get the sensor positions from the API and render the scene with the tongue avatar.

$$OptiSpeechVMT\ latency = total\ latency - API\ latency \qquad (8)$$

As we cannot directly compare the raw displacement values between the sensor, the API, and Opti-Speech-VMT, since the sensors are not calibrated, we use an oscillating trajectory, normalize the amplitudes of the trajectories, and plot them (Fig. 6). Next, we measure the latency at points in the trajectory where there is a change in direction (peaks and valleys of the oscillating trajectory). Since the oscillating movement of the real sensor is done by hand, the trajectories aren't perfectly sinusoidal. We process the video recording in Python frame-by-frame and use OpenCV [24] to track the trajectories of the sensors based on color.

Since the monitor displaying the API and Opti-Speech-VMT sensors and the camera have a refresh rate 60 Hz, the lowest latency we can measure is

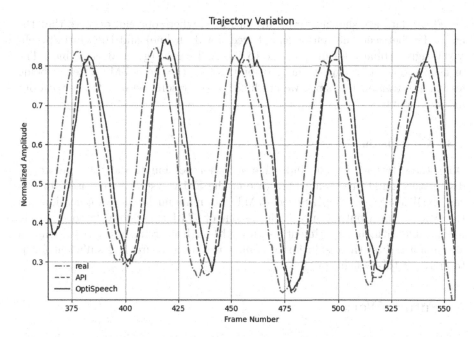

Fig. 6. Normalized amplitude of the trajectory of the Real sensor, API sensor and Opti-Speech-VMT sensor plotted against the frame number. The graph has been magnified to focus on a few periods of the oscillation to better show the temporal differences between the trajectories. (Color figure online)

1/60 s, which is 16.67 ms. The latency is directly measured in frames, and then converted to milliseconds based on the frame time (16.67 ms) (Eq. 9). We average the latency measurements from 42 samples taken at the peaks and valleys of the trajectories.

$$latency\ in\ ms = number\ of\ frames * 16.67 \tag{9}$$

4.2 Results

The results in Table 1 show a total latency of 5.238 frames (87.318 ms), out of which the API latency is responsible for 4.19 frames (69.855 ms) while Opti-Speech-VMT accounts for 1.048 frames (17.464 ms).

Table 1. Latency test results.

	Avg. total latency	Avg. API latency	Avg. Opti-Speech-VMT latency
Latency (Frames)	5.238	4.19	1.048
Latency (ms)	87.319	69.855	17.464

These data are shown graphically in Fig. 6, where one can observe that the major lag between the sensor signal (red dot-dash line) and the Opti-Speech-VMT signal (blue solid line) is due to the API signal (green dotted line). The measurements also suggest the possibility of Opti-Speech-VMT latency being less than 1 frame time, since we are limited to a resolution of 1 frame with our measurements.

4.3   Conclusion

With these results, we conclude that a major portion of the total latency is due to the signal processing hardware of the EMA system being used, in this case NDI Wavefront. Opti-Speech-VMT has minimal latency implications on the system, contributing only 17.46 ms out of 87.31 ms of total latency, barely measurable with our experimental setup. Although the refresh rate of the camera and monitor limit the resolution of latency we can measure, it is sufficient for us to arrive at this conclusion.

5   Future Work

Studies on the effects of latency on visual-feedback systems suggest that the minimum latency that can adversely effect human performance can greatly differ based on the nature of the task [21–23]. Although studies such as the one by Chesters et al. [23] investigate the effects of delayed visual feedback on speech experiments, the values of delays tested in such research are significantly higher than ours. Thus, a more comprehensive study into the effect of latency in speech visual- feedback systems in specific scenarios/speech experiments would be needed to evaluate the potential impact of Opti-Speech latencies across a variety of experimental settings.

Our findings suggest the total latency can be improved based on the EMA hardware being used or signal processing optimizations by the hardware manufacturers. At the time of this writing, the NDI WAVE system is no longer in production, with its support ending soon. Opti-Speech-VMT, while capable of receiving input from NDI WAVE, is being optimized for input from Carstens AG500 series articulography systems. These devices are more accurate, with measured dynamic accuracy of 0.3 mm during speech recording [25,26], and providing sampling rates as high as 1250 samples/sec. Such instrumentation, along with a faster API, should greatly reduce potential accuracy problems resulting from system latency lags.

A concomitant improvement we are working on is to devise a means of calibration to map distances between the real world and the virtual scene, as distances for the oscillating targets are currently estimated through approximation. We have had some success with this in a recent study [27] by scaling talker's vocal tract size as a function of maximum tongue displacement. We plan to expand these efforts to provide more effective target placement in Opti-Speech-VMT.

References

1. Katz, W., et al.: Opti-Speech: a real-time, 3D visual feedback system for speech training. In: INTERSPEECH, pp. 1174–1178 (2014)
2. Wang, J., Green, J.R., Samal, A.: Individual articulator's contribution to phoneme production. In: IEEE International Conference on Acoustics, Speech and Signal Proceedings, pp. 7785–7789, May 2013
3. Wang, J., Samal, A., Rong, P., Green, J.R.: An optimal set of flesh points on tongue and lips for speech-movement classification. J. Speech Lang. Hear. Res. **59**(1), 15–26 (2016)
4. Katz, W.F., Mehta, S.: Visual feedback of tongue movement for novel speech sound learning. Front. Hum. Neurosci. **9**, 612 (2015)
5. Watkins, C.H.: Sensor driven real-time animation for feedback during physical therapy, (Masters Thesis), The University of Texas at Dallas (2015)
6. Mental, R.L.: Using Realistic Visual Biofeedback for the Treatment of Residual Speech Sound Errors, (Doctoral Dissertation), Case Western Reserve University (2018)
7. Fazel, V., Katz, W.F.: Visuomotor pursuit tracking accuracy for intraoral tongue movement. J. Acoust. Soc. Am. **140**(4), 3224 (2016)
8. Fazel, V.: Lingual speech motor control assessed by a novel visuomotor tracking paradigm, (Doctoral Dissertation), The University of Texas at Dallas (2021)
9. Bernhardt, M.B., et al.: Ultrasound as visual feedback in speech habilitation: exploring consultative use in rural British Columbia. Canada. Clin. Linguist. Phonetics **22**(2), 149–162 (2008)
10. Preston, J.L., Leece, M.C., Maas, E.: Intensive treatment with ultrasound visual feedback for speech sound errors in childhood apraxia. Front. Hum. Neurosci. **10**(2016), 440 (2016)
11. Preston, J.L., et al.: Ultrasound visual feedback treatment and practice variability for residual speech sound errors. J. Speech Lang. Hear. Res. **57**(6), 2102–2115 (2014)
12. Haldin, C., et al.: Speech recovery and language plasticity can be facilitated by sensori-motor fusion training in chronic non-fluent aphasia. A case report study. Clin. Linguist. Phonetics **32**(7), 595–621 (2018)
13. Laporte, C., Ménard, L.: Multi-hypothesis tracking of the tongue surface in ultrasound video recordings of normal and impaired speech. Med. Image Anal. **44**, 98–114 (2018)
14. Karimi, E., Menard, L., Laporte, C.: Fully-automated tongue detection in ultrasound images. Comput. Biol. Med. **111**, 103335 (2019)
15. Mozaffari, M.H., Lee, W.-S.: Encoder-decoder CNN models for automatic tracking of tongue contours in real-time ultrasound data. Methods **179**, 26–36 (2020)
16. Shtern, M., Haworth, M.B., Yunusova, Y., Baljko, M., Faloutsos, P.: A game system for speech rehabilitation. In: Kallmann, M., Bekris, K. (eds.) MIG 2012. LNCS, vol. 7660, pp. 43–54. Springer, Heidelberg (2012). https://doi.org/10.1007/978-3-642-34710-8_5
17. Tilsen, S., Das, D., McKee, B.: Real-time articulatory biofeedback with electromagnetic articulography. Linguist. Vanguard **1**(1), 39–55 (2015)
18. Suemitsu, A., Dang, J., Ito, T., Tiede, M.: A real-time articulatory visual feedback approach with target presentation for second language pronunciation learning. J. Acoust. Soc. Am. **138**(4), EL382-7 (2015). PMID: 26520348, PMCID: PMC4608962. https://doi.org/10.1121/1.4931827

19. James, K., et al.: Watch your Tongue: A point-tracking visualisation system in Blender
20. Katz, W.F., Bharadwaj, S.V., Carstens, B.: Electromagnetic articulography treatment for an adult with Broca's aphasia and apraxia of speech. J. Speech Lang. Hear. Res. **42**(6), 1355–1366 (1999)
21. Kulpa, J.D., Pfordresher, P.Q.: Effects of delayed auditory and visual feedback on sequence production. Exp. Brain Res. **224**(1), 69–77 (2013)
22. Friston, S., Karlstrum, P., Steed, A.: The effects of low latency on pointing and steering tasks. IEEE Trans. Vis. Comput. Graph. **22**(5), 1605–1615 (2016)
23. Chesters, J., Baghai-Ravary, K., Mottonen, R.: The effects of delayed auditory and visual feedback on speech production. J. Acoust. Soc. Am. **137**(2), 873–883 (2015). https://doi.org/10.1121/1.4906266
24. Bradski, B.: The OpenCV Library. Dr. Dobb's J, Software Tools (2000)
25. Berry, J.: Accuracy of the NDI wave speech research system. J. Speech Lang. Hear. Res **54**, 1295–1301 (2011)
26. Sigona, F., Stella, M., Stella, A.P., Bernardini, P., Fivela, B.G., Grimaldi, M.: Assessing the position tracking reliability of Carstens' AG500 and AG501 electromagnetic articulographs during constrained movements and speech tasks. Speech Commun. **104**, 73–88 (2018)
27. Glotfelty, A., Katz, W.F.: The role of visibility in silent speech tongue movements: a kinematic study of consonants. J. Speech Lang. Hear. Res **2021**, 1–8 (2021)

A Systematic Study of the Influence of Various User Specific and Environmental Factors on Wearable Human Body Capacitance Sensing

Sizhen Bian[1,2(✉)] and Paul Lukowicz[1,2]

[1] DFKI, Kaiserslautern, Germany
{Sizhen.Bian,Paul.Lukowicz}@dfki.de
[2] University of Kaiserslautern, Kaiserslautern, Germany

Abstract. Body capacitance change is an interesting signal for a variety of body sensor network applications in activity recognition. Although many promising applications have been published, capacitive on body sensing is much less understood than more dominant wearable sensing modalities such as IMUs and has been primarily studied in individual, constrained applications. This paper aims to go from such individual-specific application to a systemic analysis of how much the body capacitance is influenced by what type of factors and how does it vary from person to person. The idea is to provide a basic form which other researchers can decide if and in what form capacitive sensing is suitable for their specific applications. To this end, we present a design of a low power, small form factor measurement device and use it to measure the capacitance of the human body in various settings relevant for wearable activity recognition. We also demonstrate on simple examples how those measurements can be translated into use cases such as ground type recognition, exact step counting and gait partitioning.

Keywords: Human body capacitance · Electric field sensing · Capacitive sensing · Respiration detection · Gait partitioning · Touch sensing · Ground type recognition · Step counting

1 Introduction

Electric capacitance, defined as the ratio between charge and the resulting electric potential, is a fundamental physical property. For a given object, "self-capacitance" reflects the electric potential with respect to the ground. It depends primarily on the object composition and size but is also significantly influenced by the shape and the spatial relation between the object and ground (Fig. 1). When considering the Human Body Capacitance (HBC), we have a baseline given by the body composition (which is 60% water) and a specific person's size plus components related to posture, limb motion, the contact surface to the

M. Ur Rehman and A. Zoha (Eds.): BODYNETS 2021, LNICST 420, pp. 247–274, 2022.
https://doi.org/10.1007/978-3-030-95593-9_20

ground and contact with other objects. The latter varying components make *HBC* an interesting modality for on-body sensing as they allow a single quantity to capture complex phenomena ranging from complex postures and motions, through clothing and the composition of the environment (in particular the floor) to physiological parameters such as breathing.

A well-known *HBC* application is the musical instrument Theremin [1,2] where the acoustic volume and pitch are controlled by the distance between limbs and two metal loop antennas. Besides that, *HBC* was finitely explored in specific motion-sensing applications. Arshad et al. designed a floor sensing system to monitor the motion of elderly patients [3] to various gesture monitoring systems. Marco [4] presented a textile neckband for head gesture recognition. Bian [5] showed a capacitive wristband for on-board hand gesture recognition. The background behind is the capacitance between two positions on the skin. The variation of the skin capacitance was used to deduce the neck movement. Cohn [6] took advantage of the *HBC* to detect the arm movement by supplying a conductive ground plane near the wrist.

1.1   Paper Aims

This paper aims to go from individual-specific application to a systemic analysis of how much the body capacitance is influenced by what type of factors and how does it vary from person to person. The idea is to provide a basic form which other researchers can decide if and in what capacitive sensing is suitable for their specific applications. To this end, we have designed and implemented a low-cost, low-power consumption, wearable prototype capable of monitoring the value of the *HBC* when the user is in both static and dynamic (moving, walking) states. We also briefly show in simple illustrative experiments how the property that we investigated can contribute to use cases such as ground type recognition (F-score of 0.63), exact step counting (with 99.4% accuracy, 94.3% with a gyroscope for comparison), gait partitioning (with an accuracy of 95.3% and 93.7% for stance and swing phases, respectively, 93.1% and 90.8% with a gyroscope for comparison).

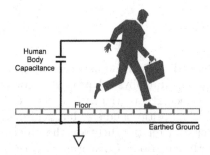

Fig. 1. Human body capacitance: the coupling between body and earthed ground/surroundings

Table 1. Human body capacitance measurement

Authors/Year	Tool	HBC value (pf)	Test condition	Variation source
Bonet et al. [7,8] 2012	Impedance analyzer (10 kHz–1 MHz)	70–110 110–180	Foot on ground Foot 10 cm above ground	Different frequency input of the analyser
Buller et al. [9] 2006	Mathematical model of body-conducive wire mutual capacitance	48.5–48.9	Static standing	Body - wire distance
Forster et al. [10] 1974	Cathode-ray oscilloscope and a shielded resistive probe	100–330	Volunteer lying on medical bed	Laboratory environment
Greason et al. [11] 1995	Mathematical model of ESD and the human body	Qualitative analysis		Grounding, charge sources, etc.
Huang et al. [12] 1997	Capacitive meter	112–113	Sitting on chair	Human body resistance, leakage resistance
Pallas et al. [13] 1991	Oscilloscope and voltage divider probe	120–520	Static standing	Interference from power line
Iceanu et al. [14] 2004	Electrometer (6517A model) and Faraday's cup	160–170 159–165	Static standing Sitting on chair	Different charging voltage from the electrometer
Jonasson et al. [15] 1998	Mathematical model Electrometer (charger sharing method) Conventional AC-bridge (AC-measurement method)	100–300 268 170	Static standing Standing with polymeric soles, linoleum floor Standing with polymeric soles, linoleum floor	Shoes and floor
Fujiwara et al. [16] 2002	Polyhedral model, power charger, analog switch (surface charger method)	120–130	Static standing	Foot-ground distance
Serrano et al. [17] 2003	Physical model, oscilloscope and voltage divider probe	110–3905	Static standing, touching surrounding	Power lines and surroundings
Haberman et al. [18] 2011	Fluke 112 multimeter and customised circuit	110–280	Standing, sitting, touching surrounding	Power lines and surroundings

1.2 Related Work

Research on the measurement of human body capacitance was mainly performed many years ago. Table 1 summarizes the result of such work by different groups. Most of the concluded value matches the definition of the human body capacitance from the Electrostatic Discharge Association (ESDA), in which a value of 100 pF is stated. However, the related explorations are either based on mathematic estimation methods [7,9,15,17], or measured in a laboratory with heavy, expensive instruments, like impedance analyzer, oscilloscope [8,12–14,16]. Besides the theoretical or laboratory methods, all those works focused on the *HBC* value with a static body state, like sitting, standing, or lying.

To understand how the body capacitance changes in real-time, we developed a wearable, low-cost, low power consumption prototype capable of measuring the value of *HBC* in real-time (in Sect. 2). We first explored the body capacitance with a static body state, sitting and standing with this prototype. Secondly, we tested the potential influence factors that could change the body capacitance, like the body postures, the wearings like the sole's height, the surroundings like the different indoor spots and ground types (in Sect. 3). Then we observed the body capacitance's real-time change while the tester was in a dynamic state, like walking around a building (in Sect. 4). Finally, we showed several potential applications either quantitively or non-quantitively with our wearable prototype, like exact step counting, gait partitioning, passive touch sensing, respiration monitoring (in Sect. 5).

2 Sensing Approach

Inspired by the Theremin [2], we designed a simple circuit that takes the body as part of it so that the body capacitance could be measured in an straightforward way. Capacitance itself usually is not easy to be measured directly, especially when the sensing unit needs to be portable and battery-powered. Thus, physical variables like the voltage, current, or frequency are adopted as a reflection of the capacitance. Here we put the body into an oscillating circuit, by measuring the frequency of the oscillator, the body capacitance could be deduced. The security is guaranteed when the body is enclosed into the circuit since the current flowing on the skin is in uA level and the voltage in mV level [19].

Figure 2 depicts the timer-based RC oscillator, where the capacitor charges through R1 and R2, discharges through R2. The trigger and threshold terminals are connected so that the oscillator will trigger itself and free run as a multivibrator. The frequency can be calculated by Eq. 1 [20]:

$$f = \frac{1.44}{(R1 + 2 * R2)C} \tag{1}$$

Where C is the capacitance of the parallelly connected $C2$ and $C4$. $C4$ indicates the capacitance of the body. To be noticed, this equation does not account for the propagation delay of the timer as well as the input capacitance of the

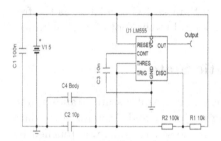
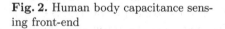
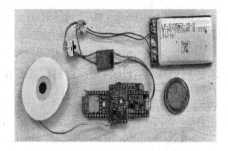

Fig. 2. Human body capacitance sensing front-end

Fig. 3. Hardware prototype

trigger and threshold terminals (around 2 pF each pin). The input capacitance is a particular value, while the propagation delay of the timer will increase with a higher frequency [21]. To address the propagation delay and the pins' input capacitance caused virtual capacitance, we put $C2$ alone in the circuit, and measured an output frequency of 335 kHz, meaning that the virtual capacitance was 10.47 pF. Then we changed $C2$ from 10 pF to 20 pF, got a virtual capacitance of 10.62 pF, which is not too much different from the previous value. Thus in the following experiment, we first read the oscillating frequency, then calculated the body capacitance enclosed into the circuit by subtracting the virtual capacitance of 10.5 pF from the result of Eq. 1.

Figure 3 shows the hardware prototype. The sensing front end is followed by a Teensy 3.6 development board from the market [22], which is capable of counting the frequency up to ten's MHz. The signal data is collected with 10 Hz sample rate and is recorded into an SD card, or transmitted by a low power Bluetooth or a USB cable to the computer. An IMU (BNO055) is also attached to the main board for supplying comparable movement data. The electrode is the universal ECG electrode that can stick on the skin. A 3.7 V lithium battery with 1050 mAh capacity is used to power the hardware after being boosted to 5.0 V. The whole design consumes 85 mA current, where the capacitance measurement part consumes only 2 mA current. The cost for the capacitance measurement part is nothing more than a normal timer as well as a few capacitors and resistors, costing less than one dollar.

A similar front end was used by Tobias [23], where he used a timer-based oscillator for capacitive cm-level proximity sensing. The difference is that the charging and discharging object in the reference was from the environment outside the circuit, namely the capacitance between the electrode and the environment. Another remarkable design was from Cheng's work [24], where the authors used a transistor-based LC oscillator (Colpitts oscillator) for capacitive movement sensing, and focused on the activity recognition. Although an LC-based oscillator enjoys a higher oscillating frequency than RC based timer oscillator, it is less sensitive to the capacitance variation than an RC oscillator, as the frequency of an LC oscillator is inversely proportional to the root of a capacitance.

3   Exploration of HBC in a Static State

We firstly explored the *HBC* while the body is in a static state: standing and sitting. As Fig. 4 depicts, we had the sensing prototype and a computer for data recording on an office desk, an electrode from the sensing unit was touched by the left hand of the volunteer while the volunteer was sitting on an office chair or standing beside. The prototype was connected to the computer by a USB cable, so they both shared the same ground. The computer was grounded through the power line so that the body was enclosed within the oscillator circuit, as the capacitor *C*4 in Fig. 2 represents. In essence, *HBC* occurs as a form of an electrostatic field, which is caused by the charge on the body and the charge from the unshielded wiring in the environment. The floor (normally composed of non-conductors like carpet, wood, concrete) itself cannot store charge. When one walks across a floor, the electrostatic charge accumulates on the body. This phenomenon does not implicate the existence of charge stored on the floor. The reason behind locates in the triboelectric effect [25]. That is to say, the dielectrics of the *HBC* include all the materials between the body and the grounded wires, namely the series of shoes and floor, instead of the shoes alone. This also matches the above mentioned literature [7–18] where all the instruments used to measure the *HBC*, like the oscilloscope, impedance analyzer, were earthed to the power lines, so as the mathematical or physical models in the literature. The human body model (*HBM*) in section 3.4.1 of ESD Handbook defined by the ESDA [26] also guarantees the grounded side in a body's physical electric model.

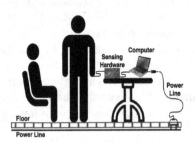

Fig. 4. *HBC* measurement in static body state

In this experiment, seven participants joined the measurement. Table 2 lists their gender, weight, and height. Table 3 lists the *HBC* of the volunteers with standing and sitting state. They wore their daily clothes and shoes during this measurement. This measurement was performed in a 4 m × 5 m working office.

Table 2. Volunteers' information

Volunteer	1	2	3	4	5	6	7
Age	31	21	25	25	19	29	28
Gender	Male	Male	Male	Female	Female	Female	Male
Weight (kg)	98	83	71	64	54	58	92
Height (cm)	185	176	168	165	157	161	180

Table 3. HBC in standing and sitting

Volunteer	1	2	3	4	5	6	7
Standing frequency (MHz)	0.0580	0.0680	0.0685	0.0680	0.0698	0.0695	0.0655
Standing capacitance (pF)	97.72	80.34	79.60	80.34	77.74	78.16	84.19
Sitting frequency (MHz)	0.0570	0.0664	0.0675	0.0678	0.0672	0.0690	0.0650
Sitting capacitance (pF)	99.80	82.77	81.09	80.64	81.54	78.88	84.99

The measured capacitance from all volunteers shows a value of 77 to 100 pF, which matches the result of previous work, where the HBC was measured by labor used heavy instruments. The capacitance value from all volunteers also shows that the HBC in sitting body state is slightly higher than in the standing state. This is reasonable since the distance from the body to the ground will be shorter by sitting down. The data also shows that volunteers with larger body form (taller and higher weight) have a higher value of HBC, like volunteers one and seven. Volunteers five and six have a smaller body form, and give a smaller standing body capacitance. However, how the body form affects the HBC is not clear at this point, since the body form related cross-objects observation is not acquired with a controlled variable method and also the observation is not common since volunteer two's body form is also big, but he had the same standing body capacitance with volunteer four.

The certain point is that factors like the environment, the wearing, will impact the electrical characteristics of a body. For example, standing against a working grounded refrigerator will form a relatively strong electric field between the body and the appliance. Thus with our simplified HBC meter, we researched the following factors that can affect the HBC by observing the HBC variation within different configurations of a single volunteer.

(A) HBC Influence Factor: Wearing

We firstly focused on the wearing, especially the type and height of sole, which is the main dielectrics that insulate the body from the grounded plane. Four types of soles with two types of material and two sets of height were prepared for the testers. Since it was not easy to find a sole with pure PVC or pure rubber, we took the maximum composition as the sole type. The height of the sole was rounded to the nearest integer number. Table 4 presents the measured HBC with different sole configuration.

Table 4. HBC of different sole height, type with the body standing (unit: pF)

Volunteer	1	2	3	4	5	6	7
bare feet	107.67	91.00	90.10	81.54	88.34	83.39	92.47
2 cm height PVC	95.72	81.54	80.34	79.60	79.46	73.43	89.21
3 cm height PVC	89.21	78.16	78.16	76.08	76.08	69.72	83.39
2 cm height rubber	93.40	77.74	79.60	76.76	78.16	70.32	86.98
3 cm height rubber	90.10	76.76	77.46	76.35	76.08	69.13	85.81

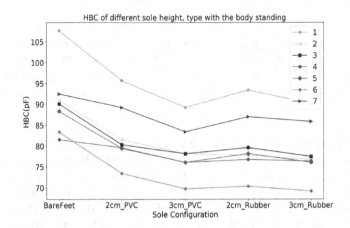

Fig. 5. Seven volunteers' HBC with different sole configuration

Figure 5 depicts a clear HBC variation with different sole configuration for each volunteer. While wearing nothing on the feet, each volunteer gives the highest value of HBC. This value decreases as they wear a thicker sole, which is reasonable since the capacitance value is inversely proportional to the distance between the two corresponding conductive plates. The material types of the sole should also have some influence on the HBC since they have distinct permittivities, but from our data, a clear and uniform difference from the sole material type can not be observed.

(B) HBC Influence Factor: Posture

Besides the wearing, the body postures also play an important role on the HBC, since the postures of the body will change the distance and the overlapping area of the two plates of a capacitor, as Table 3 represents. Besides sitting and standing, we also researched posture variations from the limbs. Table 5 lists the measured capacitance with different postures when the tested volunteer was sitting on the office chair.

The measured capacitance from the seven volunteers locates in the range of 72 pF to 107 pF and shows a uniform variation with the five postures (Fig. 6). Lifting legs will decrease the HBC, the decreased scale can be up to 10 pF, and can be as low as less than 1 pF. It should have something to do with the lifting height that the volunteers performed (unfortunately we didn't instruct the lifting height during the test). Lifting the arm will enlarge the HBC, the reason behind is the enlarged body area relative to the ground. This also explains the result of postures with different distance between the two legs, moving the leg apart will enlarge the HBC.

Table 5. HBC of different postures with the body sitting on the chair (unit: pF)

Volunteer	1	2	3	4	5	6	7
Sitting	99.80	82.77	81.09	80.64	81.54	78.88	84.99
Lift one foot	90.10	78.30	74.08	80.04	76.08	75.00	81.84
Lift two feet	86.64	77.46	73.43	79.17	72.16	73.43	80.79
Lift right arm	104.63	86.81	83.39	81.24	83.39	79.90	90.10
Two legs close to each other	93.78	78.88	74.74	76.08	76.76	77.18	82.15
Two legs apart from each other	106.48	88.34	82.15	81.84	84.19	80.34	89.56

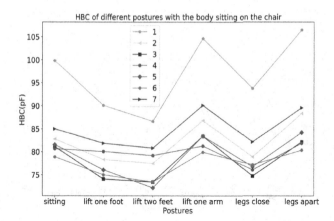

Fig. 6. Seven volunteers' HBC in different body postures

(C) HBC Influence Factor: Environment

Lastly, we tested the influence of the environment, including four ground types. All the objects wore their daily clothes and shoes, stood static in different spots in the office building. Table 6 lists the measured body capacitance value. It is evident that the environment, referring to different spots, different ground types in an office building in this paper, has a significant influence on the HBC while the body is in a static standing state. The largest HBC change was from volunteer one, where around 50 pF was raised while he stood against the wall compared to his standing state in the social hall. The smallest HBC variation was 18.28 pF from volunteer four while she stood against the wall and stood on the wood floor stair.

Table 6. HBC of different environment (unit: pF)

Volunteer	1	2	3	4	5	6	7
Office room	97.72	80.34	79.60	80.34	77.74	78.16	84.19
Against server room door	111.37	103.05	91.91	91.91	83.71	83.08	104.86
Social hall	94.55	77.88	77.74	78.88	77.46	69.72	82.92
Near wall	142.76	113.43	122.35	94.36	95.72	86.64	129.22
Textile floor	99.80	93.03	85.98	77.46	78.88	72.16	95.72
Carpet floor	116.09	102.39	88.34	84.35	84.99	81.84	112.65
Concrete floor	108.88	80.34	81.84	81.84	80.04	78.88	98.13
Wood floor	99.38	74.74	77.46	76.08	74.74	63.12	91.54

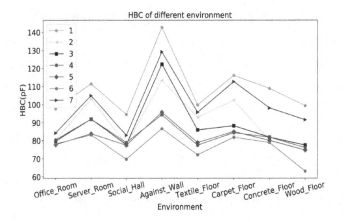

Fig. 7. Seven volunteers' HBC in different environment

Figure 7 depicts the variation of HBC in different environments. The first four spots (office room, near the server room, social hall, and near the wall) had the same textile floor. Each volunteer shows the highest capacitance value while standing against the bearing wall since the solid iron inside the wall is good-coupled with the grounded cables inside the building. The server room is occupied with grounded electric instruments, thus causes a higher HBC while the volunteers stood near the server room's door. At the social hall, all volunteers have the lowest capacitance value compared to the other three spots. The four floor types were chosen since those are pretty common types inside a building.

The textile floor and carpet floor are in the aisle, and the concrete floor locates between the elevator and aisle, the wood floor is the wood stairs between each storey. From the measured capacitance, the body capacitance on the textile floor and concrete floor are different from each other and also do not show a uniform relation among the seven volunteers. The carpet floor gives the highest capacitance value, and the wood floor shows the lowest. However, we can only compare the value measured with the body standing on the carpet and textile floor since they have the same surrounding (wall at both sides), the concrete floor is far from walls, and the wood floor is the stairs. Apparently the body on the carpet floor has higher capacitance than the body on the textile floor, demonstrating that the floor type also affects the HBC.

(D) HBC in static state: briefly summarise

The above-collected data demonstrates that the HBC is not a constant value. The volunteer's wearings, postures, environments are three critical factors that affect the HBC. For example, decreasing the distance between body and ground, enlarging the overlapping area of body and ground, wearing a pair of shoes with a thin sole, standing in an environment where good-grounded metal or wire exists, will enlarge the body's capacitance. This section's study supplied a closer look of the value of HBC in static body state with different wearings, postures, and environment configurations with the low-cost prototype.

4 HBC in Real-Time and Dynamic State

In this section, we recorded the HBC value with a dynamic body state in real-time. Firstly, we cut off the sensing hardware's earthed path so that the volunteers can walk indoors and outdoors without space limitation. Secondly, we stretched the local ground of the sensing unit to the soles with two pieces of wire and conductive tapes (attaching to the underside of the shoe sole). The hardware was worn on the upper back with the sensing electrode attached to the back neck, as Fig. 8 depicts.

4.1 HBC While Walking

Since in this wearable way, the prototype only senses the capacitance between body and underside sole, it does not indicate the value of HBC precisely. For verification, we attached the sensing electrode to the floor, and earthed the prototype through the computer, aiming to measure the capacitance between the floor and the earth by averaging the measured one-shot values from over twenty spots of the certain floor type (Fig. 9). Table 7 lists the measured averaged capacitance of different floor types, including the cement brick outside our working building. The value of HBC could be deduced by combining the floor capacitance and the capacitance of the body part measured in the wearable way (when dismissing the tiny step-caused sole-to-ground capacitance).

Fig. 8. Body part capacitance measurement in dynamic state

Table 7. Capacitance between floor and earthed ground

Floor type	Textile	Carpet	Concrete (indoors)	Concrete (exit stairway)	Wood	Cement brick (outdoors)
Capacitance (pF)	23.01	30.28	22.36	24.02	24.61	12.54

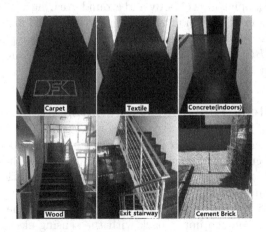

Fig. 9. Six floor surface types

To address the human body capacitance in a dynamic body state, we worn the prototype and recorded the body part capacitance while the volunteers were walking through the office building. Figure 10 shows five sessions of the recorded capacitance. In the first subplot of Fig. 10, the volunteer started walking on textile (0 s to 9.5 s, 14 s to 19 s, 22.5 s to 24 s) and carpet (9.5 s to 14 s, 19 s to 22.5 s) ground surface, followed by concrete (24 s to 36 s, 48 s to 67.5 s) surface, in between the volunteer went downstairs per wood stairs (36 s to 48 s). Then the volunteer went to the exit stairway and downstairs on the concrete surface (67.5 s to 105 s) for two floors. The outliers in between arose while the volunteer was at the exit stairway's joint spots, near the doors or windows. Finally, the volunteer walked out of the building and wandered around on cement brick ground (105 s to 129 s) for a while.

The body part capacitance of the first volunteer indoors locates in the range of 58 pF to 75 pF. When combined with the floor capacitance listing in Table 7, the HBC will be in the range of 80 pF to 110 pF, which also matches the HBC measured in a static body state. The peak-form signals in Fig. 10 is caused by the swing phase of a gait process, which is like the "lift foot" posture presenting in Table 6, causing around several pico-farads decrease in the body capacitance. Again, each volunteer shows a different value of HBC while the body is in a dynamic state. As explored in the last section, the influence factors could be their body form, postures like step scale, wearing, distance to the wall, etc.

4.2   Classification of Floor Surface Type

As Fig. 10 represents, while walking on different ground surfaces through the office building, the volunteers show regular body capacitance variation. This variation could be used for ground type recognition. We collected 28 sessions of body capacitance variation data from the seven volunteers. Each volunteer walked indoors to outdoors and back with the same path for four times. The interesting point is that the body capacitance variation mode in the exit stairway while walking from indoors to outdoors is significantly distinct with the mode while walking back, as the first two subplots depict (67.5 s to 105 s in the first subplot, vs. 28 s to 65 s in the second subplot). This observation is uniform in all sessions among all volunteers. Thus a potential conclusion can be made that the body capacitance relates not only to where the body is but also to where the body used to be, which will be quantitatively investigated in our future work.

In the HBC based dynamic body state applications, the absolute value of HBC does not matter much. Instead, the variation of the value during different activities is the decisive information. Suppose that the initial body part capacitance (standing on the textile ground surface) were known for each volunteer, so the capacitance value in each session will take the "textile capacitance" as a reference.

We performed the classification without considering the walking direction. In the beginning, we used the sliding window approach to get instances. The size of the window is 1 s, with 0.5 s overlapping. Classical approaches solving the problem of classifying sequences of sensor data involve two steps. Firstly, handcraft the features from the time series data with the sliding windows. Secondly, feed the models with the features and train the models. Different classic machine learning approaches, like k-Nearest Neighbors, Support Vector Machine, Gradient Boosting Machine, were tested, and we chose finally Random Forest model since it provided the best result. All hyper-parameters we used were the default ones by the scikit-learn [27]. We used two procedures to evaluate the classification result.

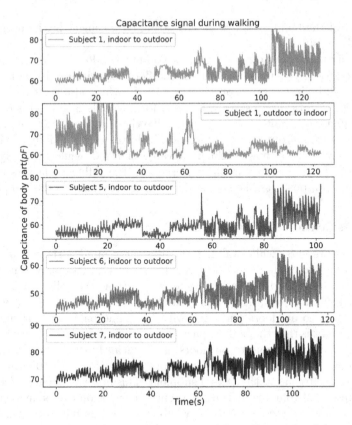

Fig. 10. Body part capacitance while walking around

- Firstly, we evaluated the model by **leaving one session out**, where each of the seven test sessions was selected from the four sessions of each volunteer. The model was then run with four-fold cross-validation.
- Secondly, to test across volunteers classification ability, we employed a **leave one user out** procedure where, for each fold, the test set contains all sessions of one volunteer, while the training set contains all sessions from the remaining volunteers. We run the models with seven-fold cross-validation with one volunteer out.

F-score and accuracy will represent the classification result. At the very beginning of the model procession, we balanced the labels with the method of SMOTE [28] since our data was unbalanced, more instances of the concrete ground type in the exit stairway than instances of the carpet ground type.

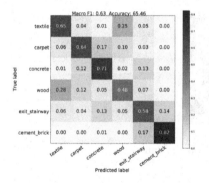

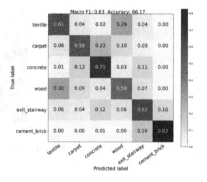

Fig. 11. Leave one session out   **Fig. 12.** Leave one user out

The performance of a machine learning model relies on the quality of the feature extraction result [29]. Within each window, we have 10×1 raw data. We summarized the following mathematical features in the time domain: mean, mad, SMA, energy, IQR, entropy, skewness, and kurtosis. We did not consider the spectral domain since all volunteers wandered with a normal walking speed. In total, we utilized eight features, so the input sample was an array of 1×8 per window. The features were then normalized to 0–1.

Figure 11 and Fig. 12 depict the recognition of ground surface types. Overall, by the Random Forest model, a combined F-score of 0.63 is achieved. In both procedures, the outdoor ground type and the indoor concrete ground type have the highest classification rate. The textile surface and wood stairs are the most easily miss-classified types between each other. Considering the HBC influence factors like wearing, body forms, this recognition result is robust and concludes that the HBC signal could be a feasible information source for ground type recognition. Further applications like indoor positioning fusing with other sensing modalities could be explored (when HBC acts as a complementing approach) to reach a higher accuracy, addressing other sensing modalities' drawbacks (like the un-robustness of RF-based approach, drift-accumulation of IMU-based approach).

5   Other Potential Use Cases

Previous sections described how much is the value of HBC in both static and dynamic body states with our sensing unit and demonstrated the prototype's feasibility for HBC monitoring. In this section, we will focus on four potential use cases with this prototype. To be noticed, the following evaluation does not aim to give efficient context recognition based on a large amount of data, but rather at presenting a significant information supplier that can be utilized in future work of human-related interaction and computing.

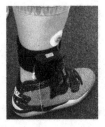

Fig. 13. Sensing unit on the calf

Since the acquisition of the absolute value of HBC is not necessary in the application field, the contribution will be mainly from how it changes in a dynamic context. Thus we simplified the deployment of our sensing unit to a more portable device. Only one conductive tap was attached to the underside sole, and the hardware was worn on the lower calf instead of the upper back, as Fig. 13 represents.

5.1   Exact Step Counting

Traditional step counting relies on motion sensor [30,31], which is widely used in current wearable devices. However, the accuracy is not guaranteed during the relatively complicated algorithms (removing the noise, abstracting the step information). Our prototype can be an effective approach for exact step counting without any signal noise processing. By wearing the prototype on the lower calf with a local-ground connected conductive tape beneath the sole, the testers walked around the building on the different types of floors. To avoid components damage from accumulated charge while walking, we used an insulated tape to cover the conductive tape. Figure 14 depicts the capacitance measured on the calf and the six axes signals from the IMU. Among the six IMU supplied motion signals, the Z axis from gyroscope supplies the most obvious step information. During each gait procedure (stance phase and swing phase), the prototype sampled an obvious capacitance variation, and this variation information could be used for exact step counting.

As Rhudy et al. [32] summarized in his comprehensive comparison paper, four different step counting techniques were applied to the data from the traditional motion sensing sensor for step counting mostly: peak detection, zero-crossing, autocorrelation method, and fast fourier transform (FFT); and it was determined that using gyroscope measurements allowed for better performance than the typically used accelerometers. Before applying the step counting algorithm, the IMU signals was firstly smoothed by a fourth-order low-pass Butterworth filter with cut-off frequency 4 Hz. Lowpass filters are commonly used in step detection algorithms to reduce undesirable sensor noise [33–35]. In our case, we use the most widely used peak detection method for step counting. Figure 15 shows the detected peaks with the capacitance and gyroscope z-axis data. For the capacitance signal, we detects the peaks simply by checking if the new sampled

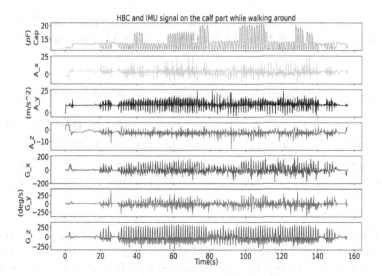

Fig. 14. Capacitance and IMU signal on the calf part while walking around

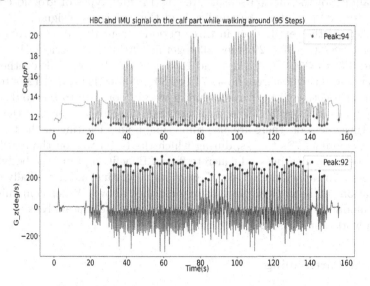

Fig. 15. Peak detection for step counting

data is 1.0 pF smaller than the sampled data 1 s ago, and is 1 s away from the last peak. The detection method can be accomplished by only one or two instructions in code. For the gyroscope signal, we tried different peak detection methods, including the same method as the capacitance one, and the *find_peaks* function from SciPy library [36] shows the best accuracy, with which we defined the prominence of the function as 200 (the prominence of a peak measures how much a peak stands out from the surrounding baseline of the signal and is defined as the vertical distance between the peak and its lowest contour line). Table 8 gives the peak detection result from the ten sessions data sets, the capacitance signal supplies the highest step counting accuracy with 99.4%.

Table 8. Step counting with signal from gyroscope and body-capacitance

Sets	1	2	3	4	5	6	7	8	9	10	Over all (accuracy)
Practical step	95	101	125	98	89	85	96	121	105	83	998 (100%)
Gyroscope z-axis	92	100	120	90	85	80	91	110	98	75	941 (94.3%)
Capacitance	94	101	126	97	88	85	95	119	104	83	992 (99.4%)

Compared with the movement sensor supplied step signals, the capacitance sensing unit supplies a more clear signal of each step firstly. As a result, the step number can be algorithmically easily captured with high accuracy. Secondly, the capacitance sensing unit supplies also the ground information, which is beyond the capability of the motion sensors. In Fig. 14, four types of ground could be derived simply by reading the amplitude of the capacitance signal. The volunteer walked on the textile floor in three periods, from 19 s to 38 s, from 43 s to 56 s, from 138 s to 151 s, 29 steps all together. Also three periods during carpet floor: 38 s to 43 s, 56 s to 72 s, and 134 s to 138 s, 19 steps all together. And three periods during concrete floor: 74 s to 80 s, 96 s to 111 s, and 127 s to 132 s, 19 steps all together. Two periods during wood floor: 80 s to 96 s and 112 s to 127 s, 22 steps all together. The steps are read directly by counting the peaks. Besides those periods, there are also some time points locating at the transition state, for example, 72 s to 74 s, during which the tester was on the textile floor (located between a carpet and concrete floor). Benefitting from the body's electric property in capacitance, tasks of exact step counting and potentially ground classification can be implemented (as we described above). When combining this sensing modality with the motion sensor, more accurate gait analysis and indoor location work would also be interesting topics.

5.2   Gait Partitioning

Gait monitoring is used widely in clinical practice for the evaluation of abnormal gait caused by disease, like Parkinson's disease [37–39]; multiple sclerosis [40–42]; attention deficit hyperactivity disorder [43–45], etc. Among the gait-related parameters, the temporal parameters (stride duration, stance duration, and swing duration) are the mostly evaluated ones because of their intensive connection to the gait abnormalities [46,47]. Whereas the stride length, gait speed is more related to estimate the walk trajectory [48–50]. The exact partitioning of the gait event is always the first step in gait analysis.

A variety of sensors can be used for gait phase partitioning, as summarized by Taborri et al. [51]. The most widely used sensor is the inertial sensor, like accelerometer [52,53], gyroscope [54,55], or IMU [56,57]. The inertial sensor wins quantitatively in the number of works because of its competitive advantages in size, cost, power consumption, and wearable capability. According to Taborri's survey, around two-thirds of gait analysis studies (among the 72 studies) relied on the inertial sensors. Anyway, to discriminate the gait event, the inertial sensor-based approach suffers from its computational load, accumulated drift over time, and also the necessary calibration procedure. Another popular gait partitioning approach is to use the footswitches [58] or foot pressure insole [59,60]. Both are based on force-sensitive sensors and require simple signal conditioning as well as post-processing. They could provide high accuracy in gait phase detection, which is reasonable since the gold standard in gait discrimination is represented by the foot's direct contact with the ground during a gait cycle. Besides those two approaches, some other sensing modalities were explored, like electromyography [61,62], ultrasound sensors [63], optoelectronic sensors [64]. Those marginally proposed approaches could give accurate partitioning results, but they are not feasible approaches for out-of-lab and long-term gait monitoring.

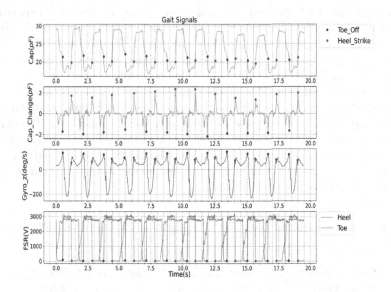

Fig. 16. Gait events detection with sensors of FSR, capacitance and gyroscope

As we described above, body capacitance variation during a walk can supply the gait event information directly and explicitly. This subsection presents a novel approach for gait partitioning (stance phase and swing phase) by utilizing the variation of human body capacitance during the walk. We firstly deployed the prototype (as depicted in Fig. 13) at the lower calf, with the sensing electrode attached to the skin and the locally grounded conductive tap beneath the shoe sole. Meanwhile, we added two FSR (Force Sensitive Sensor [65]) to the underside of the shoe sole (at the front and end position of the shoe sole), aiming to sense the contact of heel and toe to the ground and to supply the ground truth of the gait partitioning test. As described in [51], the direct measurements of the contact between foot and ground by force-sensitive sensors are often used as a gold standard for the validation of other methodologies. In this study, five volunteers walked around our office place with a regular speed for around one and a half minutes by wearing the prototype on the right calf. The sample rate of all the signals in this study is 50 Hz. Figure 16 depicts the sensed signals from FSR, z-axis of gyroscope, and the capacitance prototype. Among the six signals supplied by the IMU (three axes of the accelerometer, three axes of the gyroscope), z-axis of the gyroscope gives the most reliable source, which is also demonstrated by other works [32,51,66]. The algorithm we used to detect the heel-strike and toe-off from the gyroscope signal is a rule-based algorithm, which was described by Catalfamo et al. in [67] (with some calibration of the corresponding parameters), where the success rate for heel-strike and toe-off was over 98%. The ground truth was supplied by the two FSR, where the contact of the FSR to the ground could be easily detected by simply observing the voltage on the FSR. Once the voltage drops to zero (resistance of the FSR drops to zero), the contact happened. The gait event detection from the capacitance signal was attained by observing the change (the second subplot of Fig. 16) of the observed capacitance value (the first subplot of Fig. 16), utilizing the same algorithm described in [67]. To be noticed, the signal of z-axis of the gyroscope from Fig. 15 and Fig. 16 is not in the same pattern simply because of the prototype's orientation difference during the experiments. Overall, we recognized 523 steps from the FSR, 521 steps from the capacitance prototype, and 501 steps from the z-axis of the gyroscope with the above-described methods. To compare the performance of the gait event detection and gait phase partitioning from different signal sources, we synchronized all the detected steps from the three signal sources, meaning that the steps without the successful detection of all the three sensing approaches are discarded.

Table 9. Gait event sensing time error with signals of Cap and Gyro (FSR source as ground-truth)

Gait event and signal source	Heel strike, cap	Heel strike, gyro	Toe off, cap	Toe off, gyro
Mean(s)	−0.002	−0.022	0.043	0.040
Standard deviation(s)	0.010	0.014	0.009	0.019

Figure 17 depicted the gait event detection's time error distribution from the capacitance sensing and gyroscope sensing with a Boxplot [68]. The FSR approach supplies the ground truth. The heel-strike detection by the capacitance signal is significantly more accurate than the detection by the gyroscope z-axis signal since the majority of the time error from the capacitance signal locates in

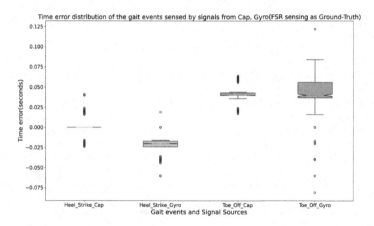

Fig. 17. Time error of Heel_Strike and Toe_Off with sensing source of capacitance and gyroscope

the field of the ground truth. For the event of toe-off, although most time errors from both capacitance and gyroscope sensors have an error of around 40 ms, the capacitance approach shows a much stable result. The same result could also be viewed by the mean and standard deviation of the errors from Table 9, where the mean error of the capacitance-based heel-strike detection is only two milliseconds. The gait event detection shows that the human body capacitance could be a reliable signal source for gait partitioning.

Based on the above analysis, we calculated the stance phase and swing phase's duration in each step after the gait partitioning by each signal source. The Boxplot in Fig. 18 shows the distribution of sensed stance and swing duration in seconds. The duration of both stance and swing phases detected by the capacitance prototype is closer to the ground truth (supplied by FSR) than the duration sensed by the gyroscope. As Table 10 lists, the mean duration of stance and swing phase from the FSR is 0.903 s and 0.674 s, respectively, the capacitance sensing gives 0.945 s and 0.632 s for each phase, with a mean accuracy of 95.3% and 93.7%, which is higher than the mean accuracy of the gyroscope-based stance and swing duration detection (93.1% and 90.8%).

Table 10. Gait phase duration with signals of FSR, Cap and Gyro

Gait phase and signal source	Stance, FSR	Stance, cap	Stance, gyro	Swing, FSR	Swing, cap	Swing, gyro
Mean(s)	0.903	0.945	0.965	0.674	0.632	0.612
Standard deviation(s)	0.041	0.040	0.045	0.035	0.036	0.038

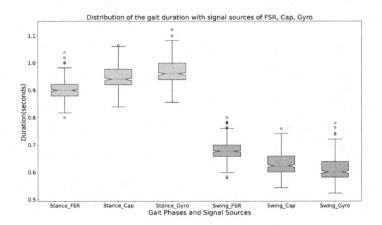

Fig. 18. Duration of stance and swing

The gait partitioning evaluation with our prototype demonstrated that the human body capacitance is a reliable signal source for gait partitioning. Our new approach is more simple (vs. force-based approach, only one small grounded electrode is needed), lower-cost (vs. force-based approach), and more accurate (vs. initial measurement unit).

5.3 Touch Sensing

Current *HBC* related capacitive sensing applications mostly focused on proximity sensing [3,69,70], activity recognition [24,71–73]. Another body-utilized capacitance application, probably one of the oldest, easiest, and most useful applications is touch sensing [74,75]. The most widely used capacitive touch sensing application is the capacitive touch button [76] and touch screen [77] for decades. Those applications are mostly based on the induced current on the sensing unit mounted on the touched object, caused by finger-touch. Different electrode layouts enlarged its touching scenarios [78]. With our prototype deployed at the lower calf (as Fig. 13 depicts), we utilized the body capacitance for touch sensing with the sensing unit on the body, approached the awareness of touch sensing at the executor side, instead of the receptor side as the previous work described.

Figure 19 shows the capacitance signal when touching the different objects within the working office. Three times handshakes caused the first three peaks (1 s to 8 s). From 9 s to 20 s, the executor touched a ground-standing metal frame, and a second volunteer touched the frame at a different position three times. The executor could sense the touch-action from the second volunteer. This sensing ability could be used for cooperation activity detection in an industrial manufactory, where the presence of the hand from a second colleague needs to be detected while processing the same objects. From 22 s to 31 s, 38 s to 44 s, 55 s to 62 s, and 69 s to 76 s, the executor touched the earthed computer, the whiteboard, the wall and the glass window for three times separately. While touching the earthed or good earth-coupled object, the prototype could perceive a visible touch signal. The wall and the window could be sensed by touching since they both are good earth-coupled through the concrete reinforcing bars and metal window frames. The deep peaks in the figure are signals of foot movement. The described touch sensing is a passive, intrusive one, and without the need of deploying the sensing unit near the touch point. Here we only present a primary observation aiming to present the potential ability of the researched object, a quantitative analysis will be presented in the future.

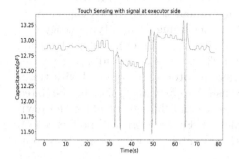

Fig. 19. Touch signal at the executor side

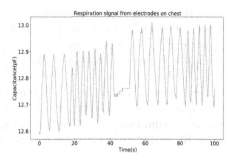

Fig. 20. Respiration signal

5.4 Respiration Monitoring

Respiration detection can be addressed by multiple ways [79], for example, by microphones, monitoring the loudness of the breath sound, or sensors that can analyze the air breathed out. Recently some novel methods were provided, like WIFI signal [80], ultra-wideband radar [81]. In our work, we use body capacitance to detect respiration, a wearable, and low-cost way. We attached the sensing electrode on the chest, and the local-ground of the prototype as a second electrode on another spot of the chest. The distance of the two electrodes was kept around 15 cm. In essence, this kind of deployment measures the local capacitance of part of the body, which was explained by Cheng [24] in detail, namely the local capacitance variation caused by the structure change inside the body.

Figure 20 recorded the capacitance signal in the level of sub-pF between the two on the chest attached electrodes. In the beginning, the volunteer breathed slowly and evenly three times, and then the respiration rate became faster. After eight times of breath, the volunteer held the breath for a while. The latter breath signal represents a repeat of the respiration in two rates. The scale of the signal variation represents the breath depth of the volunteer.

Similar applications can be explored by the same deployment but at other body parts. For example, when wearing the prototype on the wrist, with the sensing electrode attached to the finger, the local-ground electrode is also on the wrist, then the finger's movement can be observed. So as the head actions and other joint-related movements.

6 Conclusion

As one of the body's physiological variables, HBC is a pervasive signal worth further research. In this work, we first used a wearable prototype to measure the value of HBC in static and dynamic body states and got a reliable result. We also validated that the factors like postures, wearings, and environment can affect the value of HBC. Secondly, we briefly presented several body capacitance-based use cases with the wearable prototype, including ground type recognition (F-score of 0.63), exact step counting (with 99.4% accuracy), gait partitioning (with the duration accuracy of 95.3% and 93.7% for stance and swing phases, respectively), touch sensing, and respiration monitoring. Compared with traditional motion sensors, the HBC based sensing approach supplies body-related motion detection with competitive performance and the sensing ability for environmental and other physiological information. Future work will be focused on the HBC-based use cases exploration with a quantitative way, aiming to present a solid contribution of this signal.

References

1. Skeldon, K.D., Reid, L.M., McInally, V., Dougan, B., Fulton, C.: Physics of the Theremin. Am. J. Phys. **66**(11), 945–955 (1998)
2. Fritz, T.: ThereminVision-II instruction manual (2004)
3. Arshad, A., Khan, S., Alam, A.H.M.Z., Kadir, K.A., Tasnim, R., Ismail, A.F.: A capacitive proximity sensing scheme for human motion detection. In: 2017 IEEE International Instrumentation and Measurement Technology Conference (I2MTC), pp. 1–5. IEEE (2017)
4. Hirsch, M., Cheng, J., Reiss, A., Sundholm, M., Lukowicz, P., Amft, O.: Hands-free gesture control with a capacitive textile neckband. In: Proceedings of the 2014 ACM International Symposium on Wearable Computers, pp. 55–58 (2014)
5. Bian, S., Lukowicz, P.: Capacitive sensing based on-board hand gesture recognition with TinyML. In: UbiComp-ISWC 2021 Adjunct: Adjunct Proceedings of the 2021 ACM International Joint Conference on Pervasive and Ubiquitous Computing and Proceedings of the 2021 ACM International Symposium on Wearable Computers, Virtual, USA. ACM, September 2021
6. Cohn, G., Morris, D., Patel, S., Tan, D.: Humantenna: using the body as an antenna for real-time whole-body interaction. In: Proceedings of the SIGCHI Conference on Human Factors in Computing Systems, pp. 1901–1910 (2012)
7. Aliau Bonet, C., Pallàs Areny, R.: A fast method to estimate body capacitance to ground. In: Proceedings of XX IMEKO World Congress 2012, Busan, South Korea, 9–14 September 2019, pp. 1–4 (2012)
8. Aliau-Bonet, C., Pallas-Areny, R.: A novel method to estimate body capacitance to ground at mid frequencies. IEEE Trans. Instrum. Meas. **62**(9), 2519–2525 (2013)

9. Buller, W., Wilson, B.: Measurement and modeling mutual capacitance of electrical wiring and humans. IEEE Trans. Instrum. Meas. **55**(5), 1519–1522 (2006)
10. Forster, I.C.: Measurement of patient body capacitance and a method of patient isolation in mains environments. Med. Biol. Eng. **12**(5), 730–732 (1974). https://doi.org/10.1007/BF02477239
11. Greason, W.D.: Quasi-static analysis of electrostatic discharge (ESD) and the human body using a capacitance model. J. Electrostat. **35**(4), 349–371 (1995)
12. Huang, J., Wu, Z., Liu, S.: Why the human body capacitance is so large. In: Proceedings Electrical Overstress/Electrostatic Discharge Symposium, pp. 135–138. IEEE (1997)
13. Pallas-Areny, R., Colominas, J.: Simple, fast method for patient body capacitance and power-line electric interference measurement. Med. Biol. Eng. Comput. **29**(5), 561–563 (1991). https://doi.org/10.1007/BF02442332
14. Sălceanu, A., Neacşu, O., David, V., Luncă, E.: Measurements upon human body capacitance: theory and experimental setup (2004)
15. Jonassen, N.: Human body capacitance: static or dynamic concept? [ESD]. In: Electrical Overstress/Electrostatic Discharge Symposium Proceedings 1998 (Cat. No. 98TH8347), pp. 111–117. IEEE (1998)
16. Fujiwara, O., Ikawa, T.: Numerical calculation of human-body capacitance by surface charge method. Electron. Commun. Jpn (Part I: Commun.) **85**(12), 38–44 (2002)
17. Serrano, R.E., Gasulla, M., Casas, O., Pallàs-Areny, R.: Power line interference in ambulatory biopotential measurements. In: Proceedings of the 25th Annual International Conference of the IEEE Engineering in Medicine and Biology Society (IEEE Cat. No. 03CH37439), vol. 4, pp. 3024–3027. IEEE (2003)
18. Haberman, M., Cassino, A., Spinelli, E.: Estimation of stray coupling capacitances in biopotential measurements. Med. Biol. Eng. Comput. **49**(9) (2011). Article number: 1067. https://doi.org/10.1007/s11517-011-0811-6
19. Fish, R.M., Geddes, L.A.: Conduction of electrical current to and through the human body: a review. Eplasty **9**, e44 (2009)
20. TI: Texas Instrument LMC555, June 2016. http://www.ti.com/lit/ds/symlink/lmc555.pdf
21. TI: How do i design a-stable timer, oscillator, circuits using LMC555, TLC555, LM555, NA555, NE555, SA555, or SE555. https://e2e.ti.com/support/clock-andtiming/f/48/t/879112?tisearch=e2e-sitesearchamp;keymatch=lmc555
22. PJRC: Teensy 3.6. https://www.pjrc.com/store/teensy36.html
23. Grosse-Puppendahl, T.: Capacitive sensing and communication for ubiquitous interaction and environmental perception. Ph.D. thesis, Technische Universität (2015)
24. Cheng, J., Amft, O., Bahle, G., Lukowicz, P.: Designing sensitive wearable capacitive sensors for activity recognition. IEEE Sens. J. **13**(10), 3935–3947 (2013)
25. Castle, G.S.P.: Contact charging between insulators. J. Electrostat. **40**, 13–20 (1997)
26. Electrostatic-Discharge-Association: Handbook for the Development of an Electrostatic Discharge Control Program for the Protection of Electronic Parts, Assemblies, and Equipment. TR20.20-2016
27. Pedregosa, F., et al.: Scikit-learn: machine learning in Python. J. Mach. Learn. Res. **12**, 2825–2830 (2011)
28. Chawla, N.V., Bowyer, K.W., Hall, L.O., Kegelmeyer, W.P.: SMOTE: synthetic minority over-sampling technique. J. Artif. Intell. Res. **16**, 321–357 (2002)

29. Kuhn, M., Johnson, K.: Feature Engineering and Selection: A Practical Approach for Predictive Models. CRC Press, Boca Raton (2019)
30. Foster, R.C., et al.: Precision and accuracy of an ankle-worn accelerometer-based pedometer in step counting and energy expenditure. Prev. Med. **41**(3–4), 778–783 (2005)
31. Pan, M.-S., Lin, H.-W.: A step counting algorithm for smartphone users: design and implementation. IEEE Sens. J. **15**(4), 2296–2305 (2014)
32. Rhudy, M.B., Mahoney, J.M.: A comprehensive comparison of simple step counting techniques using wrist-and ankle-mounted accelerometer and gyroscope signals. J. Med. Eng. Technol. **42**(3), 236–243 (2018)
33. Do, T.-N., Liu, R., Yuen, C., Tan, U.-X.: Design of an infrastructureless in-door localization device using an IMU sensor. In: 2015 IEEE International Conference on Robotics and Biomimetics (ROBIO), pp. 2115–2120. IEEE (2015)
34. Ashkar, R., Romanovas, M., Goridko, V., Schwaab, M., Traechtler, M., Manoli, Y.: A low-cost shoe-mounted inertial navigation system with magnetic disturbance compensation. In: International Conference on Indoor Positioning and Indoor Navigation, pp. 1–10. IEEE (2013)
35. Mariani, B., Hoskovec, C., Rochat, S., Büla, C., Penders, J., Aminian, K.: 3D gait assessment in young and elderly subjects using foot-worn inertial sensors. J. Biomech. **43**(15), 2999–3006 (2010)
36. Virtanen, P., et al.: SciPy 1.0: fundamental algorithms for scientific computing in Python. Nat. Methods **17**, 261–272 (2020)
37. Sofuwa, O., Nieuwboer, A., Desloovere, K., Willems, A.-M., Chavret, F., Jonkers, I.: Quantitative gait analysis in Parkinson's disease: comparison with a healthy control group. Arch. Phys. Med. Rehabil. **86**(5), 1007–1013 (2005)
38. Salarian, A., et al.: Gait assessment in Parkinson's disease: toward an ambulatory system for long-term monitoring. IEEE Trans. Biomed. Eng. **51**(8), 1434–1443 (2004)
39. Pedersen, S.W., Oberg, B., Larsson, L.E., Lindval, B.: Gait analysis, isokinetic muscle strength measurement in patients with Parkinson's disease. Scand. J. Rehabil. Med. **29**(2), 67–74 (1997)
40. Givon, U., Zeilig, G., Achiron, A.: Gait analysis in multiple sclerosis: characterization of temporal-spatial parameters using GAITRite functional ambulation system. Gait Posture **29**(1), 138–142 (2009)
41. Benedetti, M.G., Piperno, R., Simoncini, L., Bonato, P., Tonini, A., Giannini, S.: Gait abnormalities in minimally impaired multiple sclerosis patients. Multiple Sclerosis J. **5**(5), 363–368 (1999)
42. Guner, S., Inanici, F.: Yoga therapy and ambulatory multiple sclerosis assessment of gait analysis parameters, fatigue and balance. J. Bodyw. Mov. Ther. **19**(1), 72–81 (2015)
43. Buderath, P., et al.: Postural and gait performance in children with attention deficit/hyperactivity disorder. Gait Posture **29**(2), 249–254 (2009)
44. Papadopoulos, N., McGinley, J.L., Bradshaw, J.L., Rinehart, N.J.: An investigation of gait in children with attention deficit hyperactivity disorder: a case controlled study. Psychiatry Res. **218**(3), 319–323 (2014)
45. Leitner, Y., et al.: Gait in attention deficit hyperactivity disorder. J. Neurol. **254**(10), 1330–1338 (2007). https://doi.org/10.1007/s00415-006-0522-3
46. Morris, M.E., Matyas, T.A., Iansek, R., Summers, J.J.: Temporal stability of gait in Parkinson's disease. Phys. Ther. **76**(7), 763–777 (1996)

47. Trojaniello, D., Ravaschio, A., Hausdorff, J.M., Cereatti, A.: Comparative assessment of different methods for the estimation of gait temporal parameters using a single inertial sensor: application to elderly, post-stroke, Parkinson's disease and Huntington's disease subjects. Gait Posture **42**(3), 310–316 (2015)

48. Hori, K., et al.: Inertial measurement unit-based estimation of foot trajectory for clinical gait analysis. Front. Physiol. **10**, 1530 (2019)

49. Hu, X., Huang, Z., Jiang, J., Qu, X.: An inertial sensor based system for real-time biomechanical analysis during running. J. Med. Bioeng. **6**(1), 1–5 (2017)

50. Woyano, F., Lee, S., Park, S.: Evaluation and comparison of performance analysis of indoor inertial navigation system based on foot mounted IMU. In: 2016 18th International Conference on Advanced Communication Technology (ICACT), pp. 792–798. IEEE (2016)

51. Taborri, J., Palermo, E., Rossi, S., Cappa, P.: Gait partitioning methods: a systematic review. Sensors **16**(1), 66 (2016)

52. Selles, R.W., Formanoy, M.A.G., Bussmann, J.B.J., Janssens, P.J., Stam, H.J.: Automated estimation of initial and terminal contact timing using accelerometers; development and validation in transtibial amputees and controls. IEEE Trans. Neural Syst. Rehabil. Eng. **13**(1), 81–88 (2005)

53. Han, J., Jeon, H.S., Jeon, B.S., Park, K.S.: Gait detection from three dimensional acceleration signals of ankles for the patients with Parkinson's disease. In: Proceedings of the IEEE The International Special Topic Conference on Information Technology in Biomedicine, Ioannina, Epirus, Greece, vol. 2628 (2006)

54. Formento, P.C., Acevedo, R., Ghoussayni, S., Ewins, D.: Gait event detection during stair walking using a rate gyroscope. Sensors **14**(3), 5470–5485 (2014)

55. Darwin Gouwanda and Alpha Agape Gopalai: A robust real-time gait event detection using wireless gyroscope and its application on normal and altered gaits. Med. Eng. Phys. **37**(2), 219–225 (2015)

56. Lau, H., Tong, K.: The reliability of using accelerometer and gyroscope for gait event identification on persons with dropped foot. Gait Posture **27**(2), 248–257 (2008)

57. Kotiadis, D., Hermens, H.J., Veltink, P.H.: Inertial gait phase detection for control of a drop foot stimulator: inertial sensing for gait phase detection. Med. Eng. Phys. **32**(4), 287–297 (2010)

58. Agostini, V., Balestra, G., Knaflitz, M.: Segmentation and classification of gait cycles. IEEE Trans. Neural Syst. Rehabil. Eng. **22**(5), 946–952 (2013)

59. Lie, Yu., Zheng, J., Wang, Y., Song, Z., Zhan, E.: Adaptive method for real-time gait phase detection based on ground contact forces. Gait Posture **41**(1), 269–275 (2015)

60. Kim, H., Kang, Y., Valencia, D.R., Kim, D.: An integrated system for gait analysis using FSRs and an IMU. In: 2018 Second IEEE International Conference on Robotic Computing (IRC), pp. 347–351. IEEE (2018)

61. Lauer, R.T., Smith, B.T., Coiro, D., Betz, R.R., McCarthy, J.: Feasibility of gait event detection using intramuscular electromyography in the child with cerebral palsy. Neuromodulation Technol. Neural Interface **7**(3), 205–213 (2004)

62. Joshi, C.D., Lahiri, U., Thakor, N.V.: Classification of gait phases from lower limb EMG: application to exoskeleton orthosis. In: 2013 IEEE Point-of-Care Healthcare Technologies (PHT), pp. 228–231. IEEE (2013)

63. Qi, Y., Soh, C.B., Gunawan, E., Low, K.-S., Thomas, R.: Assessment of foot trajectory for human gait phase detection using wireless ultrasonic sensor network. IEEE Trans. Neural Syst. Rehabil. Eng. **24**(1), 88–97 (2015)

64. Galois, L., Girard, D., Martinet, N., Delagoutte, J.P., Mainard, D.: Optoelectronic gait analysis after metatarsophalangeal arthrodesis of the hallux: fifteen cases. Rev. Chir. Orthop. Reparatrice Appar. Mot. **92**(1), 52–59 (2006)
65. OHMITE: FSR series force sensing resistor (2020)
66. Panebianco, G.P., Bisi, M.C., Stagni, R., Fantozzi, S.: Analysis of the performance of 17 algorithms from a systematic review: influence of sensor position, analysed variable and computational approach in gait timing estimation from IMU measurements. Gait Posture **66**, 76–82 (2018)
67. Catalfamo, P., Ghoussayni, S., Ewins, D.: Gait event detection on level ground and incline walking using a rate gyroscope. Sensors **10**(6), 5683–5702 (2010)
68. McGill, R., Tukey, J.W., Larsen, W.A.: Variations of box plots. Am. Stat. **32**(1), 12–16 (1978)
69. Braun, A., Hamisu, P.: Using the human body field as a medium for natural interaction. In: Proceedings of the 2nd International Conference on PErvasive Technologies Related to Assistive Environments, pp. 1–7 (2009)
70. Braun, A., Hamisu, P.: Designing a multi-purpose capacitive proximity sensing input device. In: Proceedings of the 4th International Conference on PErvasive Technologies Related to Assistive Environments, pp. 1–8 (2011)
71. Bian, S., Rey, V.F., Younas, J., Lukowicz, P.: Wrist-worn capacitive sensor for activity and physical collaboration recognition. In: 2019 IEEE International Conference on Pervasive Computing and Communications Workshops (PerCom Workshops), pp. 261–266. IEEE (2019)
72. Bian, S., Rey, V.F., Hevesi, P., Lukowicz, P.: Passive capacitive based approach for full body gym workout recognition and counting. In: 2019 IEEE International Conference on Pervasive Computing and Communications (PerCom), pp. 1–10. IEEE (2019)
73. Bian, S., Yuan, S., Rey, V.F., Lukowicz, P.: Using human body capacitance sensing to monitor leg motion dominated activities with a wrist worn device. In: Activity and Behavior Computing. Springer (2022)
74. Du, L.: An overview of mobile capacitive touch technologies trends. arXiv preprint arXiv:1612.08227 (2016)
75. Savage, V., Zhang, X., Hartmann, B.: Midas: fabricating custom capacitive touch sensors to prototype interactive objects. In: Proceedings of the 25th Annual ACM Symposium on User Interface Software and Technology, pp. 579–588 (2012)
76. Curtis, K., Perme, T.: Capacitive multibutton configurations (2007)
77. Leeper, A.K.: 14.2: integration of a clear capacitive touch screen with a 1/8-VGA FSTN-LCD to form and LCD-based touchpad. In: SID Symposium Digest of Technical Papers, vol. 33, pp. 187–189. Wiley Online Library (2002)
78. Baxter, L.K.: Capacitive Sensors: Design and Applications (1997)
79. AL-Khalidi, F.Q., Saatchi, R., Burke, D., Elphick, H., Tan, S.: Respiration rate monitoring methods: a review. Pediatr. Pulmonol. **46**(6), 523–529 (2011)
80. Wang, H., et al.: Human respiration detection with commodity wifi devices: do user location and body orientation matter? In: Proceedings of the 2016 ACM International Joint Conference on Pervasive and Ubiquitous Computing, pp. 25–36 (2016)
81. Li, X., Qiao, D., Li, Y., Dai, H.: A novel through-wall respiration detection algorithm using UWB radar. In: 2013 35th Annual International Conference of the IEEE Engineering in Medicine and Biology Society (EMBC), pp. 1013–1016. IEEE (2013)

Software Design and Development of an Appointment Booking System: A Design Study

Kamarin Merritt[1] and Shichao Zhao[2](✉) [ID]

[1] Northumbria University, Newcastle-Upon-Tyne NE1 8ST, UK
[2] Glasgow School of Art, Glasgow G3 6RN, UK
s.zhao@gsa.ac.uk

Abstract. This paper outlines, utilises and reflects upon effective software design and development through effectively applying current practical solutions such as use case modelling, class and sequence diagrams and by developing a prototype program which reflects the designs from said diagrams. A discussion is presented regarding the best method of approaching the Software Development Life Cycle (SDLC), justifying the selection and also concluding with a reflection on the professional, ethical and security issues in relation to the proposed design and use of software within the healthcare sector. In regards to ethical considerations, the Code of Ethics was discussed in relation to the design and development of the system and the importance of it alongside ensuring a high level of ethics and professionalism is of utmost priority when handling personal identifiable information in the development of a system. As well as this, security issues during and post development is an area of significant importance when it comes to data management, this has been discussed in general and against the software development life cycle. Additionally, in the design and development of software it is crucial to abide by world software quality standards such as International Organisation for Standardisation (ISO), and this paper reflects upon current issues and how to address these in the process of design and development.

Keywords: Systematic design · Digital information management system · Design reflection

1 Introduction

The purpose of this paper is to design and develop a program prototype solution for a case study, which will see the development of a hospital appointment booking system and develop a critical discussion on the current issues. This paper will demonstrate a Use Case Diagram which will model the functional requirements from the case study and document one primary use case. Secondly, a Class Diagram will be produced to model the systems structure, displaying various classes and their variables/attributes, relationships and procedures. Thirdly, a Sequence Diagram will be produced, illustrating

M. Ur Rehman and A. Zoha (Eds.): BODYNETS 2021, LNICST 420, pp. 275–294, 2022.
https://doi.org/10.1007/978-3-030-95593-9_21

an overview of the functional requirements for one of the primary use cases, and this will be concluded with a prototype program, showing a proposed solution using OOP language (object-oriented programming).

Furthermore, this paper will go in depth and critically discuss the Software Development Life Cycle (SDLC) methodology adopted in the solution development and critically reflect upon the professional, legal, social, security and ethical issues related to the design and development of the solution developed for the case study.

This case study is based around a hospital, who has built a new central dental unit and they now want to create a digital information management system to replace the outdated one. This will fulfil the purpose of recording, searching, updating and storing patient data. It is expected that all staff will use this system in order to support day-to-day tasks such as booking, deleting, updating, managing and recording appointments, while also allowing for the system to be utilised for other business needs. The system needs to ensure efficiency and ease of use, through two functions (booking online or via call). Additionally, the system will need to accommodate many functions.

2 Related Work

Typically, a use case is used to capture the requirements of a system and what the system is supposed to do [1]. When building this system, the first step we take in the Object-Oriented Modelling (OOM) approach is to build a Use Case Diagram. This stage is crucial as starting with a 'use case subject' allows for key functional requirements, such as logging in and out, to be defined and outlined [2]. One of the many benefits of using models to document functional requirements, is that it enables you, as the system analyst, to define clearly the details of the needs and requirements of the stake-holders, thus allowing for ease when explaining to stakeholders a system solution or proposal [3, 4]. The overall purpose of a use case diagram is to identify the Functional Requirements. Requirements identify a list of characteristics that a system must have and also describe what a system should do; in software engineering, there are two types of requirements, which are; Functional Requirements and Non-Functional Requirements [4]. Functional requirements identify potential 'features' in which the given system may have [4]. Therefore, a list has been generated, of the functional requirements which derive from, the case study: Login; Logout; Handle Login Errors; Check Account Balance; Book Appointment; Cancel Appointment; Check in Patient; Review Treatment History; Amend Appointment; Available Tools and Equipment; Transport History. The above Functional Requirements extend further in the Use Case and are discussed in the further section.

In all use cases there is a person who will use the system, this person is known as an 'actor' [3]. This actor specifies a role which is performed by the user. An actor models an entity which is outside of the system, and it is crucial to identify who these actors are as they play a role in interacting with the system, to make it work [3]. In the case study, there are various actors who fall under different categories, due to their relationship with the system. To define these actors, it is suggested that we need to ask ourselves as a systems analyst, the following: Who will supply, use or remove any information? Who will use the function (i.e., who will login, logout, etc.)? Who will support and maintain the system? What do the systems need to interact with? What does the actor need to do exactly? [2]. By following this criteria, the actors within the specific case study, and those who will interact with the use case, are: User; Patient; Staff; Doctor; Receptionist; Admin; Practice Manager; Driver. It was stated that there are two types of actors: Primary Actors and Supporting Actors [5]. All of the actors within this overall use case subject, are Primary Actors, as they are all a stakeholder who calls upon the system, to deliver one of its services. In the section below, actors are discussed in more detail regarding relationships with other actors and classes.

3 Design Process

This section will go in more depth when it comes the use case and relationships each actor and the use cases have, while also applying and documenting them via diagrams. The overall purpose of the design process is to show how each element of the process is mapped out in accordance with the earlier use case requirements. Relationships, Inheritance, Use Cases and Class Diagrams were developed in StarUML and this was then followed by a prototype solution being written in code and developed in NetBeans. StarUML is a Unified Modelling Language (UML) software tool which allows for agile and short prototyping, which is usually targeted to be used by small, yet agile teams. Additionally, NetBeans is the tool which allows for the StarUML prototypes to come to life through, as it is an open source, integrated development environment that is meant for the development of applications on various operating systems. Below, each stage has been discussed in depth and processes have been applied in depth also.

3.1 Relationships in the Use Case (Design Decisions)

There are various types of relationships when developing a use case, and these can be between actors and the use cases themselves [4]. Below, is a breakdown of the relationships which have been utilised in the Use Case shown in Fig. 1.

Actor Inheritance. It is highly common for all systems to have a generic User, in which other actors inherit attributes from [4]. The purpose of having a generic user is so that within diagrams such as the Class Diagram, classes can be illustrated simply, rather than doubling up information in a class, we can use a generalisation relationship; also known as a parent-child relationship [1]. In Fig. 1, there is an outline of the relationship between each actor, the clear headed arrow indicates a generalisation relationship.

Use Case Relationships. Within the Use Case diagram, various use cases have a relationship between them, which allows for the functionality of the system to be demonstrated clearly, for stakeholders to grasp with ease [5]. The most common relationship between use cases is the directed relationship, more specifically 'extend' and 'include' as shown in Fig. 2. In Fig. 2, we can see the use case 'Book Appointment', for example. Now in the new system being developed, patients will be able to book an appointment through two different methods, either via calling in; or booking online, the purpose of <<extend>> is to allow users within the system, a choice. However, if the patient

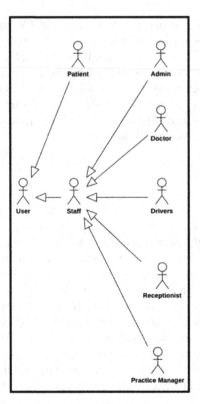

Fig. 1. Actor relationships in the case study.

is not registered, their path in the process would be different than that of an existing patient. Therefore, in order to enable this option, we would have 'Book Appointment' as a main use case and then we use the directed relationship (<<extend>>) to get to the 'Register Patient' stage in the system, which would allow us to add the patient to our system after taking relevant details, then they can follow the path of an ordinary patient by choosing their preferred booking method. As we can also see in Fig. 2, there is an <<include>> relationship, now this is a required function that needs to be undertaken, unlike the <<extend>> relationship and a user in the system cannot proceed to the next stage or use case, without undertaking this function. This has been explained more clearly, in the section below which demonstrates the 'Book Appointment' use case in more detail.

Documentation of a Use Case Using House Style. In order to demonstrate various elements of a use case within the Use Case subject, the 'Book Appointment' use case has been documented through using the House Style technique (as shown in Table 1). The purpose of documenting this particular use case is due to the fact that it is one of the key use cases within the system, also the purpose of this is to illustrate further details that may not be visible in the use case diagram.

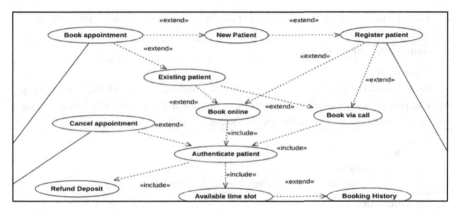

Fig. 2. Screenshot from the system use case diagram.

3.2 Class Diagram (Use STARUML)

The class diagram which illustrates the system is extremely complex and has many classes within. Therefore, no design pattern has been adopted, as it would cause confusion within the system. Using design patterns in UML may cause for confusion or lack of function [4, 6]. In the class diagram, there are various main classes, the most important one being the 'Appointment' class. The reason for this being the main class is that it is connected to most actors and requires an interaction from various aspects of the system such as payment, notifications, and actors such as doctors and admin. This class has various associations with other classes, as shown in the snippet in Fig. 3 on the left side and full diagram in Appendix B, the main type of relationship is composition. The composition relationship is similar to a parent and child [2]. The child cannot exist without the parent, just like a room cannot exist without a house [2, 4]. Therefore, by connecting other classes with the composition tool, this shows that for example, a 'Confirmation Notification' cannot exist without booking an appointment.

Furthermore, multiplicity notations have also been utilised, the purpose of this is to indicate the number of instances of one class linked to one instance of another class [4]. For example, as seen in Fig. 3 on the right side, one appointment will have one payment, but one payment can only be made from booking one appointment, thus the reason for the '1' notation at either end of the composition relationship. It has been highlighted that in a class diagram, 'multiplicity' is when the association between classes is being depicted [4]. For example between 'Account' and 'Patient', there can be one to many (1..*) patients, but only one (1) account per patient. Therefore, along the association relationship line as shown in Fig. 3 on the right side, we can see this illustrated. The diagram is not limited to the above specific relationships and multiplicities, and many others have been used and can be seen in the full diagram outlined in Appendix B.

Table 1. Documentation and structure of the 'Book Appointment' use case diagram.

Name: Book Appointment

Description:

Patient wants to book an appointment, which can be done via calling in or booking online. Admin will determine date and time, upon which a deposit will be taken, and confirmation notification will be sent to the patient.

Actors:
- Patient
- Administrator
- Receptionist (in the case of Cancelling appointment or no show)

Pre-Conditions:
- Be a registered patient
- Patient credentials have been validated (booking via call and online)
- Patient needs to book an appointment

Basic Flows:
- Use case begins when Actor contacts to book appointment
  - << extend >> Book via call
  - << extend >> Book online
- Authenticate patient
- Determine appointment date and time
- Deposit payment
- Appointment confirmation notification

Post Conditions:
- Patient successfully books appointment slot
- Administrator saves record of appointment and updates patient record
- Patient receives appointment confirmation notification

Alternative Flows:
- If patient is not registered, admin team will have to register patient before booking appointment
- If patient authentication is failed, terminate call (via call) or display error message and return user to home screen (via online)
- Call lines full – patient will need to hold the line and wait (via call)

Notes: --

Business Rules
- Patient must be registered before booking an appointment
- Patient must verify details
- Patient must have required amount of credit within their account to pay deposit (usually a notification is sent to the patient if balance is low

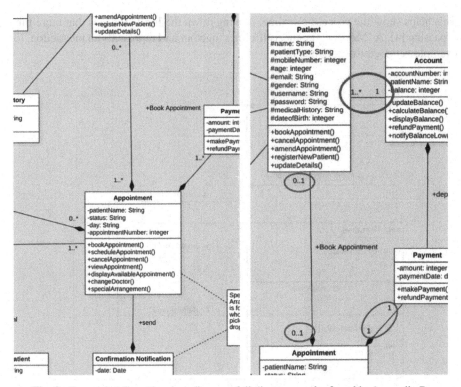

Fig. 3. Screenshot from the class diagram, full diagram can be found in Appendix B.

3.3 Sequence Diagram (Use STARUML)

In order to further demonstrate the Use Case documented earlier using the House Style documentation method, a sequence diagram demonstrating this Use Case 'Book Appointment' and the basic flows of it, has been developed in StarUML and is illustrated in Appendix C. A Sequence Diagram is a UML diagram which demonstrates how the system or the classes within a code interact with one another [1]. The new system requires a core function which is to book appointments for patients, and the sequence diagram demonstrates this through mapping out a sequence of interactions to perform this function.

This sequence diagram demonstrates the steps of the system when booking an appointment over the phone and online, however, the diagram firstly outlines a Login sequence which is paramount for when the user, in this case the Admin and the Patient, want to access the online system and when the Admin wants to use the system to record an appointment (see Fig. 4). Thus, the two main sequences are Login and Book Appointment, as booking an appointment could not happen without the Admin logging into the system. The main sequence in this diagram, however, is the appointment booking sequence which is shown in Fig. 5. In this sequence there are lifelines which are vertical dashed lines, in which various objects (i.e., Booking History; Patient Records; Account) and Actors (i.e. Patient; Admin) connected by various different interactions, are placed.

This helps show the process overtime, moving down the lifeline means that more time is passing [4]. A 'Message' connects lifelines together and represents an interaction, for example veryDetails (dob, name).

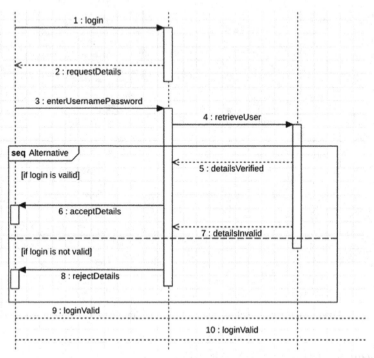

Fig. 4. The login sequence extracted from sequence diagram; full diagram shown in Appendix C.

In the Appointment Booking sequence diagram, the first step (after successfully logging in) is to book an appointment. In Fig. 5 we can see the first interaction is 'bookAppointment' illustrated by a straight line with a filled in arrowhead, this inter-action is known as a message and is sent from one actor to another to start the process. Below this is a further interaction, known as a reply and is represented by a dashed line. The first sequence is broken down into two stages, as it is only possible to book an appointment if the patient is already registered, if they are not registered, they will not be able to book an appointment and follow the normal sequence of the diagram which includes steps interactions 11–16. Therefore, an 'alternative' frame is used. This symbolises a choice between two message sequences, which are usually mutually exclusive, and this has been placed around interactions 11–19. The conditions are if the patient is registered or if they are not. A dashed line separates the two choices, the option above is called 'patientExists' and will proceed to the following sequence of booking appointment, however the below option is called 'patientNonExistent' and will extend the sequence to an alternative path to register them. The two main interactions used in the sequence diagram are message and reply message, with the design decision to use various alternative frames to navigate through different areas of the system, when a function cannot be performed.

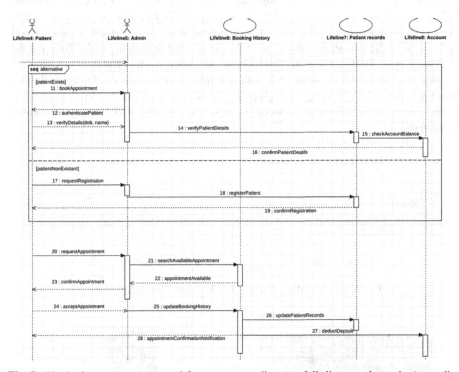

Fig. 5. The login sequence extracted from sequence diagram, full diagram shown in Appendix C.

3.4 Program Prototype

As this prototype will become extremely long due to the nature of the system, there has been a focus on the main class of 'Login' and 'Book Appointment'. The system prototype reflects how a patient would log into the system and book an appointment via the online method, outlined originally in the Use Case Diagram and Sequence Diagram.

The first JFrame (a JFrame is a container which provides a window, in which other components such as menu, buttons, text fields etc. rely on) is built around the 'Login' class. In the class diagram, the User was a generic actor and would hold the operation of being able to login to the system, upon verification of their details. In the prototype developed in NetBeans, upon inserting Graphical User Interface (GUI) components (i.e., Buttons, Text field etc.), raw code and strings were connected to them (see Fig. 6) to allow for specific credentials to be used in order for access, and if not, the user would be presented with a 'Login Failed'. This was possible due to using the code 'String name/pwd=' and setting and 'if' code to verify what name and password equal. If the login is successful, the user will be presented with a 'Login Successful' alert on the login page and an additional JOptionPane will pop up, allowing the user to progress to the next screen, this can be seen in the code too (see Fig. 6 and 7). In order to connect the login page JFrame to the next page, known as 'patientAccount', a connection had to be made. This was implemented by setting up the GUI button to register an event, creating a 'java.awt.event.MouseEvent evt' private void. In this event we had to add code to make the connection work, and this can be seen within the code. To make the transition more fluid, the use of 'this.dispose' was used, so that the previous window would close, and the user wasn't left with multiple open windows – this helps fluidity when it comes to progressing through an application so multiple windows are not left open. The use of 'this.dispose' is beneficial as it free's up allocated memory or releases unmanaged resources.

```
private void loginButtonActionPerformed(java.awt.event.ActionEvent evt) {

//login credentials, including else for failures

    String name = usernameTextField.getText();
    String pwd = new String(passwordField.getPassword());
        if(name.equals("Kamarin") && pwd.equals("User1"))
{
    JOptionPane.showMessageDialog(null, "Login successful, welcome " + name, "Successful Login", JOptionPane.INFORMATION_MESSAGE);
        new patientAccount().setVisible(true);
        this.dispose();
}
    else
        JOptionPane.showMessageDialog(null, "Login Failed" + name, "Failed Login", JOptionPane.INFORMATION_MESSAGE);
    }
}
```

Fig. 6. Login code, containing ELSE variants for login failure.

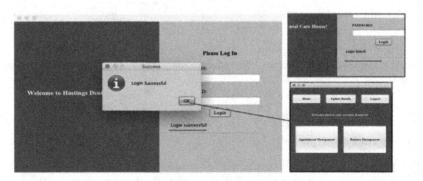

Fig. 7. Login JFrame in demonstration showing two results (Login.java).

Once at the next window known as 'patientAccount', the user is presented with options, all of which were set out the attributes/functions, both in the use case and class diagram. This JFrame included a link to the main class, 'Book Appointment' and to progress to this stage the user must simply click the Button GUI 'Appointment Management'. Again, similarly to above and the Login button, code was used to allow for the current JFrame to transition to the next (see Fig. 8).

In this JFrame, the user is presented with three options. Due to the complexity of building three different JFrames and code, only 'Book Appointment' button will take you to a working JFrame, the other two options take you to a new, but blank JFrame. This is simply just a navigation page, and uses minimal coding to progress, the coding

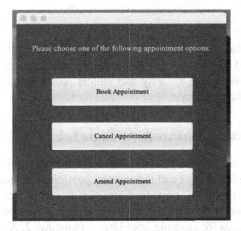

Fig. 8. Appointment management JFrame, developed in NetBeans.

for this was already demonstrated earlier. Upon clicking the 'Book Appointment' button the user is provided with the final window of the system, which is 'bookAppointment' and they are presented with appointment slots which were connected in one Panel using various Check Box swing controls and then inserted into the swing control, List. Once the user has selected an appointment time, they are then able to press 'Book appointment'. After clicking this button, a JOptionPane will pop up confirming the booking (see Fig. 9) and by clicking OK, this will end the process from the patient's side, and Admin will continue to finish the process of updating patient records/assigning doctor.

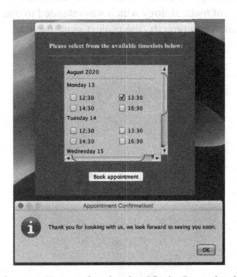

Fig. 9. Book appointment JFrame, also showing JOptionPane, developed in NetBeans.

4   Discussion

This section is going to critically discuss the Software Development Life Cycle (SDLC) methodology adopted in the above solution development and critically reflect upon the professional, legal, social, security and ethical issues related to the design and development of the above solution.

4.1   Critical Discussions: Software Development Life Cycle (SDLC)

The Software Development Life Cycle is a phased methodology which produces software to a high standard with low cost and the shortest possible time frame [1]. De-pending on the chosen model, the SDLC provides a structured order of phases which enable an organisation to efficiently produce robust software that is both well tested and ready for use [4]. These phases for example, could be: 1. Planning; 2. Analysis; 3. Design; 4. Implementation; 5. Testing; and 6. Deployment and Testing [7].

There are a plethora of SDLC models, the most popular models are Waterfall Methodology and the Agile Methodology [1]. These are used massively, in order to produce an efficient and effective robust program solution. Thus, it was paramount that the correct SDLC was adopted prior to starting the process [4]. If the correct methodology is not used, this can cause the solution to become problematic within the process and cause design flaws, lack of security and disrupt the functionality [8].

The Agile methodology consists of 6 stages, as shown in Fig. 10 and is an iterative and incremental based development, as it allows for requirements to be changeable according to needs [9]. Generally, the common issue in systems development is that there are constant requirement changes or even changes in the technology itself, however, Agile is a software development methodology which was intended to overcome this particular issue, therefore not managed correctly, the project may lose track and the process may be disrupted [10].

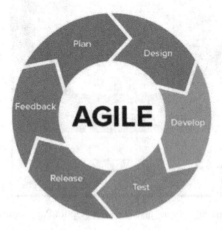

Fig. 10. Agile methodology phases, adapted from Kendall and Kendall [1].

This presenting a limitation of using the Agile method, is that the project may lose track if not managed properly and the functions are not outlined correctly [11], whereas Waterfall methodology is an easier method to manage. Due to its nature, each phase has specific deliverables and a review process [4]. With Waterfall (as shown in Fig. 11), it can be highlighted that its approach values planning ahead, keeping direction straight and accurate, however, if the requirement is not clear at the beginning, the method can become less effective, which will have a major impact on cost and implementation [12]. This presenting the major different between Agile, the fact that Waterfall approach values planning ahead but can meet more obstacles throughout the process, while Agile values adaptability and involvement and is able to change during the process [4, 11].

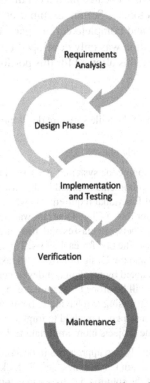

Fig. 11. Waterfall methodology, adapted from Sommerville [4].

Furthermore, Waterfall has less stakeholder involvement which causes a hands-off approach. This approach is not suitable for every product, and the majority of users/stakeholders need to be involved in the system for example, to meet the correct requirements [12]. However, Agile focuses on delivering a high quality and user-friendly product through incorporating stakeholder engagement into all stages which allows for a more structured list of requirements [1]. Thus, Agile is more suitable in the development of this system as the methodology has two core elements: Teamwork and Time – and breaks the overall project into smaller pieces with an individual time scale and 'sprints' [13]. Using such a method allows for feedback from previous phases to be planned into the next, so if a requirement is missing, or feedback has been given, this can be used, whereas in Waterfall, what is developed is based on the feedback and plans given in the first place [1].

4.2 Agile Methodology Within the Program Solution

As discussed above, Agile is one of the most robust and beneficial methodologies to use in during the SDLC. The main benefit for using this methodology in the development of the program solution is that feedback can be given per stage and requirements can change along with way. The key instrument for Agile development is iterations, and this process sets out actions which are repeated until a condition is met [4]. One of the most productive Agile development tools is Scrum. Scrum uses 'Sprints' which allow for the development team to achieve and complete certain parts of the systems functionality. Therefore, as the program solution was only developed up to the stage allowing for the patient to book an appointment, this allowed for this portion of the solution to be robust (as shown in Table 2).

Table 2. Stages of the agile software development life cycle.

Agile software development life cycle phases	
1. Plan	When developing the system, a use case diagram was developed, deriving from the requirements outlined in the case study. This allowed for the outlining of functional requirements which would be required in the system. After this, a Class Diagram was outlined showing various relationships between classes and also outlining various attributes and functions specifically, for each class. Thus, a Sequence Diagram was developed, and the Design Phase could take place It has been noted by many that if developers decide to ignore this stage, the system will be prone to 'feature creep'. This is where non crucial features keep arising and having to be implemented along the way, which while scrum is a good method to implement these along the line, it can cause for the projects more important tasks to lack time [1, 13]
2. Design	There is usually two approaches in designing the solution: 1) looking at the visual design i.e. JFrames, and; 2) looking at the architectural structure of the solution, i.e. the source code In the design phase the coding was implemented in the Phase 3, but here, the basic JFrames were developed in NetBeans, as outlined earlier in Fig. 7 and 8. In these JFrames, various GUI components were inserted per guidance of the previously developed diagrams. From making these GUI components in regards to the requirements, the system started to take place, however could not take place without building in code
3. Develop (Coding stage)	Now all GUI components were built into the JFrames, the functionality needed to be coded into the source code, in NetBeans

(continued)

Table 2. (*continued*)

Agile software development life cycle phases	
4. Testing	Unlike in the traditional SDLC approach where development and testing are individual phases, Agile connects these two phases together, allows for the testing and development team to work together as one and reduces overall costs and defects which may incur later [1] NetBeans allows a program to be run, thus the ability to test if coding works and the GUI components work when used and the JFrames connect to each other, as supposed to. Agile Testing stage is to draw out any defects and fix them as soon as possible prior to releasing [4] In the developing phase, coding appeared difficult when trying to build the various different JFrames for different users, therefore, only the Patient (Actor) portion was built. This is usually the longest process as it is writing advanced functionality of the system and allowing it to work. However, in the developing phase, there usually isn't many changes to the iterations here, this is in Phase 4: Testing During Phase 4, further iterations become apparent as the factors such as integration, operability and user testing take place
5. Releasing	As in the above phases, only the patient portion of the booking system was built. This allows for the system to be released to users initially, in order to gain any potential feedback on whether the user interface is unappealing, hard to navigate and whether there are any additional requirements that could be built into the system when the sprint for the next round starts again. From this, iterations are updated in the existing software, which introduces additional features and resolves any issues [4]
6. Feedback	Upon completing all of the previous development phases, the whole system can be reviewed. When finishing the solution in NetBeans, it was apparent that the coding and the JFrames held some functions that were not outlined in any of the Use Case, Class or Sequence Diagrams. Therefore, these were able to be updated accurately and made sense when looking at the diagrams and prototype in comparison to each other After this final phase, the Agile software development life cycle could begin again in order to extend the current booking system to other actors such as Admin, Doctors and so on

4.3 A Critical Reflection: Professional, Security and Ethical Issues

When it comes to the design and development of a system which involves a user interface and requires interaction, especially of that in the healthcare sector, there are a plethora of professional, security and ethical issues which may arise [4]. Within the development of the system, it was paramount that these issues were considered.

Ethical Issues. The term ethics refers simply to the governing, conduct and principles of people's behaviours [4]. In software development, ethical issues are massive and can be very complicated, this is due to the rise of new technologies such as machine learning, AI and Big Data. Some of these issues include privacy, transparency, accountability and diversity. However, in order to overcome these issues, it is imperative that organisations who develop and design their own software, have a Code of Ethics. Specifically, personally identifiable data in healthcare has been an arising issue in the past few years and following the Code of Ethics will allow for employees to understand and be trained on a set of acceptable behaviours in order to remain ethical and professional, when handling personal identifiable information, and organisational data in general [14], in software development, ethics is taking into consideration all of the implications which we may create as a result of software algorithms. As an organisation, it is imperative that standards are not violated and that as a software developer, systems analyst or even just an employee ethics and also morals are used interchangeably [14].

Security Issues. In the software development process, security is a constant process that involves all employees and practices within an organisation [15]. As technology advances, software environments are becoming more dynamic and complex, causing the development of systems to become more challenging. Also, with the increasing growth of the software development life cycle, the engineering behind it is under huge pressure to deliver requirements fast [15]. This causes less attention to be focused on security issues in which may arise in the system or software.

Many software applications are outsourced, and the development lacks in incorporating software security and due to this, issues arise around the growth of an organisation and availability of meeting requirements for its customers [16]. Overall, from the beginning, organisations should ensure that during the software development life cycle, security is tightly bound from the get-go. The TCSEC Glossary (Trusted Computer Systems Evaluation Criteria) defines security requirements as a set of laws and practices which govern how an organisation protects, distributes and manages any form of sensitive information [17]. It also states that security requirements should be measured during the SDLC, and can be classified into functional security requirements, non-functional security requirements and derived security requirements [18]. Thus, during the SDLC, software developers must review these specific requirements outlined in the glossary, in order to reduce vulnerabilities down the line once the system is deployed.

Professional Issues. In the design and development of software, it is crucial to abide by the world software quality standards, in which there are various professional issues that may arise, the majority of these relate to the factors which are outlined in the ISO9126, such as: Functionality; Reliability; Usability; Efficiency; Maintainability; Portability [19]. When developing software in an organisational context, it is crucial to take into consideration the user and their experience. Firstly, user experience (i.e., Functionality; Usability; Efficiency) is crucial in gaining feedback on the systems from a user perspective [20, 21]. For example, this allows developers to reflect upon system feedback and incorporate new iterations in the program to make it more usable, functional and efficient for the user – thus, professional issues generally arise in the Testing stage of the software development life cycle, particularly in the Agile methodology [1]. Furthermore, when taking into consideration a patient booking appointment system, the system should cater for all users. Thus, factors such as disabilities, visual or hearing impairments and also those who may be illiterate are a key focus when developing and designing a system; allowing for everyone to book an appointment successfully. This would also include developing the system to not solely be based on JAVA and developing it for various platforms which would allow it to reach as many users as possible.

5   Conclusion

To conclude, this paper has developed from start to finish a program solution prototype for the case study. This has included outlining the functional requirements of the system, down to coding and creating the system itself in NetBeans. Upon doing this, the SDLC was reflected upon and how, as a systems analyst we were able to approach it. Furthermore, it was apparent that due to the vast amount of Ethical, Security and Professional issues in the software engineering domain and generally in organisations, that there are many principles and legislations that need to be followed in order to overcome these.

This paper enables useful insight into developing an appointment booking system through looking into the core, and various aspects within the SDLC, choosing the correct method of approach whether this is through the waterfall or agile methodology and in general discussing the best method of approaching the SDLC, justifying it and reflecting upon various issues that may arise. This is an important element of contribution from this paper, as it approaches software design and development through effectively applying it, while also justifying and reflecting upon the effectiveness of using it within practical solutions. Additionally, this paper reflects upon current issues (i.e., ethical, security, legal, etc.) and how these can be addressed in the process of design and in general, development.

Appendix A

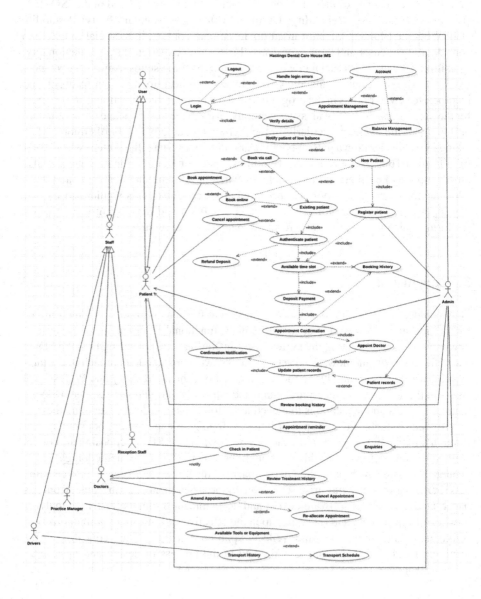

Appendix B

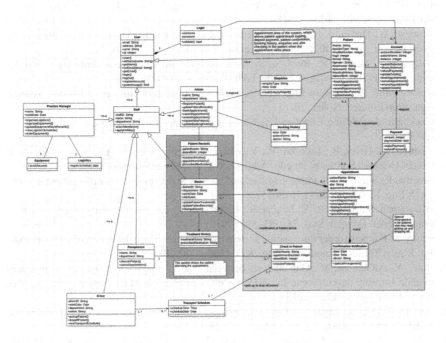

Appendix C

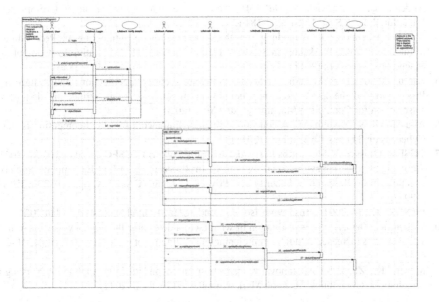

References

1. Kendall, K., Kendall, J.: Systems Analysis and Design, 10th edn., pp. 1–576. Pearson Education Limited, Harlow (2019)
2. Bruegge, B., Dutoit, A.: Object-Oriented Software Engineering Using UML, Patterns, and Java, 1st edn., pp. 11–40. Pearson Education Limited, Harlow (2014)
3. Satzinger, J., Jackson, R., Burd, S.: Systems Analysis and Design in a Changing World, 1st edn., pp. 171–200. Cengage Learning EMEA, Andover (2008)
4. Sommerville, I.: Software Engineering, Global Edition, 10th edn., pp. 119–140. Pearson Education Limited, Noida (2016)
5. Cockburn, A.: Writing Effective Use Cases, 1st edn., pp. 1–259. Addison-Wesley, London (2006)
6. Gamma, E., Helm, R., Johnson, R., Vlissides, J.: Design Patterns: Elements of Reusable Object-Oriented Software, 1st edn. Addison-Wesley, Massachusetts (1994)
7. Sharma, P., Singh, D.: Comparative study of various SDLC models on different parameters. Int. J. Eng. Res. **4**(4), 188–191 (2015)
8. Aljawarneh, S., Alawneh, A., Jaradat, R.: Cloud security engineering: early stages of SDLC. Future Gener. Comput. Syst. **74**, 385–392 (2017)
9. Andry, J.: Purchase order information system using feature driven development methodology. Int. J. Adv. Trends Comput. Sci. Eng. **9**(2), 1107–1112 (2020)
10. Rauf, A., AlGhafees, M.: Gap analysis between state of practice and state of art practices in agile software development. In: 2015 Agile Conference (AGILE), National Harbor, MD, USA, pp. 102–106. IEEE (2015)
11. Azman, N.: The development of IoT tele-insomnia framework to monitor sleep disorder. Int. J. Adv. Trends Comput. Sci. Eng. **8**(6), 2831–2839 (2019)
12. Schuh, G., Rebentisch, E., Riesener, M., Diels, F., Dolle, C., Eich, S.: Agile-waterfall hybrid product development in the manufacturing industry–introducing guidelines for implementation of parallel use of the two models. In: 2017 IEEE International Conference on Industrial Engineering and Engineering Management (IEEM), pp. 725–729. IEEE, Singapore (2017)
13. Abdelghany, A., Darwish, N., Hefni, H.: An agile methodology for ontology development. Int. J. Intell. Eng. Syst. **12**(2), 170–181 (2019)
14. Aydemir, F., Dalpiaz, F.: A roadmap for ethics–aware software engineering. In: Proceedings of the International Workshop on Software Fairness, pp. 15–21. Association for Computing Machinery, New York (2018)
15. Zarour, M., Alenezi, M., Alsarayrah, K.: Software security specifications and design. In: Proceedings of the Evaluation and Assessment in Software Engineering, pp. 451–456. Association for Computing Machinery, New York (2020)
16. Aljawarneh, S., Yassein, M.: A conceptual security framework for cloud computing issues. Cyber Secur. Threats **12**(2), 12–24 (2018)
17. TCSEC - Glossary | CSRC. https://csrc.nist.gov/glossary/term/TCSEC. Accessed 02 Jan 2021
18. Sterne, D.: On the buzzword 'security policy'. In: Proceedings of IIEEE Computer Society Symposium on Research in Security and Privacy, Oakland, CA, USA, pp. 219–230. IEEE (1991)
19. ISO/IEC 9126-1:2001. https://www.iso.org/standard/22749.html. Accessed 06 Jan 2021
20. Merritt, K., Zhao, S.: An investigation of what factors determine the way in which customer satisfaction is increased through omni-channel marketing in retail. Admin. Sci. **10**(4), 01–24 (2020)
21. Merritt, K., Zhao, S.: An innovative reflection based on critically applying UX design principles. J. Open Innov. Technol. Mark. Complex. **7**(2), 1–12 (2021)

Robust Continuous User Authentication System Using Long Short Term Memory Network for Healthcare

Anum Tanveer Kiyani[1]([✉]), Aboubaker Lasebae[1], Kamran Ali[1],
Ahmed Alkhayyat[2], Bushra Haq[3], and Bushra Naeem[3]

[1] Faculty of Science and Technology, Middlesex University London, London, UK
`AK1933@live.mdx.ac.uk`
[2] E-Learning Department, Islamic University, Najaf, Iraq
[3] FICT, BUITEMS, Quetta, Pakistan

Abstract. A traditional user authentication method comprises of username, passwords, tokens and PINs to validate the identity of user at initial login. However, a continuous monitoring method is needed for security of critical healthcare systems which can authenticate user on each action performed on system in order to ensure that only legitimate user i.e., genuine patient or medical employee is accessing the data from user account. In this aspect, the perception of employing behavioural patterns of user as biometric credential to incessantly re-verifying the user's identity is being investigated in this research work to make the healthcare database information more secure. The keystroke behavioural biometric data represents the organisation of events in such a manner which resembles a time-series data, therefore, recurrent neural network is used to learn the hidden and unique features of users' behaviour saved in time-series. Two different architectures based on per frame classification and integrated per frame-per sequence classification are employed to assess the system performance. The proposed novel integrated model combines the notion of authenticating user on each single action and on each sequence of actions. Therefore, firstly it gives no room to imposter user to perform any illicit activity as it authenticates user on each action and secondly it tends to include the advantage of hidden unique features related to specific user saved in a sequence of actions. Hence, it identifies the abnormal user behaviour more quickly in order to escalate the security especially in healthcare sector to secure the confidential medical data.

Keywords: Continuous authentication · Periodic authentication ·
Keystroke dynamics · Recurrent neural network

1 Introduction

Computer systems and networks are essential part of almost every aspect of human life. All the businesses, healthcare, banking systems, government services,

M. Ur Rehman and A. Zoha (Eds.): BODYNETS 2021, LNICST 420, pp. 295–307, 2022.
https://doi.org/10.1007/978-3-030-95593-9_22

medical, aviation, communication, education and entertainment are mainly controlled by computer systems. Each organisation is effectively using computer systems to store important information and data including confidential financial transactions, employee records, personal and business emails and medical history. However, this escalating dependence on computers has excavate new computer security threats as well. Moreover, cybercrimes have also been escalated owing to the presence of imposter users who can masquerade the legitimate user in order to get access to system resources which can result into serious exploitation and obliteration of personal, governmental and medical information. In order to preclude the imposters to steal those confidential information and files, one important factor is robust continuous user authentication (CUA) system which can validate the users' identity on each action while accessing the medical records.

The behavioural biometrics i.e., keystroke dynamics can collect the regular behavioural data about the user while interacting with system or relevant device. Hence, this type of behavioural biometric data highly depends on the specification of hardware device or background context [7].

The scholarly works, presented in literature review in domain of CUA using behavioural biometrics, mostly rely on statistical features based on mean and standard deviation of those features [2]. These approaches had considered to maintain the static database of the relevant extracted features. However, this approach has few shortcomings: Firstly behavioural biometrics tend to change gradually with time or based on configuration and specification of different hardware devices. Therefore, the main disadvantage of maintaining a static database of users populated with statistical features could affect and decrease the performance or accuracy of system over time. Secondly, behavioural data i.e., keystroke dynamics, represents a sequential events of time-series which can contain hidden information regarding the specific behaviour of user which cannot be represented with statistical feature profiles of users as well as traditional classification methods cannot mine these type of features to distinguish one user from other.

Continuous user authentication (CUA) problem is not new in the research domain, however, the preceding research conducted in this domain [1] had mostly focussed on periodic user authentication (PUA) based on fixed block of actions which can give room to imposter user to perform illicit activities. In contrast, a true CUA mechanism should authenticate the user on each action. However, keystroke sequential series, consisting of more than one action, can contain unique and hidden features related to specific user. For instance, it can be the unique behaviour of specific user to commit mistakes while typing some specific words or it might be regular user behaviour to open files on system by double clicking the mouse button instead of right clicking on file and then press OPEN option. This type of behaviour can be saved in a sequential series. In this regard, we have proposed a novel approach of integrating the CUA based on single action event and PUA based on keystroke actions sequence in order to improve the system performance.

The main contributions of this work are:

- Recurrent Neural Network (RNN) is used to exploit the time-series nature of keystroke behavioural biometric data.
- A two phase methodology is proposed to authenticate user on each action while accessing the confidential medical records.
- A novel architecture based on integrated per frame LSTM and per sequence LSTM is proposed to combine continuous and periodic user authentication.
- Robust recurrent confidence model (R-RCM) is combined with RNN to continuously authenticate user.

The rest of this paper is arranged as follows: Sect. 2 addresses the background of CUA using keystroke dynamics. Section 3 shows a proposed system model for CUA. Section 4 presents the results and assessment of system model. Subsequently, Sect. 5 discusses the conclusion of this study.

2   Background

Continuous and Periodic user authentication intend to verify the identity of user after the initial login to ensure that only legitimate user is using the system for the whole session. However, PUA validates the user's identity after fixed time intervals or fixed block sizes in contrast to CUA which can authenticate user on each activity or action. The key requirement for both PUA and CUA is that authentication process should not disturb the user while he/she is performing important tasks on system for which behavioural biometrics i.e., keystroke dynamics can be used. This section presents the background study of CUA/PUA systems using keystroke dynamics. The summary of research works performed on CUA/PUA problem with traditional machine learning methods is presented in Table 1 while the detailed results are discussed below.

Table 1. Machine learning methods works for CUA with keystroke dynamics

Work	Users	Features	Block	Method	Results
[1]	53	Duration, digraph latency	500	Neural Network	FAR 0.0152% FRR 4.82% EER 2.13%
[2]	30	Statistical features	1000	Decision Trees	FAR 1.1% FRR 28%
[14]	200	Trigraph latency	900 words	Kernel Ridge Regression	EER 1.39%
[4]	34	Digraph latency	14 Digraphs	Support vector machine	EER 0.0–2.94%
[9]	20	Hold time, Digraph	6 blocks	One class SVM	FAR = 2.05% FRR = 2%
[3]	103	Digraph latency	200	Random forest classifier	EER 7.8%
[10]	150	Digraph latency	—	Ensemble Classifier	FAR 0.10%, FRR 0.22%
[8]	75	Digraph latency	50 actions	CNN, RNN	EER 4.77%

The initial research on CUA/PUA employing keystroke dynamics had been proposed in 1995 with some insistent results [11]. Afterwards, the researchers in [1] presented a notable system model based on neural networks for CUA/PUA using Keystroke dynamics. Subsequently, block size of 500 keystroke actions had been used with digraph features and achieved the FAR = 0.0152%, FRR = 4.82% and EER = 2.13%.

Moreover, in [2] researchers had used Decision trees for the classification of keystroke data with the average block size consisting of 1000 action events and reported the FMR = 1.1% and FNMR = 28%. Another research work in [14] had used the kernel ridge regression a truncated RBF kernel along with block size of 900 words. In this work, trigraph latency features were used and reported results were EER of 1.39%.

Subsequently, support vector machine technique had also been exploited by researchers in [4] with varying digraph sets for implementing CUA and achieved the EER of 0.0–2.94% with different sets of digraphs. The researchers in [9] had implemented an architecture named Spy Hunter for CUA using KD which utilised two 1-class support vector machines classifiers. They had used a single key hold time and digraph latency to build the feature vector and block size of 6 actions are used to classify a user after each block. The resultant FAR reported was 2.05% and FRR was 2.0% Additionally, random forest classifier had been used in [3] with block size of 200 keystroke actions and the resultant EER as reported was 7.8%.

Moreover, the researchers in [10] had implemented the competitive selection ensemble classifier approach based on Random Forests (RF), Bayes Net (BN), decision trees, Support Vector Machine (SVM), Random Tree (RT) and RIDOR RIpple-DOwn Rule learner (Ridor). They showed that employing an ensemble approach as compared to stand alone classifiers can improve the accuracy of system because keystroke dynamics being a weak behavioural biometric modality suffers from behavioural invariability issue. They had reported the FAR = 0.10% and FRR = 0.22% with ensemble classifier. Researchers in [8] had employed the deep neural architecture consisting of convolutional neural network (CNN) and Recurrent neural network (RNN) on the free text dataset and achieved EER = 4.77%.

It can be observed that most of the preceding research works had considered block of actions to authenticate user which can provide a security loophole for imposter user to steal confidential data. Secondly, researchers had considered using the statistical features based on mean and standard deviation with static database which can lead to low accuracy over time since the behavioural biometrics depends on external factors such as age, hardware and background context. In contrast, this research work intended to authenticate user on each single activity and used the keystroke data as a time-series to extract the hidden features with the help of recurrent neural networks which can remember and update the user information as compared to state of art classification methods.

3   System Methodology

This section presents the system architecture of proposed CUA and PUA integrated system. For this purpose, the keystroke dataset presented by University of Buffalo [12] has been used which contains 75 users and 3 different laboratory sessions having a time difference of 28 days between each session.

3.1   Keystroke Sequence Sampling

Keystroke data can be considered as chronological organisation of key down time and key up time events which gives an illustration of sequential time series where each event $i \in I$ consists of the following properties:

- $UserId(i)$ – a user that has performed given action/event.
- $SessionId(i)$ – session id of action/event.
- $DownTime(i)$ – an absolute time when any specific key is pressed.
- $UpTime(i)$ – an absolute time when any specific key is released.
- $KeyCode(i)$ – a key code for any specific key which is pressed and released by user.

Formally, each of these events containing $(UserId', SessionId', DownTime, UpTime, KeyCode)$ are assembled into a group of events to make a keystroke sequential time series as follows:

$Sequence(UserId', SessionId') = \{i|\forall i \in I, s.t.Where$
$UserId(i) = UserId',$
$SessionId(i) = SessionId',$
$DownTime(i) = DownTime,$
$UpTime(i) = UpTime,$
$KeyCode(i) = KeyCode',$
$\}$

3.2   System Model

Two types of system architectures are formulated for continuously authenticating a user. Both architectures consists of two-Phase methodology framework where recurrent neural network is the first phase while robust recurrent confidence model (R-RCM) as proposed by authors in [6] is the second phase of proposed framework.

A recurrent neural network (RNN) is mostly used for the problems containing time-series data thereby it can be employed for keystroke dynamics data owing to its sequential nature consisting of organised timestamps for each action. Moreover, robust recurrent confidence model (R-RCM) tends to calculate the confidence of users' genuineness on each action and it decides whether the user can continue using the system or should be locked out.

Phase 1: Long Short Term Memory (LSTM). The refined form of RNN named as Long short term memory (LSTM) [13] is used in this work to eliminate the problem of diminishing gradients of basic RNNs. In contrast to basic RNNs, LSTM works on loop structure and contains memory cell thereby can store and modify the previous information on each time-step hence it can update the keystroke behavioural data with time. The cell architecture of LSTM is shown in Fig. 1.

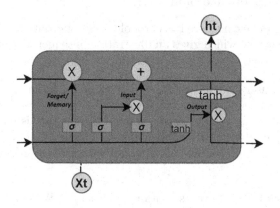

Fig. 1. The LSTM cell structure

Phase 2: Robust Recurrent Confidence Model (R-RCM). Robust Recurrent Confidence Model (R-RCM) is the second phase of both proposed architectures. The classification output from LSTM goes into the R-RCM as an input and confidence value increases or decreases based on this input and few other hyper parameters as described in [6]. Two types of thresholds i.e., alert threshold and final threshold are used where if the current confidence of user decreases than alert threshold then RCM works more robustly to identify the imposter user as quickly as possible. Moreover, if the current confidence goes down the final threshold then user is locked out of system.

Architecture 1: LSTM per Frame. The architecture of LSTM per frame is illustrated in Fig. 2. The raw keystroke data per action/frame is sent into feature extraction unit to generate key monograph and digraph features which afterwards are fed into LSTM unit containing dense layers. The probability of current action is further fed into R-RCM unit to compute the confidence in the genuineness of user and if new calculated confidence is less than the final threshold set by R-RCM, then user would be lock out of system or vice versa.

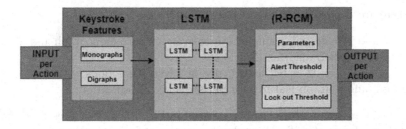

Fig. 2. Architecture 1: LSTM per frame

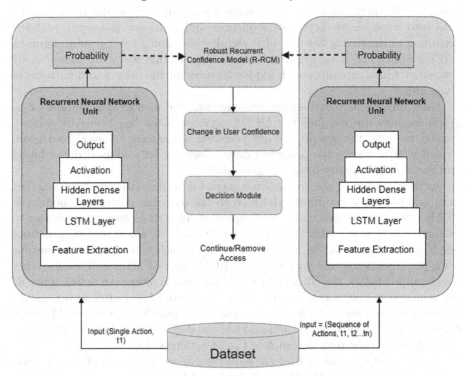

Fig. 3. The system architecture

Architecture 2: Integrated LSTM per Frame and LSTM per Sequence.
The proposed architecture integrates the two classification approaches to get the
probability based on per action as well as per sequence.

Let's assume, there is a sequence of $M + U$ keystrokes where U is the context
length and M is the length of keystroke sequence. Sequences of a defined length
$M + U$ have been sampled to generate input features and target user ids with
T *time steps* in total.

There are two setups in practice:

- $U = 1$ and $T = M = 1$, a single keystroke action with monograph and digraph features for per frame classification.
- $U = 1$ and $T = M = 64$, a sequence of keystroke actions with monograph, digraph and n-graph features for per sequence classification.

The system architecture has been shown in Fig. 3. The first presented model based on per frame classification takes the input data as each action and extracts the action based features containing monographs and digraphs. On the other hand, the second model based on sequence classification segregates the keystroke data into fixed length keystroke sequences and generates the input patterns according to the timing features of keystrokes containing monographs, digraphs and n-graphs. The fixed length sequences used in this study are based on 64 time-steps which contain enough hidden features for the behavioural patterns of given user.

Later on, the prepared sequence comprising the monograph, digraph or n-graph features are fed into the LSTM network which has been efficaciously trained to mine the unique hidden behavioural patterns of user from given sequence. Afterwards, the processed data is sent to fully coupled dense layers and the final probability output is generated.

As shown in Fig. 3, the probability output for both models i.e., per frame(left side) and per sequence (right side) goes to the recurrent confidence model (R-RCM) which further processes these inputs along with its hyper parameters to calculate the new confidence level of user. It must be noted that output from per frame LSTM would go into the R-RCM on each action, while the output from per sequence would go into the R-RCM after 64 actions. Therefore, per frame output makes the changes in user's confidence after each action whereas per sequence output makes the change in confidence of user after 64 actions. In a case, when the user's confidence becomes low than the final threshold before the user has completed the 64 actions then the user would be lock out of system without waiting the user to complete the 64 actions sequence.

The core notion of integrating the sequential approach with per frame method is that model can learn the hidden behavioural features from a given sequence and generates an output according to the unique behavioural pattens which cannot be extracted through per frame and also it tends to authenticate the user on each frame hence escalating the system security as well.

Formally speaking, this architecture combines the continuous and periodic authentication owing to classification based on per action and per sequence strategies respectively. It combines the advantage of per action features which specifies the user behaviour on each action with per sequence features which can depict the unique hidden user behaviour based on general computer usage habits.

4   Results and Discussion

The performance metrics described in [5] for CUA system have been used in this research which are Normalised Average Number of Imposter Actions (ANIA) and Normalised Average Number of Genuine Actions (ANGA).

Suppose there are total U users, each of U cases is allotted two attributes in which first shows if $ANGA = 100\%$ or not, while the second one checks if $ANIA > 40\%$ or not. Based on these two attributes, four user categories are outlined as follows:

- Very Good, $ANGA = 100\%$ and $ANIA \leq 40\%$
- Good, $ANGA < 100\%$ and $ANIA \leq 40\%$
- Bad, $ANGA = 100\%$ and $ANIA > 40\%$
- Ugly, $ANGA < 100\%$ and $ANIA > 40\%$

Figure 4 presents few extracts of the results based on 512 actions, however in practical, testing is done on whole testing set. It shows the results of LSTM per frame architecture where genuine user is tested with its own training sample (left) and it can be observed that genuine user is not falsely locked out by system even once. Similarly, an imposter user is tested with the same genuine user training set (Fig. 4 right side), it can be observed that imposter user is locked out by system after performing only few actions marked as L1. After each lockout, it is assumed that imposter user gained access to genuine users' system and its confidence is again set at 1.00. However, on each attempt, imposter user is locked out by system after only performing few actions.

4.1   Aggregated Results of Architecture 1: Per Frame Model

The aggregated results for all the users are presented in tabular form and Fig. 5 shows the results in percentages. Table 2 shows the results of stand-alone LSTM per frame model approach. It can be observed that 66 users are falling in very-good category which means these 66 users have never been falsely locked out of system while 9 users are falling in Good category. There are no users in bad and ugly categories. System's ANIA is 0.04 with this approach and ANGA is reported as 0.98.

4.2   Aggregated Results of Architecture 2: Integrated Model

The collective results of Architecture 2 have been listed below in Table 3 and Fig. 6 shows the results in percentages. It can be observed that only 3 users have been falsely locked out of system and imposter users have been detected by system after performing only 0.016 portion of actions.

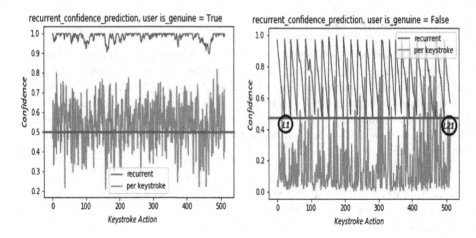

Fig. 4. A genuine user tested with its own template (left) and with imposter set (right)

Table 2. Architecture 1 (setting III): aggregated results of LSTM-robust RCM

Category	Users	ANGA	ANIA
Very good	66	1.00	0.04
Good	9	0.88	0.05
Bad	0		
Ugly	0		
System total	**75**	**0.98**	**0.04**

Table 3. Architecture 2: aggregated results of integrated LSTM per frame and per sequence

Category	Users	ANGA	ANIA
Very good	72	1.00	0.016
Good	3	0.91	0.03
Bad	0		
Ugly	0		
System total	**75**	**0.99**	**0.016**

4.3   Discussion of Results for Architecture 1 and Architecture 2

If both experimental settings are compared, then it can be observed that architecture 2 has locked out the imposter users on 0.016% of actions which is quite less than the architecture 1 results (ANIA= 0.04%), hence the imposter users are quickly caught by architecture 2 and also only 3 genuine users are falsely locked out as compared to Architecture 1 where 9 users are falsely locked out

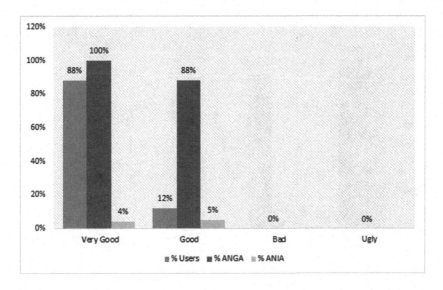

Fig. 5. LSTM-robust RCM results presented in percentage

by system. System's ANGA and ANIA are improved with architecture 2 which has combine CUA and PUA approaches to continuously authenticate user.

4.4   Results in Terms of EER

Equal error rate (EER) has also been calculated to evaluate the results with previous research works. EER is a metric which assesses the data classification performance for any model. In this work, EER has been calculated for both proposed architectures and the results are shown in Table 4 below:

Table 4. Results in terms of EER

Methodology	EER %
LSTM per frame	3.2%
LSTM integrated per frame-per sequence	1.04%

If the results of this research work are compared with previous scholarly works given in Table 1, then it can be observed that most of the research works have used the block size of actions and the researchers in [14] achieved the EER of 1.39% but they had utilised the block size of 900 words instead of single keystroke action or sequence size comparative to 64 actions as used in our research to authenticate the user. Moreover, another notable work presented in [8] had also used the RNN for authenticating the users but researchers had used the sliding window approach consisting of sequence of block actions i.e., 50 actions, 100

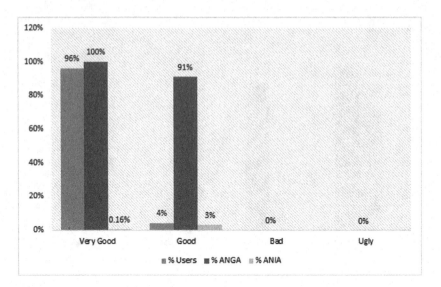

Fig. 6. Integrated LSTM per frame and per sequence results presented in percentage

actions to achieve the EER of 4.77%. In contrast, the results provided in our research have used the single action (Architecture 1) to achieve 3.2% while we have achieved the lowest error rate (EER) of 1.04% (Architecture 2) precisely with sequence consisting of 64 actions.

5   Conclusion

A robust continuous user authentication model is proposed and implemented which can authenticate user on each action in order to escalate the security of system resources and confidential information in healthcare sector. Since one time validation of user's identity, at the start of session, using usernames and passwords is insufficient to provide optimal security to important medical history and information. In this paper, keystroke dynamics is used as a behavioural biometric modality to continuously authenticate the user on each key press and key release actions while accessing the medical records. In contrast to previous scholarly works, keystroke biometric data is treated as a sequential time-series which can contain hidden unique behaviours patterns of user and these patterns cannot be represented with static database containing mean and standard deviation of features. In this aspect, LSTM model is used which can proficiently learn the time-series data along with the robust recurrent confidence model (R-RCM) that can authenticate user based on each action. Two different architectures based on LSTM per frame and LSTM per Frame-per Sequence are formulated which have considered the behavioural keystroke dynamics data as a set of chronological time-series in order to utilise all the hidden properties of data. The novel proposed integrated architecture, named as per frame-per sequence LSTM model, investigated the effect of combining true continuous user authentication and periodic user authentication on system performance. It has been observed that proposed integrated model has performed well to identify imposter users in only few actions and also avoided the false lockout of genuine users to a greater extent.

References

1. Ahmed, A.A., Traore, I.: Biometric recognition based on free-text keystroke dynamics. IEEE Trans. Cybern. **44**(4), 458–472 (2013)
2. Alsultan, A., Warwick, K., Wei, H.: Non-conventional keystroke dynamics for user authentication. Patt. Recog. Lett. **89**, 53–59 (2017)
3. Ayotte, B., Banavar, M., Hou, D., Schuckers, S.: Fast free-text authentication via instance-based keystroke dynamics. IEEE Trans. Biomet. Behav. Identity Sci. **2**(4), 377–387 (2020)
4. Çeker, H., Upadhyaya, S.: User authentication with keystroke dynamics in long-text data. In: 2016 IEEE 8th International Conference on Biometrics Theory, Applications and Systems (BTAS), pp. 1–6. IEEE (2016)
5. Kiyani, A.T., Lasebae, A., Ali, K.: Continuous user authentication based on deep neural networks. In: 2020 International Conference on UK-China Emerging Technologies (UCET), pp. 1–4. IEEE (2020)
6. Kiyani, A.T., Lasebae, A., Ali, K., Rehman, M.U., Haq, B.: Continuous user authentication featuring keystroke dynamics based on robust recurrent confidence model and ensemble learning approach. IEEE Access **8**, 156177–156189 (2020)
7. Kiyani, A.T., Lasebae, A., Ali, K., Ur-Rehman, M.: Secure online banking with biometrics. In: 2019 International Conference on Advances in the Emerging Computing Technologies (AECT), pp. 1–6. IEEE (2020)
8. Lu, X., Zhang, S., Hui, P., Lio, P.: Continuous authentication by free-text keystroke based on CNN and RNN. Comput. Secur. **96**, 101861 (2020)
9. Manandhar, R., Wolf, S., Borowczak, M.: One-class classification to continuously authenticate users based on keystroke timing dynamics. In: 2019 18th IEEE International Conference On Machine Learning And Applications (ICMLA), pp. 1259–1266. IEEE (2019)
10. Porwik, P., Doroz, R., Wesolowski, T.E.: Dynamic keystroke pattern analysis and classifiers with competence for user recognition. Appl. Soft Comput. **99**, 106902 (2021)
11. Shepherd, S.: Continuous authentication by analysis of keyboard typing characteristics. In: European Convention on Security and Detection (1995)
12. Sun, Y., Ceker, H., Upadhyaya, S.: Shared keystroke dataset for continuous authentication. In: 2016 IEEE International Workshop on Information Forensics and Security (WIFS), pp. 1–6. IEEE (2016)
13. Tse, K.W., Hung, K.: User behavioral biometrics identification on mobile platform using multimodal fusion of keystroke and swipe dynamics and recurrent neural network. In: 2020 IEEE 10th Symposium on Computer Applications & Industrial Electronics (ISCAIE), pp. 262–267. IEEE (2020)
14. Wu, P.Y., Fang, C.C., Chang, J.M., Kung, S.Y.: Cost-effective kernel ridge regression implementation for keystroke-based active authentication system. IEEE Trans. Cybern. **47**(11), 3916–3927 (2016)

When Federated Learning Meets Vision: An Outlook on Opportunities and Challenges

Ahsan Raza Khan[1], Ahmed Zoha[1(✉)], Lina Mohjazi[1], Hasan Sajid[2], Qammar Abbasi[1], and Muhammad Ali Imran[1]

[1] James Watt School of Engineering, University of Glasgow, Glasgow G12 8QQ, UK
`ahmed.zoha@glasgow.ac.uk`
[2] Department of Robotics and Artificial Intelligence, SMME National University of Sciences and Technology (NUST), Islamabad, Pakistan

Abstract. The mass adoption of Internet of Things (IoT) devices, and smartphones has given rise to the era of big data and opened up an opportunity to derive data-driven insights. This data deluge drives the need for privacy-aware data computations. In this paper, we highlight the use of an emerging learning paradigm known as federated learning (FL) for vision-aided applications, since it is a privacy preservation mechanism by design. Furthermore, we outline the opportunities, challenges, and future research direction for the FL enabled vision applications.

Keywords: Federated Learning · Vision analytics · Edge computing · Decentralized data · Internet-of-Things · Collaborative AI

1 Introduction

According to international data corporation, there will be more then 80 billion devices (IoT sensors, smartphones, wearable sensors) connected to wireless networks by end of 2025. These devices will generate approximately 163 zeta bytes of data globally, which is 10 times of data generated in year 2016 [1,2]. The adoption of these devices are fueled by the advancements in wireless communications especially 5G technology. This overwhelming availability of data, advancement in deep learning, and unprecedented connectivity speeds offered by 5G will enable near real-time response for artificial intelligence (AI) driven applications.

The large-scale model training involves many stakeholders and entails many risks, which includes user privacy, data sovereignty, and data protection laws. The two common security attacks on a machine learning (ML) model are the poisoning attack (training phase) [3], and the evasion attack (inference phase) [4]. In the poisoning attack, the malicious user internally corrupts the training data, whereas in the evasion attack, the model accuracy can be manipulated by injecting adversarial samples. Therefore, different governments have introduced data

© ICST Institute for Computer Sciences, Social Informatics and Telecommunications Engineering 2022
Published by Springer Nature Switzerland AG 2022. All Rights Reserved
M. Ur Rehman and A. Zoha (Eds.): BODYNETS 2021, LNICST 420, pp. 308–319, 2022.
https://doi.org/10.1007/978-3-030-95593-9_23

protection regulations to ensure user privacy. To overcome this challenge, existing solutions are equipped with various privacy preserving techniques including differential privacy and modern cryptography techniques [5].

In recent times, differential privacy, coupled with powerful and advance wireless communications inspired many researchers to utilize the relevant data for many emerging AI driven applications [6,7]. However, the conventional cloud-centric model training approach requires transferring a large amount of raw data from the edge node to third-party servers. This however, has several limitations including:

- Data is privacy sensitive and highly protected under the legislation by General Data Protection Regulation (GDPR) [8].
- Latency issues incurred due to long propagation delays which are not acceptable in time-sensitive applications like smart healthcare, and self-driving cars [9].
- Inefficient bandwidth usage, higher communication and storage cost which also results in substantial network footprints.

This leads to the emergence of a new learning paradigm, termed as federated learning (FL) [10], which aims to bring computations to edge devices without compromising their privacy. Google being the pioneer, makes extensive use of FL algorithms to improvise their services like Gboard and next word prediction [11].

Though, FL was initially introduced with special emphasis on edge device and smartphone applications, but the combination of FL with IoT sensors and powerful AI tools has numerous applications in industry 4.0, digital health cares, smart cities, smart buildings, pharmaceutical drug discovered, video surveillance, digital imaging, virtual or augmented reality (VR/AR), and self-driving cars [12]. For instance, vision processing is an emerging technology, especially for healthcare and smart city applications. The vision sensors generate a large amount of data and it is challenging for the current wireless network architecture to process this data for time-sensitive applications. The key bottleneck is the communication cost and unprecedented propagation delays caused by the network congestion [1]. The 5G connectivity coupled with FL, is enabling a plethora of vision-aided applications, especially in smart healthcare, live traffic monitoring, and incident management [13]. The majority of these applications are privacy sensitive and latency intolerant. Therefore, the prospect of 5G connectivity and privacy by design of FL is envisioned to be a promising solution for vision-aided applications. Vision processing enabled by FL is an emerging field, therefore, it is very difficult to cover all related aspects. To this effect, in this article, we will discuss some of the possible verticals, system architecture, challenges, and future research directions of vision-aided applications.

The rest of the paper is organized as follows. Section 2 provides a brief overview of FL. Section 3 covers the possible vision-aided applications and review some of the use cases, whereas in Sect. 4, the detail of challenges and future research directions will be discussed. Finally, Sect. 5 will concludes the paper.

2   Preliminaries and Overview

FL is an algorithmic solution for collaborative model training with the help of many clients (smart phones, IoT sensors, and organizations) orchestrated by the centralized server, which keeps the training data decentralized [10]. It embodies the principle of relevant data collection and has the privacy by design. The concept of FL was initially introduced with special focus on smartphone and edge device applications, however, due to its decentralized nature of model training, it is also gaining popularity in other fields [12]. Therefore, keeping the common abstractions of different applications in mind, FL can be categorized based on the scale of federation, data partitioning, and privacy mechanism as shown in Fig. 1 [14].

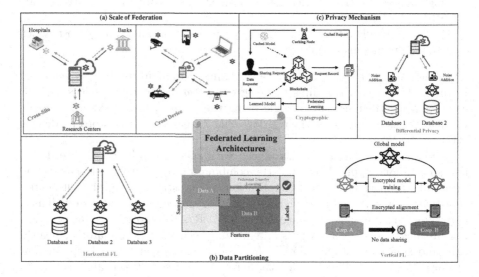

Fig. 1. Overview of different FL architectures.

2.1   Scale of Federation

The scale of federation is highly dependent on the number of edge nodes participating in the training process. When the clients in the training process are big organizations (hospitals, banks, and government institutions etc.), the number of participants will be small and this setting is called as cross-silo FL as shown in Fig. 1(a). Conversely, in cross-device FL settings, large number of users (smartphones, wearable sensors, and IoT sensors) participate in the training of a global model on a highly decentralized data-set [14]. The typical examples of cross-device and cross-silo FL are google Gboard and Nvida Clara for brain tumor segmentation respectively [10,15]. In vision-aided applications, the scale of federation is highly dependent on the nature of data and user's intent.

For instance, in brain tumor segmentation, the data was stored on central servers placed in different geographical locations, and as a result, the cross-silo mechanism is used for model training. In the smart cities video surveillance scenario, anomaly detection to identify the unusual activity in the environment is one of the of the examples. In this case, the cross-device mechanism may be used because this setting involves a large number of vision sensors placed in different locations.

2.2 Data Partitioning

FL is extremely useful in collaborative training where the data is distributed among a large number of users. In the era of digitization and big data, every click of user is captured to derive useful statistical information which may belong to similar or different application domains. Therefore, data partitioning plays a key role in FL where it is broadly divided in horizontal, vertical and transfer learning [14]. In horizontal FL, participants have similar features at different instances and vary in terms of data samples, whereas in vertical FL, common data of unrelated domains is used for model training. In vertical FL, users can have similar data but differ in terms of features. The classical example of horizontal FL is Google Gboard with the assumption of honest consumers and secure centralized server for global model training [10]. On the other hand, a real-world use case for vertical FL may be a scenario where the credit card sales team of a bank train its ML model by using the information of online shopping. In this case, only common users of the bank and e-commerce website will participate in the training process. With this liaising of secure information exchange, banks can improve their credit services and provide incentives to active customers [16].

In transfer FL approach, a pre-trained model is used on a similar datasets to solve a completely new problem set. The real-time example of transfer FL could be similar to vertical FL with small modifications. In this approach, the condition of similar users with matching data for model training can be relaxed to create a diverse system to serve individual customers [17]. It is a personalized model training for individual users to exploit the better generalization properties of global model which can be achieved by either data interpolation, model interpolation, and user clustering [18].

3 Vision-Aided Applications Enabled by FL

In recent times, vision processing has many practical applications in healthcare, smart transportation systems, video surveillance, and VR/AR. Conventional model training relies on server-led training solutions, however, video data is not only privacy sensitive but also incurs large communication cost as well [1]. FL mechanisms, on the other hand, are privacy-aware by design and significantly reduce the communication cost by exploiting the edge processing capabilities. Therefore, it is a very challenging task to build vision-aided solutions in a centralized server-led model. In recent times, FL is an exciting solution for decentralized model training, which is gaining attention in both academia and industry. As a result of that, many FL enabled applications have surfaced. An overview of vision-aided applications enabled by FL for smart healthcare (cross-silo), smart transportation system and smart homes is presented in Fig. 2. It is very difficult to cover the entire liaison of FL applications, therefore, in this section we will focus on some of the vision-aided applications.

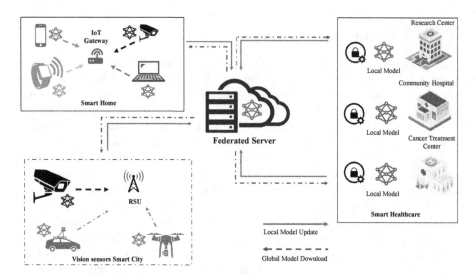

Fig. 2. Overview of vision-aided applications enabled by FL.

3.1   Smart Heath-Care System

In healthcare systems, data-driven ML is a promising approach to develop a robust model for learning features from large curated data for knowledge discovery. Even in the age of big data and advanced AI, the existing medical data is not yet fully exploited for model training due to privacy [19]. Most of the data is stored in secured locations i.e. a data island with restricted access. Furthermore, collecting, curating, and maintaining good quality data is both time consuming and expensive. Therefore, to improve the quality of health-care, collaborative learning without data share is a need of the hour and this platform is provided by FL. It is a promising solution to improve the healthcare data analytic, especially bio-medical imagining. FL can be applied on various domains of health-care but the key application areas involving vision data analytics are:

- Magnetic resonance imaging (MRI) to find neurological disease or disorders.
- Brain tumor segmentation.
- Human emotion detection to identify the mental health of patients.
- Cancer cell detection.

In [20], a FL framework is proposed to analyze the brain images to investigate neurological disorders. This framework used both synthetic as well as the real dataset, showing the potential of medical imaging in future applications. The authors in [21] presented a deep learning model for brain tumor segmentation using FL. In this study, multi-institutional collaboration is used which achieved the accuracy of 99% without sharing any data. Similarly, the authors in [22] exploited the client-server architecture of FL to train a differential privacy preserved deep neural network for brain tumor segmentation. In this study, the results show that there is a trade-off between privacy protection and model performance. In [23], a human emotion monitoring system is proposed using facial expression and speech signals to create an emotion index, which is used to find the mental health of individuals. Using FL, the proposed method showed promising results by detecting the depression of individuals without compromising the users' privacy.

3.2 Smart Homes

In smart homes, safety and security is highly dependent on vision processing solutions. Unfortunately, it is very difficult to deploy these solutions due to the privacy, latency, and high cost of video transmission. By addressing the privacy concerns effectively, real-time video analytic has many applications in smart homes. For instance, the combination of wearable sensors and real-time activity inference on indoor vision sensor feeds can help in fall detection and trigger corrective measures [24,25]. Similarly, for smart home safety, an alert can be triggered by visual instance detection which can identify the possible threat i.e., fire hazard. In [26], a visual object detection model *FedVision* is presented which can be used to develop vision-aided solutions for safety monitoring in smart homes, cities, or industries. In this work, horizontal FL architecture is exploited to train the ML using the image data owned by a different organization to develop a warning mechanism for safety hazards. The experimental results showed improvement in operational efficiency, data privacy, and reduced cost.

3.3 Smart Cities

FL has a huge potential of effectively managing the assets, resources and services of smart cities using vision data analytics collected by vision sensors (smartphone cameras, CCTV, and dash-cams) [27]. With the challenge of privacy and high cost, cloud-centric approach also involves long propagation delay and incurs unacceptable latency for time sensitive applications like traffic and emergency management, self driving cars, disaster management [12]. For example, in smart transportation systems, a fleet of autonomous cars may need an up-to-date information of traffic, pedestrian behavior, or unusual incident (accident) to safely operate. Similarly, the video captured from individual smartphones or dash-cam can provide the live street view, which can be used for delivering the information of hospitals, popular restaurants, or providing insights on real-time behaviour of pedestrians and fellow drivers. However, building accurate models in these scenarios will be very difficult due to the privacy and limited connectivity of each device. As a result, this can potentially impede the development of new technologies for smart cities [12,13]. Therefore, to reduce the transmission cost, and latency, FL can be used to locally process the information and only send the model parameter updates to the cloud. Using the FL paradigm, the following are the application domains of vision-aided solutions for smart cities.

– Smart transportation systems for real-time traffic management and navigation, incident detection, and automatic license plate/tag recognition.
– Self driving cars (automatic driving management and driver assistance).
– Safety and security of public places using the CCTV images and videos.
– Drone video surveillance for crowd management on special events.
– Natural disaster management using satellite imagery and drone footage.

In [28], a FL framework is proposed using unlabelled data samples at each user participating in the training process for two different application domains. The authors have demonstrated the application of FL and obtained promising results in natural disasters analysis and waste classification. Similarly, vision-aided applications enabled by FL also have a huge potential to improve the model training in some other domains like VR/AR, gaming, agriculture and smart industries, etc. The details of the used cases along with the area of applications are given in Table 1.

Table 1. Summary of vision aided applications enabled by FL.

Ref	Domains	Area of application	FL approach
[20]	Health-care	Neurological disorder	Cross-silo/Horizontal
[21]	Health-care	Brain tumor segmentation	Cross-silo/Horizontal
[22]	Health-care	Brain tumor segmentation	Cross-silo
[23]	Health-care	Human emotion detection	Cross-device/Horizontal
[26]	Smart homes	Visual object detection	Cross-device
[28]	Smart city	Disaster and waste classification	Cross-silo

4 Challenges and Future Research

FL is an emerging yet very effective and innovative learning paradigm for collaborative model training. Despite of recent research efforts to address the core challenges, FL is still prone to many limitations, especially in vision-aided application that hinder it to be adopted in different domains. In this context, we will discuss some of the challenges and future research directions.

4.1 Privacy and Security

In vision-aided applications, ML models are trained using highly sensitive data. Although, data never leaves the edge device during the training process, it is worth mentioning that FL does not address all the potential privacy issues. For instance, the FL trained model may indirectly leak some information to a third party user by model inversion, gradient analysis, or adversarial attacks [29]. Therefore, counter measures like adding noise, adding differential privacy is needed in cross-device architecture [12,14].

Level of trust among the participants in the training process is also a very big challenge in FL applications. In cross-silo structures, the clients are usually trustworthy and bounded by collaborative agreements, which reduces the trust deficit. As a result, there is a less possibility of privacy breach, which can help to reduce sophisticated counter protective measures [30]. However, in the cross-device architecture, the training process is done on a highly distributed dataset and it is almost impossible to enforce collaborative agreement. Therefore, trust deficit is a very big problem among the participants, and it is necessary to have some security strategies to ensure security and protect the end-user interests [19]. Similarly, privacy vs. performance trade-off is also a huge challenge in decentralized training, because it impacts the accuracy of final model [7].

4.2 Data Heterogeneity

The data captured by vision sensors is highly diverse, since it is collected by devices having different computational, storage, and network capabilities. For instance, an image or video captured by a smartphone or a dash-cam may have different pixel qualities [7]. Similarly, medical imaging data may also have distinct features and dimensions due to acquisition differences, quality and brand of the device, and local demographic bias [19,22]. Therefore, this non-identically distributed data poses a substantial challenge, which leads to the failure of a FL enabled solution under specific conditions. Data heterogeneity also leads to a situation where there is a conflict in the optimal solution and demands a sophisticated method to reach a global shared model. Therefore, data heterogeneity is still an open research problem and needs attention based on specific applications.

4.3 Asynchronous Aggregation Mechanism

Communication architecture for model aggregation is also huge challenge and is currently an active area of research. In cross-device model training, each device has different storage, computation and communication capabilities. Furthermore, device dropout is also very common in the training process due to connective and energy constraint [30]. These system level characteristics pose a critical challenge in model aggregation process. The traditional FedAvg algorithm uses the synchronous model aggregation mechanism, thus prone to the straggler effect in which FL server waits for all devices to complete their local training for global model update as shown in Fig. 3(a). This aggregation method slows down the training process as it depends on the slowest device in the network. Further-more, this mechanism does not account for a user who joins the training pro-cess halfway. On the other hand, asynchronous aggregation updates the global model as it receives the local update Fig. 3(b). One of the advantage of using asynchronous aggregation mechanism is its ability to deal with the straggler effect.

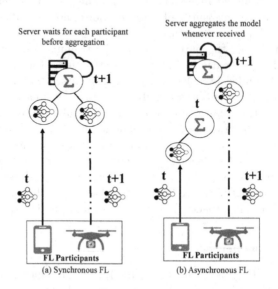

Fig. 3. Comparison of synchronous and asynchronous communication mechanism for FL.

4.4   Scale of Federation

The scale of federation is highly dependent on the number of participants in the training process for a specific application. For example, in health-care appli-cations, cross-silo architecture is usually adopted for model training, where the edge nodes are hospitals and government institutes [19,30]. The participants in the training process are trust-worthy and equipped with secure communications, powerful computational resource. This is quite a straight forward training process and each client is bounded by the collaborative agreement. However, in smart city, cross-device architecture can be used for applications like transportation system and self-driving cars. The fully decentralized model training has many challenges including communication and propagation delays, trust deficit among client, model convergence and aggregation, and agreement of optimal solution [19]. This aspect of vision-aided application is unexplored.

4.5   Accountability and Incentive Mechanism

Data quality in ML-driven applications is essential because the performance of the system is highly dependent on the data. In FL model training, the data quality has more significance. In non-trusted federation, the accountability of clients is very important to improve the performance of the model. This information can be used to develop a revenue model to give incentives and encourage the participants with relevant data to participate in the model training and improve the global model accuracy.

5 Conclusions

Data-driven solutions have led to a wide range of innovations, especially in the domain of vision-based applications and services. However, a lot of intelligence still remains untapped because of inaccessibility of user-centric information due to privacy challenges. Federated learning mechanism has led us to an exciting research paradigm that allows us to collect and analyze the massive amount of information without compromising on privacy and network resources. In this paper, we have provided an outlook on FL-enabled vision-aided applications. Furthermore, we have set the scene for vision applications in the era of 5G connectivity through FL paradigm and highlighted a number of fundamental challenges and future research directions.

References

1. Lim, W.Y.B., et al.: Federated learning in mobile edge networks: a comprehensive survey. IEEE Commun. Surv. Tutor. **22**(3), 2031–2063 (2020)
2. Zhu, G., Liu, D., Du, Y., You, C., Zhang, J., Huang, K.: Toward an intelligent edge: wireless communication meets machine learning. IEEE Commun. Mag. **58**(1), 19–25 (2021)
3. Muñoz-González, L., et al.: Towards poisoning of deep learning algorithms with back-gradient optimization. In: Proceedings of the 10th ACM Workshop on Artificial Intelligence and Security, AISec 2017. ACM Press (2017)
4. Nasr, M., Shokri, R., Houmansadr, A.: Comprehensive privacy analysis of deep learning: passive and active white-box inference attacks against centralized and federated learning. In: IEEE Symposium on Security and Privacy, pp. 739–753 (2019)
5. Bae, H., et al.: Security and privacy issues in deep learning. arXiv preprint arXiv:1807.11655
6. Li, T., Sahu, A.K., Talwalkar, A., Smith, V.: Federated learning: challenges, methods, and future directions. IEEE Signal Process. Mag. **37**(3), 50–60 (2020)
7. Li, P., et al.: Multi-key privacy-preserving deep learning in cloud computing. Futur. Gener. Comput. Syst. **74**, 76–85 (2017)
8. Custers, B., Sears, A.M., Dechesne, F., Georgieva, I., Tani, T., van der Hof, S.: EU Personal Data Protection in Policy and Practice. TMC Asser Press, The Hague (2019)
9. Yang, K., Jiang, T., Shi, Y., Ding, Z.: Federated learning via over-the-air computation. IEEE Trans. Wireless Commun. **19**(3), 2022–2035 (2020)
10. McMahan, H.B., Moore, E., Ramage, D., Arcas, B.A.: Federated learning of deep networks using model averaging. arXiv preprint arXiv:1602.05629 (2016)

11. McMahan, B., Moore, E., Ramage, D., Hampson, S., Arcas, B.A.: Communication-efficient learning of deep networks from decentralized data. In: Artificial Intelligence and Statistics, pp. 1273–1282 (2017)
12. Aledhari, M., Razzak, R., Parizi, R.M., Saeed, F.: Federated learning: a survey on enabling technologies, protocols, and applications. IEEE Access **8**, 140699–140725 (2020)
13. Deng, Y., Han, T., Ansari, N.: FedVision: federated video analytics with edge computing. IEEE Open J. Comput. Soc. **1**, 62–72 (2021)
14. Mothukuri, V., Parizi, R.M., Pouriyeh, S., Huang, Y., Dehghantanha, A., Srivastava, G.: A survey on security and privacy of federated learning. Futur. Gener. Comput. Syst. **115**, 619–640 (2021)
15. https://resources.nvidia.com/en-us-federated-learning/bvu-ea6hc0k?ncid=pa-srch-goog-84545
16. Yang, S., Ren, B., Zhou, X., Liu, L.: Parallel distributed logistic regression for vertical federated learning without third-party coordinator. arXiv preprint arXiv:1911.09824 (2019)
17. Chen, Y., Qin, X., Wang, J., Yu, C., Gao, W.: FedHealth: a federated transfer learning framework for wearable healthcare. IEEE Intell. Syst. **35**(4), 83–93 (2020)
18. Mansour, Y., Mohri, M., Ro, J., Suresh, A.T.: Three approaches for personalization with applications to federated learning. arXiv preprint arXiv:2002.10619 (2020)
19. Rieke, N., et al.: The future of digital health with federated learning. NPJ Digit. Med. **3**(1), 1–7 (2020)
20. Silva, S., Gutman, B.A., Romero, E., Thompson, P.M., Altmann, A., Lorenzi, M.: Federated learning in distributed medical databases: meta-analysis of large-scale subcortical brain data. In: IEEE 16th International Symposium on Biomedical Imaging, pp. 270–274 (2019)
21. Sheller, M.J., Reina, G.A., Edwards, B., Martin, J., Bakas, S.: Multi-institutional deep learning modeling without sharing patient data: a feasibility study on brain tumor segmentation. In: Crimi, A., Bakas, S., Kuijf, H., Keyvan, F., Reyes, M., van Walsum, T. (eds.) BrainLes 2018. LNCS, vol. 11383, pp. 92–104. Springer, Cham (2019). https://doi.org/10.1007/978-3-030-11723-8_9
22. Li, W., et al.: Privacy-preserving federated brain tumour segmentation. In: Suk, H.-I., Liu, M., Yan, P., Lian, C. (eds.) MLMI 2019. LNCS, vol. 11861, pp. 133–141. Springer, Cham (2019). https://doi.org/10.1007/978-3-030-32692-0_16
23. Chhikara, P., Singh, P., Tekchandani, R., Kumar, N., Guizani, M.: Federated learning meets human emotions: a decentralized framework for human-computer interaction for IoT applications. IEEE Internet Things J. **8**(8), 6949–6962 (2021)
24. Wu, Q., Chen, X., Zhou, Z., Zhang, J.: FedHome: cloud-edge based personalized federated learning for in-home health monitoring. IEEE Trans. Mob. Comput. (2020)
25. Sozinov, K., Vlassov, V., Girdzijauskas, S.: Human activity recognition using federated learning. In: IEEE International Conference on Parallel & Distributed Processing with Applications, pp. 1103–1111 (2018)
26. Liu, Y., et al.: FedVision: an online visual object detection platform powered by federated learning. In: Proceedings of the Conference on Artificial Intelligence, vol. 34, no. 08, pp. 13172–13179 (2020)
27. Zheng, Z., Zhou, Y., Sun, Y., Wang, Z., Liu, B., Li, K.: Federated learning in smart cities: a comprehensive survey. arXiv preprint arXiv:2102.01375 (2021)
28. Ahmed, L., Ahmad, K., Said, N., Qolomany, B., Qadir, J., Al-Fuqaha, A.: Active learning based federated learning for waste and natural disaster image classification. IEEE Access **8**, 208518–208531 (2020)

29. Wang, Z., Song, M., Zhang, Z., Song, Y., Wang, Q., Qi, H.: Beyond inferring class representatives: user-level privacy leakage from federated learning. In: IEEE INFOCOM IEEE Conference on Computer Communications, pp. 2512–2520 (2019)
30. Kairouz, P., et al.: Advances and open problems in federated learning. arXiv preprint arXiv:1912.04977 (2019)

Author Index

Printed in the United States
by Baker & Taylor Publisher Services

Printed in the United States
by Baker & Taylor Publisher Services